A Time
To Be Born

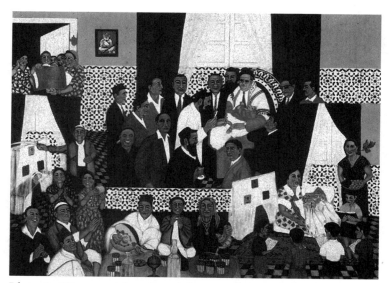

Plate 1: Circumcision in a Moroccan Jewish family.
Gabbay, M., *Roots, Judaism: Tradition and the Folklore of the Moroccan Jews* (Beer Sheba, Israel: 1988). Courtesy of the artist.

A Time To Be Born

Customs and Folklore of Jewish Birth

Michele Klein

The Jewish Publication Society
Philadelphia 1998

Manufactured in the United States of America

Library of Congress Cataloging in Publication Data

Klein, Michele, 1950–
A time to be born: Customs and Folklore of Jewish Birth/Michele Klein.
p. cm.
Includes bibliographical references and indexes.
ISBN 0-8276-0608-7
1. Childbirth—Religious aspects—Judaism. 2. Jews—Folklore.
I. Title.
BM538.H43K58 1997
296.4'4—dc21   98-2518

05 04 03 02 01 00 99 98   10 9 8 7 6 5 4 3 2 1

JPS gratefully acknowledges support for the publication of this volume.

*This book is dedicated
to the memory of*

Bernard G. Segal

*Jurist, Humanitarian, Scholar, Leader
whose vision
fashioned the future,
whose integrity
paid honor to his past.*

I dedicate this book to my parents, to Jacob,

to Aluma, Allon, Shira, and Tom,

with love

Contents

Illustrations

Preface

The birth of a child is not necessarily a mere physiological sequence initiated by sexual intercourse and culminating in birth. It is a long process that can have religious and spiritual significance for those involved, whether or not they adhere to a religious tradition. There is something wondrous about the kicks a pregnant woman feels in her belly, and about the first cry that turns the newborn from blue to pink. There is something miraculous about how a sperm merges with an ovum to grow into a full fledged baby and eventually into an intelligent, thinking human being. However much is explained by microscopic cameras and genetic codes, the birth of a child makes one realize the existence in our universe of a power, or even a world, beyond our understanding. Judaism calls this power "God." Childbirth is the prerequisite for perpetuating God's world. In this sense, it is religiously significant. In Jewish tradition, fertility is a divine blessing and God is a partner in conception, supervising pregnancy and the safe arrival of a child. Childbirth is a spiritual experience for those who recognize this partnership. In addition, the birth of a child is significant for Jews not only as individuals, but also as a people, because the arrival of a new child promises their continuity.

HOW THE PROJECT BEGAN

The idea for this book came to me as my neighbor and I were discussing our recent experiences of childbirth. Both of us had given birth a few months earlier, each to our third child, and we were discussing the emotions of our pregnancies. My neighbor pointed out that the books she had read about pregnancy and the medical treatment she had received had ignored this aspect of her pregnancy. We agreed that most contemporary, nonreligious childbirth literature makes no mention of the mystical experiences aroused by the discovery of having conceived, by feeling the baby kick, by holding the baby for the first time in our arms, or at any or every other moment in the childbearing process. I then realized that most of the Jewish literature on childbirth similarly ignores the emotional and spiritual aspects of this process. This literature is mainly in the Orthodox domain, concerned with the Jewish laws regarding pregnancy and birth. This is not what I, my neighbor, or the large percentage of Jewish parents who do not adhere to halakhah (Jewish Law) relate to when thinking about childbirth. Nor do the many books on Jewish ethnography and folklore go into much detail on childbearing other than the topic of circumcision, which is amply documented. For these reasons, I resolved to explore in depth the emotions, beliefs, customs, and traditions of childbirth among Jews.

INTERVIEWEES

I set out to research the attitudes toward childbirth held by Jewish women and men, born in all corners of the Jewish Diaspora and in Israel, as well as their family customs and community traditions, by interviewing two hundred people—pregnant women, mothers, fathers, grandmothers, and elderly midwives—living in Israel.

My interviewees ranged from ultra-Orthodox to completely secular, with many falling somewhere in between. Whereas Orthodox women, who adhere to halakhah, continue to maintain many of the attitudes and traditions that Jews have observed since earliest times, I learned that secular Jews are often ignorant of the Jewish child-birth-related customs and values of their own families and communities of origin.

The advantage of interviewing in Israel was that, in 1984, when the interviews were conducted, Israel was at the end of the transition from the old world of folk management of childbirth to modern Western medicine. Thus, some elderly women were able to recall customs prevalent when they had given birth fifty years earlier, in areas where Western medicine was unknown, customs practiced for generations but made obsolete by modern medicine.

Israeli women, like Jewish women throughout the Diaspora, who had suffered infertility spoke bitterly of their misery and loneliness and of the social pressures from family and friends to have a child. Women who had miscarried spoke of their sense of loss and depression, especially when they suffered repeated miscarriages. When their doctors could not explain the reason for their loss, the women often blamed their own actions, or even their thoughts. In addition, some of the women I interviewed refused to consider contraception; others reported that, although their husbands would not hear of it, they discreetly practiced one or more methods to prevent conception. Some of the women I interviewed had undergone abortion to terminate an unwanted pregnancy, but many had succeeded in planning their pregnancies.

Whereas some women clearly enjoyed being pregnant, many did not, feeling ungainly and unattractive. Some pregnant women suffered physically, and some reported marital tension over sex, or over insufficient help and attention from their partner. Interestingly, many reported that they dreamed more during pregnancy than at other times, and they often interpreted their dreams to gain insight into their feelings about the fetus, or about maternal fears. Most of the women I interviewed spoke of their fear of giving birth, often quoting the biblical phrase, "In pain shall you bear children." Although they knew that Eve had suffered in giving birth, and that most women experience pain in childbirth, they never imagined that it would be as bad as it proved to be for them. Some women also described their unexpected postnatal depression.

Most of my interviewees had close relationships with their mothers, which were enhanced during pregnancy. These women related their expectation of help from their mothers after the birth of the baby. A few mentioned the importance of having a son, rather than a daughter. In addition, many described the celebrations performed after their babies' arrivals.

Although the women I interviewed came or descended from communities from all corners of the earth and expressed many different attitudes, they shared many ideas, traditions, and stories from their common Jewish heritage. For example, many women quoted Jewish sources as their reason for shunning contraception and for their suffering during birthing. Some women quoted family traditions regarding the interpretation of omens during pregnancy and the manner of naming the newborn. Old wives' tales that were passed from one generation to the next were quoted hesitantly, in embarrassed awareness that these are no longer relevant today—for instance, tales about how to predict the sex of a baby, about the importance of satisfying pregnancy cravings, and about foods that encourage milk flow.

SOURCES

Once I sat down and collated the material collected in these interviews, my next step was to search for source material on the origins, historical development, and dissemination of what I had heard. For centuries, the mysteries and suffering of childbearing have been interpreted by Jews within the framework of religion and mysticism, and the literature is considerable.

First and foremost, the Bible, the Talmud, the later Codes of Jewish Law, and the huge body of rabbinic commentaries and responsa set down Jewish laws and recorded traditions concerning conception, pregnancy, birth, and the postnatal period. These texts, which constitute the framework for all aspects of Jewish life, provide a practical guide for bringing a child into the world. Their minute and meticulous details are part of a vast system of prescribed forms of conduct: their attention to these details is one way in which Jews acknowledge their relationship with God. Judaism considers the intimate act of conceiving a child and bringing that child into the world as a process involving God. To experience the holiness within this process requires paying attention to detail in one's daily conduct. The laws and traditions of this literature are familiar to Orthodox Jews. Although an in-depth examination of these texts is not the primary focus of this study, they dictate the religious significance that childbearing has for Jews and are therefore of primary relevance.

Another Jewish source, devotional literature, spans the whole of Jewish history because prayer is the way in which people communicate with God. In biblical times, prayers were often spontaneous expressions of fears, hopes, feelings, and desires. In the Bible, Isaac and Hannah both pray to God for the divine blessing of a son. By talmudic times (second to sixth centuries), prayer had become congregational, mandated at fixed times of the day, week, month, and year. Private prayers could be inserted into the petitionary benedictions (of the *Amidah*) recited every weekday except for Sabbath and festivals. A group prayer, or a prayer for someone else, was considered more effective than a personal petition, and the atmosphere in the synagogue, where everyone prayed together, was conducive to the concentration necessary to commune with God. Thus, a husband's supplications for his wife, recited in synagogue and supported by the presence of the congregation, was thought to be much more effective than a woman's praying on her own. In the gaonic period (sixth to eleventh centuries), in Babylonia, prayers for the postnatal rituals were formalized. In medieval times, especially in Provence, Spain, and Germany, a new depth of meaning, a mystical dimension, was infused into prayer and soon spread to Jewish communities almost worldwide. This change came about as medieval intellectuals interested themselves in the earlier Jewish mystical literature and developed philosophical concepts of God. In the sixteenth century, private prayers for childbearing were formulated, using the standard format of Jewish prayer. These prayers were written in the vernacular as well as in Hebrew, making them accessible to everyone, including women, and "men who were like women" in that they could not read

Hebrew. Kabbalists—Jewish mystics—encouraged private, intensely emotional prayer. All prayers written for childbearing were emotional, reflecting the importance as well as the fears and dangers of bringing a baby into the world and stressing the Jew's repentance, his or her turning toward God, the desire for God's attention and response, and appreciation of God's mercy and loving kindness.

The extensive Jewish mystical literature, especially the thirteenth-century Zohar and the sixteenth-century (and later) Lurianic Kabbalah, addresses the spirituality of childbearing, that is, the divine manifestations in the process of bringing a child into the world. Stressing the importance of fulfilling the commandments, prayer, and repentance, the mystical literature also emphasizes the holiness of the act of conception and considers the divine origins of the soul and its descent into the body.

Some prayer books document local customs and traditions. Registers kept by circumcisers, community records, and memoirs also provide fascinating material related to Jewish childbearing customs and experiences. Moreover, *sifrei minhagim* (books of local customs) are also illuminating, as are some tomes about Jewish life written by non-Jews. In addition, over the last hundred years, ethnographers and anthropologists have been documenting the practices of different Jewish communities, sometimes including information on the beliefs and traditions connected with childbearing. In contrast to the duties (commandments) observed in every Jewish community, customs are norms of behavior that may be localized in just a few communities. Some of these customs, such as designating a chair for Elijah for the circumcision ritual, became widespread even though they were not duties, whereas others, such as the employment of a Jewish midwife by a community, or girl-naming customs, depended on cohesiveness and social pressures within the community. When Jews moved from one place to another, as happened countless times throughout history, customs not generally practiced by Jews in the new environment were sometimes abandoned. I have not, of course, been able to include every local custom observed by Jews worldwide. What I have chosen are those customs observed by many Jewish communities, in particular those customs of significance to individual or group Jewish identity.

Manuscripts on the use of magic, Hebrew encyclopedias, pharmacopoeia, midwifery handbooks, gynecological and obstetrical treatises, and remedy books, both in manuscript and in printed form, also contain considerable material relevant to childbearing practices among Jews. Many remedies appear to be pure quackery or black magic, having no Jewish content or meaning. Others include advice and ingredients not specific to Jews. I have chosen to quote only those with some Jewish significance, for example, in their link with biblical personages or incidents, or in their numerical interpretation through the use of Hebrew letters (*gematria*).

Finally, the oral tradition of legends, folktales, and songs from the many different Jewish communities is of great interest. Jews have always been good at telling stories. The long hours of vigilance, often by candlelight, with a woman in or after childbirth or before circumcision, were well suited to telling tales reflecting fears, hopes, or experiences. I have quoted widely from tales of biblical figures, of witches and wonderworking rabbis, of despair, and of dreams come true. These stories inspire, teach, and heal. They often contain a specifically Jewish moral or lesson, to strengthen the faith and fiber of those gathered together. They also reveal the concerns of every-day life in past centuries.

Because Jewish laws and Jewish history were written by men, it is diffi-cult to find historical sources from the woman's point of view. Notable exceptions are two wills dating from the eleventh century, composed by pregnant women lest they die in childbirth. In addition, the Babylonian sage, Abbaye, who lived around 300 C.E., was familiar with aspects of childbearing and related remedies from his foster mother. The Babylonian Talmud credits this woman as the source of his knowledge. In addi-tion is a thirteenth-century Judeo-Arabic text, entitled *The Book of Dinah on All the Problems and Diseases of the Womb*, with no explanation of the title. Was Dinah an infor-mant, the wise woman who advised the author? Or was she the midwife for whose eyes or ears the text had been composed? Some of the Yiddish personal prayers (*tkhines*) that women have recited for pregnancy and birth are also believed to have been written by women. Thus, Sore bas Toyvim, who allegedly lived in the Ukraine, probably in the seventeenth century, was said to have written such prayers, although she may have been legendary and not an actual person. Gluckel of Hameln, who died early in the eighteenth century, provided descriptions of her childbearing experiences in her memoirs. It became more common for women to write and publish in the nineteenth century, so there are many female sources from the last hundred and fifty years, including prayers, folktales, and lullabies.

SCOPE OF THIS BOOK

As I pursued my research, I delighted in the many continuities in the beliefs and behaviors connected with childbearing from the different periods of Jewish history and the many parts of the world where Jews have lived. Nonetheless, there are long periods in local Jewish history about which little is known of the ideas and customs concerning pregnancy and birth. Thus, in the documentation of such communities as those of Ethiopia and India, little or nothing is said about childbearing practices and traditions before the nineteenth century, except for practices involving halakhah.

Some customs common to non-Jews among whom Jews lived were incorporated into local Jewish life over the centuries. Thus, Jews often legitimized the use of common folk remedies (for barrenness, for avoiding miscarriage, and for eas-ing delivery) by giving them a Jewish interpretation. Non-Jewish sources from ancient Babylonia, from Greek and Arabic cultures, and from medieval Germany and Spain provided the raw material for the fear of evil spirits, before conception and dur-ing and after birth, as well as for the measures Jews took to protect mother and new-born. Similarly, local customs also influenced the baby-naming rituals practiced by Jews in Spain, Alsace, and Iraq.

Realizing the necessity to choose some cut-off point for my study, I have not attempted to trace systematically the origins of all childbearing behaviors prac-ticed by Jews throughout history. Nor have I compared these practices with those from other cultures, except where they are particularly relevant or interesting. I have simply accepted that Jews believed and behaved as reported in my interviews and sources, and have sought the earliest expressions of these ideas and customs. I have pointed out continuities among Jews in distant corners of the earth and, whenever possible, I have tried to understand the purpose and reasoning behind these beliefs and behaviors. Many of these practices were abandoned under the influence of the Jewish Enlightenment in the nineteenth century and later, when many Jews took an active interest in secular studies, including recent discoveries in medicine and science. The Jewish Enlightenment contributed significantly to the assimilation of Jews into local culture and the secular management of childbirth, dictated by the advent of modern medicine.

The focus of my work is on the beliefs, attitudes, and customs of Jews when bearing children, rather than on Jewish laws connected with childbearing. I do spell out some of these Jewish laws to show their fundamental ideals and values because these laws inevitably provide the deep structure behind the diverse ideas and practices. In my pursuit of the emotional context of childbirth experiences, however, I have often highlighted customs and practices outside the mainstream concerns of Judaism. Traditional Jewish methods of coping with despair over infertility, fear of miscarriage, and death in childbirth, such as supplicatory prayers, repentance, and charity, have sometimes been unable to reduce the anxiety and danger inherent in conceiving and bearing children. Women in almost every Jewish community have therefore resorted to childbirth amulets and have accepted the clearly magical child-bearing advice offered in many Hebrew remedy books. These amulets and remedy books bear witness to beliefs and behaviors frowned on by many rabbis but that nonetheless played an important role in the Jewish childbearing experience.

Although some aspects of the traditional Jewish experience of childbirth are familiar to those observant of tradition, many other aspects belong to a world that no longer exists. I point out alternative beliefs and practices still available today, without explaining modern medical procedures that can be found in secular books and popular articles on the subject. I do discuss recent efforts to instill Jewish meaning into the experience of childbirth, such as new prayers for those who have suffered miscarriage and welcoming ceremonies to give girls a more acknowledged role in Jewish society. The scope of this book is thus to examine when and how Jews act as Jews in the lengthy process of childbearing, from conception through to the postnatal ceremonies.

HOW THE BOOK IS ORGANIZED

In organizing this book, I have arranged my material—ideas, tales, prayers, and remedial advice from different periods and different communities—into the four major phases of the childbearing process: conception, pregnancy, birthing, and the postnatal period. My intent has been to create a kaleidoscopic impression of how Jews relate to childbearing. The material included here was selected for its Jewish content, meaning, and interest. Just as a kaleidoscope projects a different design when viewed from different angles, no doubt someone else researching this topic could portray a different image. Furthermore, it is impossible to generalize about the emotions of childbearing among Jews throughout the centuries and in the many lands where Jews have lived and continue to live, because every pregnancy and birth is unique.

In addition, every Jew experiences his or her Jewishness differently. I hope that the variegated picture of childbirth presented here will give all readers, even those remote from traditional Judaism, a positive view of Jewish life.

The introductory chapter examines the main characteristics of childbirth practices among Jews and looks at Jewish ideals and values regarding childbearing. The first part of the book then examines the importance in Jewish tradition of having children. Procreation is understood as both a blessing from God and a commandment that must be fulfilled. The desire for fertility is reflected in many aspects of the Jewish marriage celebration, and a preference for boys has led to plentiful advice for the unhappy parents of many girls. Those who cannot have children have suffered bitterly in the past, just as today. Cures for infertility have depended on the perceived causes of the problem. Traditional Jewish attitudes toward contraception and abortion also derive from the age-old importance of having children, as well as from the Jewish emphasis on the sanctity of human life.

The second section deals with pregnancy. Jews have long pondered how conception occurs and how the embryo develops into a baby with a vitality of its own. They have always recognized that God is responsible for creation and for the soul and that the parents also influence the development of the fetus. Many experiences of pregnancy are explored—those of the baby in the womb, those of the mother, and those relating to marriage. Seeking predictions helps women to cope with anxieties and fears. Women take precautions against the dangers thought to affect the safe arrival of a baby. When pregnancy ends in misfortune, however, it is always a heavy blow. Judaism does not prescribe a ritual for mourning pregnancy loss and parents find their own ways of expressing their grief.

The third part of the book is about birthing. Infants are usually delivered with the help of a midwife, who offers emotional and physical assistance. Thus, one chapter in this section looks at the functions and status of a midwife and some of the dangers that Jewish midwives faced in the past. The subsequent chapter examines how Jews interpreted the pain of childbirth and the methods they used to ease delivery. Another chapter is devoted to the topic of death in childbirth, once common. In the past, a mythic demon, Lilith, was thought to be the cause of death during or just after birth; the story of Lilith and measures taken to keep her away comprise another chapter.

The last part of the book addresses the postnatal period. A baby's safe arrival is cause for celebration. Even though the mother and child require special care during the early days, celebration is still in order if both are well. To carry out such celebration, Jewish parents, and at times the entire community, enact several postnatal rituals prescribed by the Bible: the circumcision of a newborn boy, the redemption of a first-born son, and the mother's purification. The community also celebrates the birth of a girl, although this festivity differs from the ceremonial welcome accorded to a boy. In addition to welcoming the child into the community, these celebrations also allow parents to express their hope that the child will grow up to be a good Jew and live a long and full life. Such hopes are usually expressed in a traditional blessing still cited today when naming a newborn. Another way that parents have expressed their hopes and fears for their baby's future is through lullabies.

The final chapter considers the possibilities of Jewish expressions relating to childbirth today. In addition, traditional family roles, Jewish community involvement, and Jewish medical ethics relating to childbirth are viewed in the context of the modern secular world. In closing, it discusses the significance of childbearing for the Jewish people as a whole, now and in the future.

It is not necessary to read this book from beginning to end. Readers may read or skip chapters as their fancy dictates. Thus, expectant parents may wish to begin with the section on pregnancy and only later glance at the earlier chapters, whereas those contemplating having a child could start at the beginning and move on to the closing section. The important thing is to familiarize ourselves with the traditions of our ancestors to give Jewish meaning to life-cycle events such as pregnancy and childbirth because, despite the gradual disappearance of the rich Jewish folklore surrounding childbirth, the experience still involves the same feelings of happiness and disappointment, pride and pain, hope and anxiety, responsibility and commitment. For the many modern Jews who do not experience childbirth religiously or observe the Jewish laws, a look at the traditions and folklore connected with new life may help to clarify—or even change—their thoughts about childbearing and about Jewish life in general.

Acknowledgments

This book was conceived over midmorning coffee with Mrs. Nili Sneh. I thank her for the coffee and for the inspiration I drew from our conversation. Another friend, Mrs. Zahava Weinstock, helped me word the questionnaires that I used when interviewing pregnant women. Professor Dov Feldberg and Dr. Yehezkel Bluman arranged for me to start the pilot interviews. Professor Danon, Chief Scientist for the Israel Ministry of Health in 1983, enabled me to interview pregnant women in mother-baby clinics. I am especially grateful to all the men and women who agreed to share with me their experiences of childbearing.

The gestation period of this manuscript was long. I would like to thank Dr. Elliot E. Philipp, Dr. Chico Moreno, and Professors Ron Barkai, Meir Benayahu, Mark Cohen, Gershon Hundert, Samuel Kottek, Chava Turniyansky, and Chava Weissler, who each opened up new research paths for me by pointing to sources of which I had been unaware.

Many people helped to fill in details concerning childbearing practices in specific Jewish communities. In particular, I would like to thank Hadassah Assulin at the Central Archive for Jewish History, Mrs. Estelle Fink at the Sir Isaac Wolfson Museum, Rachel Gissin at the Rishon Lezion Museum, Dr. Elliott Horowitz at Ben Gurion University, Bat-Sheva Idah at the Babylonian Heritage Museum, the staff of the Edelstein Library, Dr. Haskell Isaacs at the Taylor-Schechter Genizah Research Unit at the Cambridge University Library, Miriam Russo-Katz and Esther Muchawsky-Schnapper at the Israel Museum, Dr. Zvi Langerman at the Jewish National University Library, as well as the staff in the Microfilms, Rare Books, and Manuscripts Departments of the Jewish National University Library, Dr. Michal Saraf at the Haberman Institute, Professor Menachem Schmelzer and Sharon Liberman-Mintz at the Jewish Theological Seminary, and Dr. Bracha Yaniv of the Hebrew University Center for Jewish Art, for information they shared with me.

In addition, Havah Batinko told me of customs among village Jews during her childhood in Eastern Europe; Rabbanit Kappach of Jerusalem and Hannah Aqua explained the procedures and beliefs regarding childbearing in Yemen; Mrs. Havah Karlan of Rishon Lezion related her midwifery experiences in Palestine in the late 1920s and 1930s; Mrs. Selimah of Or Yehudah told of her midwifery practice in Baghdad; Mrs. Ada Nissim sent me material regarding Italian Jews; Dr. Shalva Weil and Mrs. Flora Samuel informed me of customs among the Jews in India; Lily Magal described the traditions among Georgian Jews; Mrs. Etti Alkanli reported ceremonies observed among Jews in Turkey. Mrs. Malka Attias introduced me to the research on childbearing carried out by the Centre for Oriental Jewish Studies. Dr. Isasschar Ben-Ami, Dr. Yedidah Stillman, and Haviva Fenton told me of birth customs in Morocco. Mr. and Mrs. Mendel Metzger illuminated customs of medieval Jewry. Dr. Kinneret Shiriyon told me of birth rituals in a Reformed Jewish community, and Mrs. Yoheved Har-Paz and Mrs. Yaffa Eizen helped me with Yiddish. I am especially grateful to Rabbi Akiva Garber and his wife Deena, who commented on an earlier draft of this manuscript and who have always been willing to answer my questions about Judaism.

I enjoyed my work at Beth Hatefutsoth, The Museum of the Jewish Diaspora, Tel Aviv, which sponsored picture research on the topic of childbearing in Jewish tradition. I am particularly grateful to David Silber, who first took on this project, for the encouragement of Joel Cahen, and for the consistent encouragement of Sarah Harel-Hoshen at the Museum. Itzhak Einhorn and Bill Gross kindly showed me many items relevant to the topic of childbearing in their private collections of Judaica, some of which I have referred to in this book.

I am grateful for having been able to use the exceptional facilities of the Cambridge University Library, the Department of Near Eastern Studies of Princeton University, and especially, the Jewish National University Library in Jerusalem.

I thank Dr. Hagit Matras, Hannah Manne, and Dr. Peter Castle for their comments on an early draft of the manuscript, as well as Dr. Ora Wiskind-Elper, Shelly Allon, of Yad Elisha, Wendy Blumfield, of the Israel Childbirth Education Centre, Dr. Dan Lewinthal, and Dr. Elliot E. Philipp for reading and commenting on individual chapters as well as Professor Benny Shilo for help with one paragraph. I am deeply indebted to Norma Shneider for asking the right questions and helping me to shape my work into a readable manuscript. I am especially grateful to Dr. Ellen Frankel for her enthusiasm, warm heart, and professional guidance. I thank also all the others at the Jewish Publication Society who have helped to produce this book.

More than anyone else, my husband, Jacob, has helped me with this book. He has encouraged me all along, enabled me to pursue my goal, advised me on small details, and shown care and concern when helping me with big, important decisions.

All biblical quotations are from *Tanakh: The Holy Scriptures* (Philadelphia: Jewish Publication Society, 1985) and are reprinted by permission of the Jewish Publication Society.

CREDITS

All talmudic references preceded by B. are from *The Babylonian Talmud,* translated and edited by I. Epstein (London: Soncino Press, 1935 to 1938), in 35 volumes. The author gratefully acknowledges The Soncino Press for permission to use selections from Tractate *Oholoth* 7:6, p. 178 and Tractate *Berakhot* 3lb. pp. 192 and 194. Talmudic references preceded by J. are from *The Talmud of the Land of Israel,* (The Jerusalem Talmud) translated by J. Neusner (Chicago: University of Chicago Press, 1982 to 1986), in 33 volumes.

All references to Midrash Rabbah are from *The Midrash Rabbah*, translated and edited by H. Freedman and M. Simon (London: Soncino Press, 1951), volumes 1 to 10, unless otherwise specified.

All references to the Zohar are from English translation, *The Zohar* (London: Soncino Press, 1931), volumes I to V, unless otherwise specified.

The following borrowed material is acknowledged:

Chapter 2: "Barren," by Rachel Bluwstein, from *Memoirs of the Pioneer Women of Palestine*, edited by R. Katznelson-Shazar (New York: Herzl Press, World Zionist Organization, 1975), translated by Maurice Samuel. Reprinted by permission of Herzl Press, World Zionist Organization. Copyright by the author, ACUM, Israel, 1996.

Chapter 3: "Abortion: A Fundamental Right in Jeopardy," in *Commission on Law and Social Action*, March 1981. Reprinted by permission of the American Jewish Congress.

Chapter 6: "Healing after a Miscarriage," by Merle Feld, in *Response* (Spring 1985), and *Four Centuries of Jewish Women's Spirituality* (Boston: Beacon Press, 1992). Copyright 1985 by Merle Feld.

Chapter 9: *First Encounter*, Bella Chagall, translated by Barbara Bray. English translation copyright 1983 by Ida Chagall. Reprinted by permission of Schocken Books, published by Pantheon Books, a division of Random House, Inc.

Chapter 9: "To My Child," by Abraham Sutskever, translated by C.K. Williams, in *The Literature of Destruction*, edited by D.G. Roskies (Philadelphia: The Jewish Publication Society, 1989). Reprinted by permission of The Jewish Publication Society. Copyright by the author, ACUM, Israel, 1996.

I have taken care not to ascribe a gender to God; however, the Divine Being is often referred to in masculine form in the biblical, talmudic, and midrashic quotations cited here.

Introduction

So many aspects of childbearing have changed in our century that our experience today differs radically from that of our grandparents. We can still learn by looking back at the Jewish customs, legends, and memories central to their world, however, because just as the leaves shed by a tree nourish germinating seeds in the earth below, so, too, the customs of previous generations form the bed of tradition that nurtures new ways of viewing our Jewish heritage.

What values, ideas, and behaviors characterize childbirth among Jews? In addition to the physiological dimension of bearing a child, Jews have also traditionally endowed the experience with spiritual and cultural significance. New life is celebrated and sanctified within the framework of God, Torah, and community. All Jewish attitudes toward birth rest on these three central pillars of Jewish life. Throughout the ages, Jews have developed many different birth traditions, such as biblically prescribed postnatal rituals, customs associated with Eve, Rachel, Hannah, or famous rabbis, or practices handed down from generation to generation within a particular community. In addition, Jews have injected their own special flavor into contemporary theories and myths to explain the mysteries of childbirth.

Do such religious approaches to childbirth still exist among Jews today? Although many Jews still experience childbirth within the framework of tradition, many others have abandoned all Jewish birth traditions, except possibly the circumcision of their newborn sons. Nevertheless, growing numbers of Jews are seeking new ways of expressing their spiritual feelings about childbirth, formulating their own prayers and blessings, writing Jewish poetry, creating novel celebrations, and founding Jewish support groups.

TRADITIONAL JEWISH ATTITUDES TOWARD CHILDBEARING

God

Traditionally, Jews have believed that childbirth depends on a partnership with God, the creator of life, who forms the infant's soul, supervises pregnancy, and determines the outcome of birth. From ancient times to the present, Jewish parents have acknowledged and confirmed this partnership through their prayers and postnatal rituals.

This partnership is not one among equals, however. Parents recognize God's supremacy. Not only do human beings love God unconditionally, but also they fear God as the One who metes out justice, rewarding the righteous and punishing the wicked. In line with this belief, traditional Judaism frames childbearing experiences in terms of God's distribution of justice: righteous persons, like the biblical matriarchs, are blessed with sons who are particularly endowed with God's favor, whereas sinners such as Eve suffer the pain of travail. Barrenness, miscarriage, and death in childbirth have also traditionally been interpreted as divine retribution for sin.

This understanding of divine justice causes serious theological problems. Why then do the righteous suffer? Why do the wicked prosper? Why is it that some pious people cannot have children while others, less pious or even downright wicked, can? Why are some innocent babies born handicapped? Why do some women suffer unduly in birthing? Why does childbirth sometimes end in tragedy?

Solutions to this apparent theological contradiction appear in many Jewish tales as well as philosophic treatises. The most common explanation is that the righteous suffer in this world for every small sin, so they may reap their full reward in the World to Come. The wicked prosper for the few good deeds they have performed but will receive their full measure of punishment in the next world.

Alternatively, the suffering of the righteous has been regarded as a trial through which the righteous are tested to develop their faith. Thus have rabbis traditionally explained the barrenness of the biblical matriarchs. For yet others, divine justice is simply beyond human comprehension. Through their childbirth prayers, Jews express their belief in divine determinism.

Jews also sometimes have attributed the suffering of the righteous to sources of evil, such as demons and harmful spirits. Jewish tales tell of demon pregnancies and infant deaths, especially at the hands of the demon Lilith, who is said to prey on women in childbirth and their newborns. Jewish women have long protected themselves during delivery and lying-in with an amulet said to be effective in warding off this demon.

In addition, most Jews recognize that suffering does not always come directly from God. Barrenness and miscarriage and physical suffering during labor and delivery can result from physiological conditions, not divine punishment.

Even though parents recognize that they cannot always understand or control the forces—physical and divine—working in childbirth, they nonetheless feel compelled to do something to effect a favorable outcome. They may pray to God to reverse barrenness or to lessen pain. Husbands may pray on their wives' behalf. Many seek intercession from a *tzaddik*, a righteous Jew who has a special relationship with God. Jewish folklore is filled with legends of such extraordinary help.

Because Jews regard God as the ultimate creator of life, and the human soul as divinely created and immortal, they have always maintained a profound respect for human life. This view has determined Jewish attitudes toward contraception and abortion, as well as the manner in which Jews have managed difficult births. Partnership with God is thus at the heart of Jewish attitudes toward birth.

Torah

Throughout the ages, Jewish childbirth practices have been remarkably uniform in the different communities where Jews have flourished, largely because of the centrality of Torah and halakhah (Jewish law) in their lives. Together with faith in God, these sources of accepted authority have determined many dimensions of Jewish life. Torah and its evolving rabbinic interpretation form the basis of the codified laws guiding a Jew's daily life, including laws concerning childbirth.

Traditionally, Jews have accepted that the Torah represents a divinely revealed design for the world, covering all dimensions of human behavior: doctrine and practice, religion and morals. The Torah represents far more than a basis for social, political, and religious life, however: it is ultimately holy, a supreme value in itself.

Although its spiritual teachings may be gleaned through study and speculation, or through emotional responses to the text, most of the Torah, in its fullest interpretation, comprises a practical guide for everyday Jewish life. A religious Jew believes that by observing the Torah's laws and by dedicating himself to God's will he is not only living a holy life but he is also helping to perfect the world. Even the smallest details of how a person behaves can affect the community as a whole. Transgressing a law of the Torah is thus more than a social and religious infraction; it is a rebellion against God's design.

Confronted by the Enlightenment following on the heels of the French Revolution, some European Jews began to question their unqualified adherance to Torah. Whereas the existence of God, providence, and the immortality of the soul could be deduced through reasoning, other parts of the Torah were not amenable to such analysis. Nineteenth-century reformists endeavored to adapt Torah to "the spirit of the age," maintaining that Judaism was no more than a religion, not a blueprint for social behavior. Because Jews were no longer a nation, they argued, all laws and ceremonies that differentiated Jews from their non-Jewish neighbors should be abolished. So, for instance, these modern Jews advocated abandoning the archaic ritual of circumcision. However, this age-old rite of passage was too central to Jewish identity to be abandoned by many Jews, no matter how progressive. Other rituals did fall by the wayside, however. The degree to which individual Jews were willing to compromise with tradition eventually led to the formation of several new groups of Jews, positioned along the continuum between Orthodoxy and radical Reform, each varying in its interpretation of Torah.

Community

Jews have always had a strong sense of being a people. Because children ensure the continuity of the people, childbearing has always played a central role in Jewish communal life. Jews have linked the emotions of infertility and the experiences of birth with significant events in our people's past: difficult labor reminds women of Eve's punishment for her disobedience; childless couples recall the trials of Rachel and Hannah. "Tried and proved" folk remedies have also provided links with the past, bringing ancient and modern communities closer: the mandrake or ruby associated with Rachel, a special fruit connected to Eve in the Garden, amulets passed down for generations. Even traditional lullabies remembered from a young mother's own childhood reinforce the fabric of Jewish continuity.

Names, too, join the generations and are sometimes significant in Jewish communal life. Names such as "Cohen" or "Levy" hark back to priestly descent. Hebrew names link child to parent. Children of Ashkenazi background carry the names of deceased family members. Sephardic parents pass on their own names to their children.

Special rituals welcome Jewish children into the community. A newborn boy becomes a member of the Jewish people when he is circumcised. Although tradition provided no parallel initiation for newborn girls, Jews in modern times have created new ceremonies to assert the Jewish identity of their daughters.

One reaction to the growing assimilation of European Jews in the nineteenth century was a dramatic increase in Jewish spiritual nationalism, especially in Russia. Galvanized by new forms of anti-Semitism, many Jews united in the belief that they needed their own country; both religious and secular Jews rallied to the call for a Jewish state. Zionist pioneers learned to speak Hebrew, the traditional language of prayer and sacred study, in their daily lives, and worked together to build a new nation in the land of Israel. They viewed childbearing as a community obligation. With the exception of a small number of Orthodox pioneers, these Jews raised their children in a communal and nationalistic Judaism, divorced from religious practice.

Today, again except in the Orthodox communities, the communal dimension of childbearing has all but disappeared among Jews. Regarded as a private experience shared by the couple, birth and its celebration no longer necessarily involve the Jewish community. The couple consults a doctor instead of the rabbi. The midwife who assists in the birth usually is not employed by the Jewish community. Even though postnatal celebrations sometimes take place in the synagogue, more often such celebrations are private affairs attended only by family and close friends.

JEWISH IDEALS AND SOCIAL REALITIES

What are the Jewish ideals regarding the bringing of a child into the world? Jewish tradition has stressed that children are a fulfillment of marriage and has recommended contraception and abortion only when human life is at risk. Some couples, pregnant women, and birth helpers have not always upheld these ideals under the pressures of daily life, however.

Judaism teaches that women naturally desire to have babies, but that men sometimes have to be reminded of their duty to procreate. To demonstrate this belief in women's natural desire for children, the tradition points to the intense longing for children expressed in the plaintive laments of barren women. The experience of a difficult childbirth can sometimes turn a woman away from the desire for more children, however. Moreover, in some communities, a negative attitude toward the birth of daughters can sour a parent's sense of fulfillment. In addition, in some cases, postnatal breakdown, well documented in the literature of psychiatry, threatens a woman's sense of self.

Facing problems in childbearing, Jews have turned to traditional Jewish remedies such as supplication, repentance, and charity, as well as "tried and proved" folk remedies. When these have proved ineffective, however, Jews have freely resorted to almost any successful popular remedy, even those ritually suspect or forbidden, to save a life. Although sorcery and witchcraft are strictly forbidden in the Bible and Talmud, popular Jewish remedy books have included nonkosher magic potions. Furthermore, evidence indicates that instructions for avoiding and terminating pregnancy were sometimes followed not only in life-threatening situations.

Jewish tales tell of rabbis who overpowered sorcerers with their own supernatural powers. Throughout the ages, amulets, charms, and incantations have been authorized as "tried and proved" for use by Jews in childbirth. Such measures were not only tolerated, but were even legitimized. One account tells of an eminent Talmudist suspected of invoking a false Messiah in the childbirth amulets he wrote for women.

Because childbirth has been so important to Jewish communities throughout the ages, rabbinic authorities have been willing to bend or update Jewish laws to accommodate changing needs and social pressures. So, for instance, medieval rabbis differed in their approaches to levirate marriage (a man's obligation to marry his deceased brother's widow and produce an heir) and bigamy for the purpose of producing children. Although such marriages were forbidden in Ashkenazi communities, they were permitted in other communities until recently.

Sometimes rabbis adapted secular practices to try to make them more acceptable. Thus, folk remedies were interpreted in the light of Jewish traditions; bacchanalian postnatal visits were tamed into evenings of prayer and religious reading. Rabbis also actively opposed practices regarded as contrary to Jewish morality, such as liberalized abortion, vasectomy, artificial insemination, and surrogate mothering. Today, rabbis seek to reconcile modern medical and secular remedies for infertility with ancient Jewish solutions and ethical teachings.

This pull and push between tradition and change has always been a dynamic of Jewish life. Today, perhaps more than ever before, it is an ongoing challenge in the Jewish world.

Part I
Conception

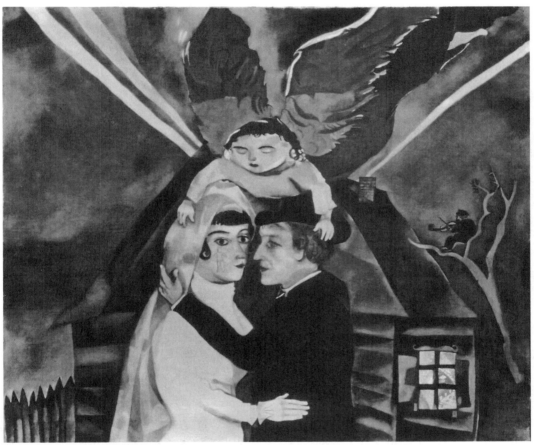

Plate 2. *The Wedding.* 1917, Marc Chagall.
Oil on canvas, 100 × 119 cm. Pushkin Museum, Moscow. Photo: Giraudon, Paris.
Copyright: ADAGP, Paris.

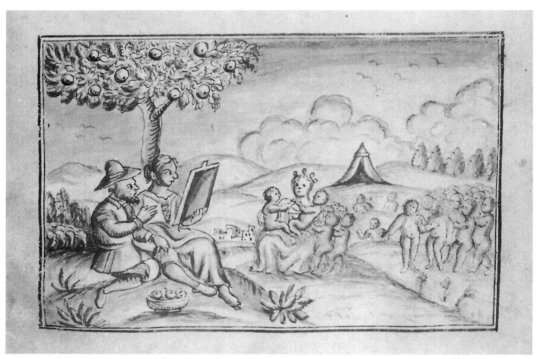

Plate 3. "I let you grow like the plants of the field" (Ezekiel 16:7). Vienna Haggadah, 1748.
Gross Family Collection, Ramat Aviv.

Chapter One

Fertility

"Be fertile and increase"

THE BLESSING

In the Bible, God creates the world for habitation and blesses Adam and Eve with the words "be fertile and increase" (Genesis 1:28). The biblical phrase contains both the blessing of fruitfulness and a commandment to reproduce. God offers the same blessing to Noah, after the Flood, when again the world requires populating.[1] Later, God promises Abraham many descendants; the same blessing is passed on to his children, then to Jacob and his grandsons.[2] After the Exodus from Egypt, Moses repeats God's promise to the Israelites, and the Prophets and Psalms reiterate time and again that children are a divine blessing.[3] The Bible uses beautiful imagery from nature to emphasize God's commitment: "I will ... make your descendants as numerous as the stars of heaven, and the sand on the seashore" (Genesis 22:17); "I let you grow like the plants of the field" (Ezekiel 16:7).

The blessing of progeny is not unconditional, however; God's promise applies only to those who live according to the laws of Torah, not to those who disobey the Commandments.[4] The Israelite prophet Hosea begs God to punish the iniquity of the people by giving them wombs that miscarry.[5]

Elaborating on the same theme, sages of the talmudic period also stressed the moral implications of God's blessing. Some proposed that, in the beginning, God created a fixed number of souls, to provide for the birth of all future generations. According to this view, once these souls have all been born, the order of the world as we now know it will change and the Messiah will come. Therefore, one who does not have children delays the arrival of the Messiah.[6] In this view, the blessing of children enables eventual Jewish national redemption. Other rabbis, who through the ages espoused different ideas about when souls were formed, have taught that procreation is an act of faith in God that guarantees the future of the Jewish people. According to Jewish tradition, each new Jewish life is sacred and serves to build up the world. Furthermore, children are the reason that God gave Jews the Torah.[7]

Rabbis in talmudic and medieval times pointed out that, unlike all other mammals, who also have genitals for procreation and breasts for nursing, only humans have the intellectual ability to take responsibility for perpetuating God's image and laws from one generation to the next.[8] A man who remains childless, these rabbis warned, nullifies the image of God as much as one who has murdered, because in both cases he has forfeited a life that has a right to exist.[9] Such behavior threatens the fabric and the future of the Jewish people. The Talmud declares that one who does not procreate "despoils the holy covenant in all of its dimensions" (B. Yevamot 63b).

In addition to the moral implications of this blessing, Jews have recognized the practical consequences, because a child provides parents with security for their old age. In Jewish tradition, parents, who may have struggled to provide for their babies, expect their adult children to care for them when they become infirm.[10] Although children may seem as much a burden as a blessing, especially when money is scarce, or when women are exhausted from childbearing, later in life parents appreciate the love and attention of their children. In the early eighteenth century, for instance, a widowed grandmother, who had borne thirteen children, recalled her suffering when she was burdened with a household of small children. "No one," she thought, "had such a heavy burden as I, and suffered as much as I through offspring. But I, foolish one, did not know how well things were with me when my children were like olive branches about my table."[11]

Jews have added yet another dimension to this blessing. Parents also can reap benefit from their offspring after they die; a person who has a child receives a reward in the next world and merits the World to Come.[12] Jewish parents have believed that a son's piety may have a redeeming influence on the souls of his departed parents and may thus guarantee repose of their souls. Since the early gaonic period, Jewish liturgy has included a special prayer for the repose of the soul—the Kaddish prayer. In the sixteenth century, a physician living in Ancona noted that a Jew had traveled all the way from Constantinople to obtain a remedy for his wife's barrenness, because he needed a son to recite this prayer when he and his wife died, so their souls might enter heaven. This custom of reciting Kaddish for a departed parent continues to this day in most Jewish communities.[13]

Although any child provides evidence that a marriage has been blessed by God, the "child of old age," the last child, is regarded as a special blessing. The Bible reports that Sarah was ninety years old when she gave birth to Isaac, and legend tells that another mother, Jochebed, was one hundred thirty years old when she gave birth to Moses.[14] Births to such geriatric mothers imply the help of a divine hand.

A child born unexpectedly late in a woman's life has always received special attention in Jewish families. In Yiddish-speaking communities, the youngest child has long been known as mezhinik (literally, the child of old age). A record of Jewish life in the shtetl tells that such a child always won the tiny Sabbath loaf baked from the scooped-up leftovers of dough after the large loaf was made and earned the name "the scooped-up." The Jews of Baghdad referred to such an infant, in Judeo-Arabic, as the fruit of old age, bazr el-shaib, in a local proverb admitting that it is no shame to spoil this child. They referred to this baby metaphorically as the "rinser of the belly," ghesal albitune; because, after this child, a mother's belly would no longer carry another.[15]

THE COMMANDMENT

Blessed with fertility, animals reproduce instinctively, but humans have choices: we can use our generative organs for pleasure alone and not for procreation; we can destroy these organs and render them incapable of functioning; or we can use these organs in perverse ways. For humans, therefore, "be fertile and increase" is not only a blessing, but also a commandment.

Through the ages, rabbis faced many practical problems relating to the performance of this duty, and some rabbinic rulings were codified into Jewish law.[16] Does bearing two sons fulfill this obligation, or is it necessary to have a child of each sex? Is it enough to have just one child, if there are grandchildren? Does the birth of an illegitimate child count toward satisfying the commandment? Does the responsibility for having children apply equally to men and to women? If a woman has suffered terribly in childbirth, must she continue to bear more children? Can one delay marriage to postpone conception? Can one forgo having children in certain circumstances? These are not academic issues, but rather, problems in real life. A widower's decision to remarry and a woman threatened with divorce on account of her barrenness could be affected by the answers to these questions.

Rabbis have differed in their answers to such questions. For example, some of the early sages maintained that a son and a daughter comprised minimal satisfaction of the duty, because the couple has "replaced" itself, whereas others thought that two sons were actually sufficient. Rabbis have generally agreed that offspring must be viable and fertile, however, with the potential to reproduce themselves eventually. Children may die before their parents, but if only one child survives to maturity, grandchildren count toward the observance of this duty. In addition, since ancient times rabbis have stressed that a man has a moral obligation to continue fathering children beyond minimal fulfillment of the commandment, if possible. Traditional Judaism has viewed procreation as a lifelong obligation.[17]

Rabbis have also differed about whether the duty to have children applies to men only or to women too. Some rabbis have included women in the obligation to procreate, because without some cooperation from his wife, a husband cannot carry out his duty. Others have maintained that only men are duty bound. A rabbi's opinion on this issue would be relevant when counseling a woman who wishes to prevent pregnancy or one who desires to wed an infertile man.[18]

The commandment to have children has often been difficult to enforce. Many of the questions addressed to rabbis through the ages have concerned marital conflicts arising from a couple's lack of offspring. In the Middle Ages and until modern times in some Jewish communities, especially in Arab lands, but also occasionally in Europe, some childless husbands took a second wife for the purpose of procreation. Rabbis, who often participated in litigation and divorce petitions, may have taken into consideration the personal circumstances of both husband and wife when endorsing divorce or bigamy for the sake of obtaining a child, but frequently they were unable to please all parties involved. Usually, rabbis could not and did not try to enforce the procreative duty. They have not wanted to break up forcibly a happy but childless marriage or to insist that an elderly widower take a young, fertile woman into his bed as a new wife.

In 1985, this traditional duty was cited by the Israeli Minister of the Interior in seeking approval for allowing life prisoners private visits with their wives, for the purpose of procreation. "We intend to see that all those serving sentences . . . have the opportunity to fulfill God's law," announced the Interior Ministry spokesman, insisting on the rights of Jewish prisoners to carry out their religious obligations. The Police Ministry, shocked and barely coping with the overcrowding of the jails, responded that on no account would it allocate facilities for private visits involving sexual relations.[19]

MARRIAGE BLESSED WITH CHILDREN

The blessing to Rebekah before she married Isaac, "May you grow into thousands of myriads" (Genesis 24:60), has become part of the traditional Jewish wedding ceremony, pronounced when the groom lowers the veil over the face of his bride. The words of Psalm 128 express the same hope that a marriage will be blessed with children: "Your wife shall be like a fruitful vine . . . your sons like olive saplings around your table . . . [may you] live to see your children's children." These and other Jewish blessings of fertility, taken from Genesis and the Book of Ruth, have adorned wedding contracts and have been included in songs and letters to convey to new couples that children are the natural and expected fulfillment of marriage.[20] Jews have repeated these blessings at nuptial celebrations worldwide and have engraved, painted, and embroidered them on wedding gifts.

Fertility Motifs at Weddings

In addition to the fruitful vine, wheat, pomegranates, fish, and fowl have also served as Jewish symbols of fertility. Like the fruitful vine, these symbols over the centuries have acquired Jewish meaning by association with Jewish sources. They are featured in the decoration of wedding contracts and clothes (such as a bride's headdress) and in the food served at marriage celebrations.

The most common symbol of fertility is the fish. Until recently, fish was served at weddings in North African and Iraqi Jewish communities and among the Sephardic Jews in the Holy Land.[21] Fish has featured in wedding celebrations in other ways, too. In the Balkans, traditionally a bride jumped over a platter with a large fish, accompanied by shouts that she should be blessed with as many children as a fish, and in Libya, the groom threw fish at his bride's feet.[22] In Morocco, "the day of the fish" referred to the eighth day after a wedding because the husband bought a fish for his wife on this day, his first outing after his marriage.[23] The association of fish with fertility stems from Jacob's blessing to his grandsons, Ephraim and Manasseh, "may they be teeming multitudes upon the earth" (Genesis 48:16). The Hebrew word for "teeming" derives from *dag*, a fish; Jacob hoped his grandsons would multiply like fish.[24]

In talmudic times, wedding participants threw roasted grains and nuts at the new couple, as a reminder of God's promise that humankind's offspring would be as plentiful as the seeds of new life in the plant world. This custom continued until modern times in Eastern and Central Europe, Kurdistan, and Djerba, sometimes accompanied by shouts of "be fertile and increase."[25] Other customs expressing the hope for children are of later origin. For example, Italian Jewish brides have recited a prayer before immersion that included the hope that their marriages would be blessed with children. Sephardic women have baked special breads or cakes to serve as symbols of fertility at a celebration with the bride after her immersion in the ritual bath on the eve of her wedding. Hasidic brides and grooms from Eastern Europe have performed a special dance, Koilich Tanz, with a twisted white loaf (*koilich*) and some salt, for the same purpose.[26]

Although many Jews now tactfully refrain from alluding to procreation at the wedding, most couples still expect to have a child in the course of their lives. When recently asked why they married, several Jewish women responded with age-old views: "So that there will be a future to our home"; "We got married in order to build a family."

PREFERENCE FOR SONS

A preference for sons over daughters is evident throughout Jewish history, as expressed in the Bible, Talmud, in medieval Jewish texts, in the later commentaries, prayers, and ethical texts, in proverbs and sayings common in Jewish communities worldwide, in blessings pronounced during pregnancy and after a birth, and in welcoming songs and lullabies. Accordingly, the social and religious customs practiced during the first week after a child's birth have differed for girls and boys. Festivities in honor of a boy's birth, culminating in the lavish circumcision celebration, have always been more ostentatious and joyous than postnatal celebrations for girls. Such a double standard is typical of a patriarchal society with male-dominated attitudes and values.

During the talmudic period, a father anticipated honor and happiness from his sons but lost sleep worrying about the future of his growing daughters. Sons represented a man's self-fulfillment and were a good spiritual and financial investment; they could gain a parent entrance into the World to Come and could increase the family's wealth, strength, and status. They would study, become pious and righteous, perform good deeds, and care for their parents in old age. They would father another generation of sons who would continue to study the Torah and uphold the family name.

Daughters, on the other hand, were a burden. A father had to keep an eye on his daughters and labor to provide a dowry for their weddings. After her marriage, a girl traditionally left the family home to live in her husband's home.[27] The Talmud admitted that both sexes were necessary for Jewish survival, yet concluded that "happy is he whose children are males [and] woe to him whose children are females" (*B. Pesaḥim* 65a). A talmudic legend told of a "town of males" called Kfar Dikhraya where women gave birth only to sons. Couples wishing for a son would settle there and those who wanted a daughter moved away.[28]

Omens

The situation for girls was not entirely bleak, however; parents have cherished daughters, too. Rabbi Hisda (third century), who himself had seven sons and several daughters, remarked that, for him, daughters were dearer than sons. A first-born daughter, he said, was a good sign that sons would follow, an adage that has given much comfort through the ages.[29] In contrast, another talmudic sage, analyzing the roots of the Hebrew words for male and female, deduced a different omen from a girl's birth: when a boy is born, peace comes into the world and his provision comes with him, whereas a girl brings nothing.[30] Continuing this tradition, medieval scholars found that the numerical value of the Hebrew letters in *zakhar*, "male," is equivalent to that of *b'rakhah*, "a blessing."[31] North African Jews pointed out that the equivalent of *nekevah*, "female," is *nezek*, "harm" or "indemnity"; parents were heartbroken at the birth of a daughter, as if harm had occurred in the family.

In the twelfth century, a midrash interpreted the biblical blessing "the Lord bless you and protect you" (Numbers 6:24) to mean "May God bless you with sons and watch over your daughters."[32] In those days, even a business letter to some-one who had no son included the hope for a male child to continue the family name. Whereas letters of congratulation on the birth of a son quoted psalms extolling the value of sons, Jews did not write such letters when a daughter was born; instead, a correspondent congratulated a new father on his wife's deliverance from the dangers of childbirth.[33]

Ethnographic accounts of Jewish communities dating from the late nine-teenth and early twentieth centuries document the preferential reception of newborn boys compared with girls, including the mocking of parents who had only daughters.[34]

Yiddish proverbs common in the shtetl warned "many daughters, many troubles, many sons, many honors" and "if you have daughters you have no use for laughter."[35] Similarly, Sephardic Jewish proverbs revealed an unambiguous bias: "One who raises a son, weaves gold; one who raises a daughter, weaves anxieties"; "When a girl is born, the walls weep"; "When there are no daughters, there is one pain; and when there are daughters, there are one hundred pains."[36] In Bukhara, Dagestan, Georgia, and the Caucasus, Jews preferred sons to daughters and named a daughter born after a few others Kamaria, meaning "enough."[37] Traditionally, Jews have expected mother and daughter to become friends and a first-born daughter to help her mother raise the younger siblings. Sephardic Jews nevertheless have a saying that a mother without a daughter has no friend.[38]

A Folktale

A Sephardic folktale, told by a Jew from Salonika, depicts the frustration of having daughters only and the good luck that can come with many sons. Once there were two brothers. One was very rich and had many daughters, but no sons, whereas the other was extremely poor and worked hard to provide for his wife and children. Each year, the wife of the poor brother bore him another boy. The wealthy wife was jealous of her in-laws for having many sons, and each time the poor brother came to ask for a little money or food, she refused and sent him away empty-handed.

When yet again the wealthy wife was delivered of a girl, the other couple produced another boy. In anger, the jealous woman went to the *mohel* (circumciser) and bribed him with a huge sum of money not to circumcise her newborn nephew. The poor brother was determined to fulfill the religious duty of circumcision, however, and he carried his newborn to a synagogue in another town early on the following morning. On his way home, he found his town buzzing with the news that thieves had stolen much silver and gold from the king's palace.

He delivered the newly circumcised infant to his wife to nurse, and when she changed the baby's diaper, she was amazed to find the soiled diaper full of silver and gold coins. Each time they changed the child's diaper, the couple found more of these coins and thanked God for performing miracles.

When the rich wife heard of her brother-in-law's change of fortune, her jealousy and anger greatly increased. She suspected him of the robbery at the king's palace and promptly reported that her in-laws were the thieves. The king's men hastened to the modest home of the suspects and saw with their own eyes that the newborn's diaper was filled with silver and gold coins at every change. They realized that the wealthy woman had lied and issued her death warrant. The good Jew and his wife continued to bless God and lived happily while raising their many sons.[39]

Although most parents no longer uphold the historical bias in favor of sons, in some Jewish communities it persists to this day. For example, recently, an eleventh daughter was born to a thirty-six-year-old father in Israel, who welcomed her with the announcement that he hoped their twelfth child would be a son. Why not? The wife of a Baghdadi rabbi bore a son only after thirteen daughters.

Advice for Obtaining a Son

Spiritual Methods

Assuming that God determines the sex of the embryo, talmudic sages advised praying for a son until the fortieth day after conception, by which time they thought that the sex of the fetus was formed.[40] A husband may have petitioned quietly during the daily public recitation of prayers (after the last of the intermediary benedictions of the *Amidah*). If a woman prayed, she may have begged God for a son when she ritually immersed herself after her menstrual period, because she hoped to conceive that very evening, and she may have prayed for a son on a Friday night when she lit the Sabbath candles. We do not know the exact words of such prayers in ancient times, but by the Middle Ages, devout Jews recited their private devotions in Hebrew, in the general style of Jewish prayers.

By the sixteenth century onward, printed collections of private prayers included prayers attributed to Nahmanides (Moses ben Nahman, 1194–1270) for reciting at the bedside before sexual intercourse, instead of in the synagogue between other benedictions.[41] Such prayers included pleas for potency and pure thoughts, pure and healthy seed, righteous male offspring, and specified all the ways in which seed could be blemished.

Also in the sixteenth century, some private prayers were translated into the vernacular, to make them more accessible to women who could not read the holy language. Expecting to conceive shortly after her immersion, a wife recited her prayer at the ritual bath, the *mikveh*, as well as when lighting the Sabbath candles and, sometimes, like her husband, after reciting the *Shema* prayer, before joining him in bed. In the eighteenth century, a Yiddish-speaking woman pleaded that God decree the seed to become a righteous and pious man, who would keep God's commandments, study Torah day and night, would never be shamed in the rabbinic academy, and would not err over matters of Jewish law. The woman praying was willing to accept her destiny that she bear a daughter and not a son, but pleaded that she be tidy and not impudent and that she learn to accept reproof from all who instruct her.[42]

Other Ashkenazi women in the eighteenth century requested, in a combination of German, Yiddish, and Hebrew, a baby son, a scholar of Talmud, a beautiful person with all good attributes, but, fearing evil influences, they pleaded that Satan leave the baby undisturbed.[43] Italian Jewish women at that time also recited a prayer for a son; they petitioned for a baby boy with a pure, unblemished soul and specified their fear of the desecration that a rebellious or undesirable child would bring them.[44]

In the late nineteenth century and early twentieth century, Jewish women in Austria, Germany, and New York who were acutely aware of the social pressures that favored boys recited the following prayer. Here, in an English translation from about 1900, a wife accuses her husband of pressing her to deliver a son, but admits that she herself desires the same:

> Lord and God! Thy goodness is infinite, and is the man unsatisfied; Thou overwhelms us daily with innumerable kindnesses, and yet have we always new wishes. Alas God forgive our dissatisfaction! . . . Thou hast blessed me, Oh God, with the rich blessing of thy fatherly hand. I feel happy as the wife of a man who deserves my love. Thou hast given me children who fill my heart with joy, in whom my sight hangs with pleasure, in whom I fully enjoy the sweetness of a mother. And yet, my Father, I cherish a wish, a sincere and warm wish, which often pains me and for the fulfillment of which I fervently pray to thee. I say it with blushing, my God, that my heart longs for a manly child, my heart desires a boy child who should plant our name further in the world. Oh Lord, grant me this wish! Forgive the weak mother who would use her motherly love to a boy, who would willingly bring up a boy to the weal of mankind, a worthy citizen, who would once help faithfully and work for his fellow creatures and gain for himself an honorable place under the sons of the native country. God, keep and guard my dear daughters whom Thou hast given me . . . but do not keep back from my loving heart the pleasure that I may give them a brother, upon whom they may point with pride and in whom they may find the replanting of their father's house. God and Lord may the sincerity with which I cherish this wish be acceptable to thee and enjoy thy Fatherly sanction. Oh listen to thy weak maid who prays to thee. Amen.[45]

Eighteenth-century Hasidim encouraged prayers for divine necessities only and not for mere personal requests. The prayer of one who had no male heir was indeed of divine consequence. When the prayer proved ineffectual, such a person may have called on an intercessor to petition for a son, the custom among Hasidim in other circumstances, too, when prayers appeared to remain unanswered. An intercessor was a holy man who knew how to commune with God and was known to be successful in achieving the goals of his prayers. There was another reason for seeking his help: Jews disapproved of egotistic tendencies in prayer. Although many Jews have uttered petitionary prayers for themselves, the Talmud taught that it is always better to pray for another who has the same need, in expectation of benefit for oneself, too.[46]

In the early twentieth century, Jews in Persia or Iraq obtained a written prayer for a son from a rabbi on an amulet, with magical seals and invocations for added power.

Many Jews have believed that death releases a righteous soul from a person's body, freeing it to return to God. Thus, Jews have prayed at the tomb or grave of a righteous person, or deposited on the tomb a written petition, in the hope that the spirit of the dead would communicate to God their pleas for a son. Parents have named a boy born after such a visit after the holy man who had interceded.[47]

A Woman's Sexual Fulfillment

Because some women have indeed been delivered of girl after girl despite their prayers, Jews through the ages have offered other advice for obtaining the desired son. The talmudic sages taught that when a couple unites in love and the wife reaches her fulfillment first, a son will result. If, however, the husband is hasty and precedes her in his fulfillment, the couple should expect a daughter.[48] The sages derived this recommendation from an interpretation of a Hebrew word in a verse of Leviticus (12:2), "when a woman at childbirth [*tazri'a*] bears a male."[49] The italicized word literally means "brings forth seed." In those days, no one understood human ovulation, and some people imagined that women emitted seed as a man does. The verse therefore could read that a woman's prior emission of seed favored male offspring. One of the talmudic rabbis, Rabbi Kattina, boasted that he could make all his children male; he always allowed his wife to bring forth her seed first.[50]

Biblical commentaries and marital handbooks written in the Middle Ages expanded on this talmudic hypothesis of sex determination and emphasized the importance of a woman's enjoyment and well-being in sexual relations for conception of the desired son. A marriage manual, *The Holy Letter*, attributed to the thirteenth-century Spanish Jew, Nahmanides, offered advice on the nature, time, intentions, and techniques of sexual intercourse and stressed the holiness of the act. Allowing a wife to reach fulfillment first, it taught, reveals a husband's consideration. The birth of a son was fitting reward for such commendable behavior.[51] This treatise explained another talmudic prescription for a son: the advice to place the bed in a north-south direction.[52] Extreme cold suffered in a north-facing bed in winter is as harmful as the extreme heat in a bed facing south in summer. The manual recommended placing the bed such that the couple is comfortable and not exposed to these extremes, taking into consideration not only their physical comfort, but also their emotional and spiritual well-being, so both are joyful in their union. Copied into the ethical writings of later Spanish rabbis (for example, Meir Aldabi in the fourteenth century and Isaac Aboab a century later), these ideas were popular and widely accepted.

Folk Remedies

In the early twentieth century, many customs believed to help influence the sex of a future baby involved magical ideas. For example, Jewish women in Georgia and Kurdistan who wanted a son took a prominent role in a circumcision ceremony, whereas, in Morocco, such women swallowed the circumcised foreskin. Sephardic women in Palestine imbibed a potion made of the burned and powdered umbilical cord of another woman's newborn son.[53] In Eastern Europe, Jewish women secretly attempted to bite off the stem of the citron (*etrog*) that was used ritually during Sukkot, on the last day of the festival; whoever succeeded believed she would give birth to a boy.[54] Sukkot is celebrated at the end of the summer, when the first autumn rains are expected to renew the earth's fertility. Jews have ascribed beneficial effects to the *etrog* at other times in childbearing, too, and have included other ritual items used in this festival in fertility potions. Medieval Jews believed that on the last day of Sukkot the verdict that God passes on the Day of Atonement was "sealed"; therefore, on this day God decided whether a woman would bear a male or a female child.[55]

Many recipes for male offspring in Jewish folk medicine include characteristically male ingredients (such as an animal's testes), thought to have contagious effects, that have no religious significance.[56]

Generation after generation continues to seek solutions to the same ancient concerns, but ours may be the nearest to discover how to determine the gender of our children. With the mapping of genes, micromanipulation of sperm injected directly into the human egg, and in vitro fertilization (in which the egg is fertilized in a glass dish), it has become possible to determine not only the gender, but also the genetic makeup of an embryo. These methods of conception are available only in highly specialized infertility clinics for couples with problems in conceiving or with family histories of genetically inherited syndromes. The use of these methods in any other circumstances raises serious ethical problems for all of us, not only for Jews.

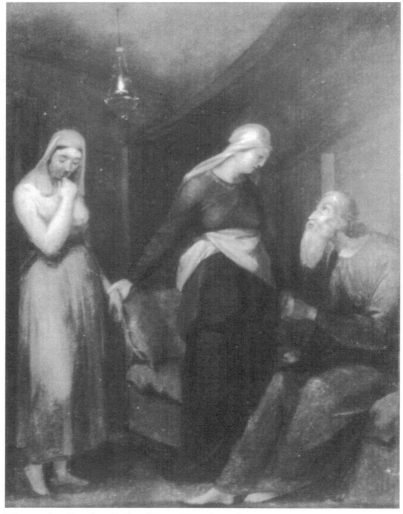

Plate 4. *Sarah Offer Her Handmaid Hagar*. c. 1824, Moritz
Oppenheim.
Oil on paper, 52.8 × 4 cm.
Collection and photo copyright, Israel Museum, Jerusalem.

Chapter Two

Barrenness

SUFFERING OF THE CHILDLESS

The Jewish picture of the childless couple is painful and sad. It depicts their suffering, their physical and spiritual destitution, the stigma, and the threat of marital breakdown that they face. It also stresses the harm to the Jewish people as a whole when an individual does not fulfill his procreative duty.

Spiritual Destitution

In the Bible, Rachel pleads, "Give me children, or I shall die" (Genesis 30:1). Distressed by her childlessness, she saw no point in living if she did not conceive. The Bible tells also of Sarah, the matriarch who suffered the pain of barrenness and gave her handmaid to her husband so he might obtain an heir. It also speaks of Hannah, who wept all the time over her wretched infertility. She was taunted by her husband's second, fertile wife, Peninnah, and was utterly depressed.[1]

In biblical times, a married man who was childless could try to have offspring with a handmaid or with a second wife. If, however, a man died childless, his wife was to marry his brother, in expectation of a baby who would be the heir of the deceased man; this arrangement was known as the levirate marriage. A releasing ceremony, called *halitzah*, in which the surviving brother relinquished this marital duty, legitimized the woman's contempt for the man who deprived her of a child and of her rights on her husband's estate in the absence of an heir.[2]

Childlessness brought about the withering of one's self and the destruction of one's family. In biblical Hebrew, a barren woman (*akarah*, meaning "uprooted") is like a tree torn out of the land, torn away from the family and left to wither without offspring. The biblical word for a man without an heir bears similar negative connotations, having the same root as the Hebrew word meaning "destroyed" (*ariri*).[3] A barren woman was a biblical metaphor for distress.[4]

Accusations about who is to blame inevitably lead to distress, when infertility is felt as a humiliation. Sarah reproached Abraham for her suffering, and Jacob was angered by Rachel's complaints concerning her barrenness.[5] A husband's admission of love was worth little when he spent his nights with another woman who was fertile. Isaac was the only patriarch who did not do this, leading rabbis to wonder whether perhaps Rebekah's failure to conceive a child was not her problem, but his.[6]

In contrast to the Bible, which shows both awareness and understanding of the suffering of the barren wife, the rabbis of the talmudic period stressed instead

15

the plight of the married man who had not fulfilled his duty to have children. These rabbis were concerned mainly with the spiritual destitution of childlessness: they taught that a person without children is cut off from all communion with God and is accounted as dead.[7] As if this were not enough, the childless man was not allowed to sit on the rabbinic council, a proscription that deprived him of status in the Jewish community and stigmatized him socially.[8]

Threat of Divorce

The Mishnah and Talmud permit a man to divorce his wife if he remains childless after ten years of marriage, so each can remarry and try again. A charming story, dating from the sixth century, tells of a couple who, after ten years of childless marriage, came to see Rabbi Simeon bar Yohai (who lived in the Holy Land in the second century) to request a divorce. The sage advised them that just as they had always lived festively together, they should not part without festivity. The wife therefore prepared a grand farewell dinner. In a good mood from copious food and wine, her husband told her that she could take with her to her father's house anything she wanted from their home. She waited for him to fall asleep and then ordered the servants to lay her husband on her bed and carry him on this to her father's house. He woke at midnight and wondered where he was. His wife explained: "You are in my father's house. Did you not tell me to take anything I cherished with me when I left? There is nothing in the world I care for more than you." Within a year, they were rewarded with a child, with the rabbi's blessing.[9]

The message of this tale—the birth of a child as a reward for a woman's true love—may have given hope to some childless couples. To this day, many childless Jews continue to visit Simeon bar Yohai's grave in Israel to pray for a blessing like that of the couple in the tale.

Sometimes, a husband has insisted on divorcing his wife for the sake of procreation, even if she has not agreed. In medieval times, a ruling, attributed to Rabbi Gershom of Mainz (tenth century), attempted to put an end to this practice by forbidding divorce against the wife's will. Rabbi Gershom also decreed against polygamy. Ashkenazi communities have observed these rulings ever since. Thus, Ashkenazi courts have not enforced divorce and remarriage for procreation. They have also favored *halitzah* to release childless widows from levirate marriage.[10] Nevertheless, some Ashkenazi men have divorced to remarry a younger woman in the hope of having children; usually, such a man offers his wife a compensation payment that she does not refuse.

A true story, about a man who was happily married but childless for fifty years, provides a good example. His name was Reb Gavriel, and he lived in Belorussia in the early nineteenth century. He was past middle age, wealthy, and unhappy that he did not have a son who would continue his name and provide continuity for the Jewish people. He weighed his options and, ignoring his wife's protests, went to his rabbi to ask for a divorce. The rabbi, however, ruled that, although Jewish law permits such a divorce after ten years of barrenness, Reb Gavriel had waited five times as long and it was now too late.

Reb Gavriel was greatly angered. He had offered ample provision for the wife of his youth and had hoped to do as he wished. Unwilling to give up, he took his case to many other rabbis and eventually found one who was prepared to arrange the divorce and also to marry him to a sixteen-year-old orphan. Reb Gavriel's wife of many years maintained her pride, however: she refused to accept either the bill of divorce or the huge sum that he provided for her every comfort in her old age.

The compliant rabbi nevertheless prepared the wedding canopy. After pronouncing the wedding blessings, he suddenly raised his hands to heaven and announced: "If this marriage is against God's will, may it prove barren as the sands of the desert! If, however, this union is the will of the Almighty, may it be blessed with many children and may even you, Reb Gavriel, together with your wife, live to marry off the youngest of your offspring!" Awestruck, the wedding guests whispered "Amen."

Everyone watched the young bride closely during the weeks that followed, and even more so when it was rumored that she no longer visited the ritual bath. Soon her pregnancy was confirmed. Only then did the old wife take the bill of divorce, because she recognized the rabbi's declaration that this marriage was the will of God. She took the money that was her due and went to die in the Holy Land. The young wife bore Reb Gavriel ten children, and he indeed lived to see his youngest child married.[11]

Another true story, from Frenda, Algeria, is about a Jewish woman, Juliette, who was divorced in the late nineteenth century on account of her barrenness. She was able to remarry and hoped for a child with her second husband, but she did not conceive and was eventually divorced again. By this time, her infertility was taken as proven, and her third offer of marriage came from Moshe, a widower who was unable to cope with five small children. He needed a wife who would mother his orphaned children and make a happy home for all of them. He did not need more offspring, and therefore Juliette was just the wife he wanted. To everyone's amazement, nine months after their marriage, she gave birth to a son, soon followed by four brothers and sisters. Moshe's feelings about his profusion of children were not recorded, but Jewish tradition would assume that he was a proud and happy man.[12]

Suffering in the World to Come

The medieval idea that a person suffered for his childlessness not only in this world, but also in the next world, appeared in a cautionary folktale, recorded in the sixteenth century. It told of a wealthy man who had a very beautiful wife, whom he loved dearly. Both had sinned, however; they were evil and had no children. Opening into their courtyard was a door where demons danced; people said this was the entrance to Gehenna (a place of torment for the wicked after death). Regardless of the husband's warnings and precautions, the wife was lured into this netherworld. Her distraught spouse set out on a long journey to find her. Eventually, he found a faithful person to whom he promised his whole fortune if this person would make contact with his wife. The messenger indeed met the wife in Gehenna, where she confessed to him her many misdemeanors. She told him of the horrors of the place and mourned for the son she had never conceived, whose *Kaddish* prayer would have redeemed her. She begged him to persuade her husband to repent of their sins, to redeem them both from this fright-ful fate. The messenger returned to the husband with the wife's ring as proof that he had fulfilled his mission and related the wife's request. The husband spent the rest of his days in synagogue repenting and asking for mercy. God noticed his atonement and gave him a share in the World to Come when he died.[13]

The woman suffered for her sins in the next world because she had no son to redeem her. On the other hand, her husband learned in time that it was not too late for him to change his own destiny by repentance. The moral of this tale is that repen-tance pays off. It teaches that when there is no possibility of repentance or redemption, the punishment of childlessness is suffered not only in this world, but in the next as well.

In the early eighteenth century, a Sephardic rabbi taught childless women how to gain credit in the World to Come. He encouraged a barren woman to agree to her husband's request of divorce (and remarriage) or bigamy (in Moslem lands only) for an heir, with the assurance that such a mitzvah would benefit her in the next world. Furthermore, this rabbi praised her for sacrificing her own interests to those of the Jewish people because, by enabling her husband to fulfill his procreative duty, she hastened the coming of the Messiah.[14]

A Misfortune

As we have seen, the Talmud enables the dissolution of a childless mar-riage, yet, in post-talmudic times, many Jewish communities permitted a man to take a second wife in order to produce an heir, without the need to divorce his first wife. This was the case in Babylonia during the gaonic period, in the Mediterranean Jewish communities in the Middle Ages, in Sephardic communities after the expulsion of Jews from Spain, and among Jews living in Arab lands until recent times.

The Hebrew word for a wife in a bigamous marriage is *tzarah*, which also means "a problem" or "misfortune" because each wife competes for the husband's love and attention. In this connection, a rabbi in Spain wrote in the thirteenth cen-tury that he knew of only two or three cases of bigamy, each on account of the first wife's infertility, and none was a happy marriage.[15]

In 1985, an Israeli great-grandmother of Yemenite origin, who had been recently widowed, talked about her family with calm acceptance of her circum-stances. Her husband had been a rabbi and circumciser, but his first wife had suffered difficult pregnancies, and only one daughter had survived. After ten years, he married a second wife, a sixteen-year-old girl (now the widow in her seventies). She referred to the first wife as "mother," as did the seven children she bore him, whereas she her-self was known by her given name. The first wife cared for the second as if she were her daughter, and the trio lived together under the same roof for fifty years.[16]

Simulated Pregnancy

A barren wife could simulate pregnancy to avoid marital tensions for a few months and delay the threat of divorce. With no objective pregnancy tests, a husband could not be sure that his wife had conceived, especially if she kept him out of her bed with claims of feeling nauseated and weak. One day, however, such a deception would have to end. Although in real life the ending to such deception was tragic, fantasy could provide a happy ending.

Elderly North African and Iraqi Jews today tell several tales about a barren wife who pretends she is pregnant: an old woman in the house might tell such a tale to a young couple, still childless a few years after their wedding, to give them hope. For example, there is a farce about a queen who feigned pregnancy and on the day of the "birth" obtained a large fish and put it in the cradle. The fish lay swaddled and covered so no one would know. On the seventh day, the queen left for the bathhouse, instructing her maid not to allow anyone, even the king, to enter her room until she returned. The maid was not careful enough, however, because a large cat smelled the fish, snatched it, and escaped onto the flat roof outside. Horrified, the maid jumped out of the window to follow the cat. Suddenly, she heard a baby cry and found a newborn abandoned in a corner of the roof. Relieved that the cat had left the baby after all, the maid quickly returned it to the cradle in the queen's room. Hearing the baby crying for the first time, the king delightedly sent for the queen at the bathhouse. She rushed home, panic-stricken that her trick had been discovered. A wet nurse was found immediately, and the king's long-desired heir grew up.[17]

In the early twentieth century, sometimes a Jewish woman in Morocco might claim that she was pregnant, but that her baby was asleep in her womb and therefore was not moving.[18]

Oh, If I Had a Son

Jewish women who want children and find that they cannot do so suffer as much today as in past generations. They may still identify with the emotions of the childless matriarchs. Earlier this century, Rahel Bluwstein (1890–1931) yearned for a child and wrote the following poem, entitled "Barren":

> Oh, if I had a son, a little son,
> With black, curled hair and clever eyes,
> A little son to walk with in the garden
> Under morning skies,
> A son,
> A little son!

> I'd call him Uri, little, laughing Uri,
> A tender name, as light, as full of joy
> As sunlight on the dew, as tripping on the tongue
> As the laughter of a boy—
> "Uri!"
> I'd call him.

> And still I wait, as mother Rachel waited,
> Or Hannah in Shiloh, she, the barren one,
> Until the day comes when my lips will whisper,
> "Uri, my son!"[19]

EXPLANATIONS OF BARRENNESS AND RELATED REMEDIES

The picture is painful and sad, but not bleak, because women sometimes conceive even after many years of barrenness. Jews have studied the biblical stories of Sarah, Rebekah, Rachel, and Hannah and have hoped for a similarly happy solution to their own predicament. They have believed that both God and a person's behavior contribute to infertility. Until modern times, many Jews believed that evil spirits could also lend a hand. Until modern science furthered our understanding of the physical causes of infertility, Jews used remedies that were spiritual, behavioral, and magical, as well as medicinal, to lift the curse of barrenness.

God Has a Role: Prayers

Biblical tales teach that God grants and withholds the blessing of fertility. Thus, after many years of barrenness, God eventually decided that Sarah should have a child and sent three angels with the good news. Sarah's daughter-in-law, Rebekah, also conceived only when God acceded to Isaac's entreaties.[20] A generation later, when Jacob grew angry at Rachel's demand of him to give her children, he remonstrated her with: "Can I take the place of God, who has denied you fruit of the womb?" (Genesis 30:2). He pointed out to her that God, not he, was preventing her from conceiving. In the same vein, the Bible notes that Hannah was barren because "the Lord had closed her womb" (1 Samuel 1:5). Eventually, in response to her prayers, and perhaps also thanks to the intercession of Eli, the priest, Hannah bore a son, Samuel. Yet another biblical couple, Manoah and his wife, welcomed the arrival (by divine blessing) of Samson, only after a long period of barrenness.[21] Puzzled by the long suffering of the biblical women, the sages of the talmudic era proposed that God first wanted to hear prayers and to see proof of their piety before enabling them to have children.[22]

Jewish tradition has maintained that God holds the key to the womb.[23] Childless Jews have therefore addressed God in prayer, repenting and asking forgiveness for whatever sins they may have committed and supplicating for mercy and beneficence. Jewish men who have prayed for their wives to conceive have had as their role model Isaac, who remained childless for many years and prayed, instead of fathering a child through a concubine.[24]

In talmudic times, a husband inserted his own personal petition during his daily prayers; only in the late Middle Ages was a specific prayer written for a childless man to recite before going to bed. Jewish women have also prayed for a child, often with prayers that use words attributed to Hannah. The wording of prayers for a child has reflected the traditional Jewish values attached to having children and the intellectual preoccupations of the supplicant. For example, one prayer rationalizes that if God made the generative organs for reproduction, they should be used for this purpose. Another reflects the importance of reproduction for national continuity and perpetuation of Torah. A kabbalistic prayer stresses the effect of procreation in promoting the unity of God. A fourth prayer for offspring admits that a woman's sins may cause barrenness and expresses fear for what will become of her soul in the World to Come.

Perhaps in their private communion with God, individual Jews have thought of other arguments to persuade God to grant them the blessing of fertility.

The Bible reports that the childless Hannah prayed silently for a long time, vowing that if God granted her request for a son, she would give him to the priesthood.[25] Her prayer is formulated by the sages in the Talmud:

> Sovereign of the Universe, of all the hosts and hosts that Thou has created in Thy world, is it so hard in Thy eyes to give me one son? A parable: To what is this matter like? To a king who made a feast for his servants, and a poor man came and stood by the door and said to him, give me a bite, and no one took any notice of him, so he forced his way into the presence of the king and said to him, Your Majesty, out of all the feast which thou hast made, is it so hard in thine eyes to give me one bite? . . . Sovereign of the Universe, among all the things that Thou hast created in a woman, Thou hast not created one without a purpose, eyes to see, ears to hear, a nose to smell, a mouth to speak, hands to do work, legs to walk with, breasts to give suck. These breasts that Thou has put on my heart, are they not to give suck? Give me a son, so that I may suckle with them (*B. Berakhot* 31b).

Following this passage, the sages taught that God rewarded Hannah with a son on account of her piety.

Prayers for conception often mention Hannah's name or state that God answered the prayers of the barren matriarchs, to tie the experience of the barren woman to biblical history.[26] In the following nineteenth-century prayer, written by a woman, a childless wife pleads with God to ensure the continuity of the Jewish people. Only at the end of the prayer does she ask for a child for personal reasons, to relieve her suffering:

> I entreat you, Oh God, who graciously remembered our mothers Sarah and Hannah. Have mercy upon my lamentation, and remember me with the blessing of fruitfulness. Let our union be blessed with a strong and healthy child, in whom we may replant your holy religion. Hallow our life with your attention to this lofty matter. God, you know our pains; you know the painful empty heart of the childless. Have mercy and redeem us from this pain. Amen.[27]

A woman recites such a prayer after immersing in the *mikveh* or when lighting the Sabbath candles.[28]

Nathan Nata Hannover (d. 1683) drew on kabbalistic sources when he composed his "midnight prayers," including one for a husband to recite "in holiness, purity and cleanliness, next to the bed on the night of intercourse," for success in obtaining offspring. The prayer petitions for potency, healthy and blessed seed, physical and spiritual purity during the act expected to result in conception, and for God's cooperation and beneficence in providing the seed with vitality and good qualities. It also supplicates against damage or deficiency in body or soul to the embryo and begs for a son, not a daughter. The text includes special mystical letter combinations (*kavanot*) on which the man is to meditate, to help the prayer reach God's supernal domain, and an Aramaic incantation against Lilith, a female demon who was thought to lurk in the marital bed and to conceive demons from the seed of man. It concludes with a mystical formula that declares that the act of marital intercourse is performed for the sake of the unity of the Godhead. This declaration endows the act of coupling with religious status. This prayer was published in a book entitled *The Gates of Zion*, in Amsterdam in 1662; the book has been reprinted over fifty times in the last three hundred years, in Holland, Italy, Central and Eastern Europe, and eventually in the United States.[29]

A Yiddish book of supplications for women, published in Vilna in 1910, also includes a prayer for the childless. In this prayer, the woman blames herself for the transgressions that she was unable to rectify and complains of the bitterness and sadness of her life. She hopes that God will accept her sorrow as atonement for her "bitter sins" and allow her soul a share in the World to Come.[30]

One more example of a prayer for those desiring a child can be found in *New Prayers and Supplications*, in Hebrew and Yiddish, printed in Hamburg in 1729. This book contains fifteen pages of prayers and supplications for conception and for sons and daughters who would grow up to be pious and upright, healthy, and God-fearing, to continue the traditions of the matriarchs and patriarchs, to marry well and bear children of their own. Thus, these prayers for children were not merely requests for conception, but rather, they had a longitudinal perspective. Those who prayed perceived their goal not merely as conception and the subsequent birth of a healthy child, but as a long process that included birthing, nurturing, educating, and raising children who would be the pride of their parents, whose good deeds would be redeeming, and who would eventually provide grandchildren.[31]

When their supplications have appeared to be unsuccessful, childless Jews in the last three hundred years, and perhaps in medieval times, too, visited holy men blessed with divine favor who were known for having their prayers fulfilled. The Prophets of antiquity were regarded as such intercessors, healing the sick and even enabling a barren woman to have a son.[32] By the talmudic period, there were no more prophets; instead, the righteous were seen as endowed with the powers of blessing: "Just as God makes barren women fertile, so the righteous can make barren women fertile."[33] Childless men and women traveled hundreds of miles to request the intercession of a holy man. Indeed, many people alive today have done exactly this, especially in hasidic Jewish communities.[34]

The custom of visiting a holy man for help in obtaining offspring is featured in many Jewish folktales.[35] The wonderworking Baal Shem Tov, Rabbi Israel ben Eliezer (c. 1700–1760), who lived in Podolia, Poland (now western Ukraine), and the Maggid of Koznitz, Israel ben Shabbetai Hapstein (d. 1814), were well known as particularly successful intercessors, consulted by many childless couples in their day. They themselves were both born to their elderly parents after many barren years.[36]

A story is told about a couple who traveled from a distant village to visit the Maggid of Koznitz, to beg him to pray that they might have a son. The sage stated that for this he would charge fifty-two gulden, because fifty-two is the numerical value of *ben*, the Hebrew word for son. The couple was very poor and had only ten gulden, but the rabbi stuck to his price. The distraught pair went home, gathered all their meager possessions and sold them in the marketplace. They added to their purse all the coppers they received and returned to the Maggid. Tipping the coins on to the table, the sage counted them: only twenty gulden. He still refused to lower his fee. At this point the villager became upset, collected his money, and said to his wife:

"Come on, let's go. God will help us without the rabbi's prayer."

"And so God has helped you," said the rabbi. And he was right.[37]

This story reinforces the hasidic premise that the role of a spiritual leader is not to solve other people's problems for them, but to help them find the solution for themselves. Thus, at their second meeting, the Maggid either divined that the woman was already with child (although the couple were as yet unaware of this), or he foresaw that she would conceive and so did not want to take their money. In any case, the couple's visit to the holy man proved worthwhile, for a son was born to them.

The reputation of holy persons who succeeded in having their prayers answered has lived on after their death; the childless have visited their graves to pray for offspring. Childless persons have hoped that the soul of the dead holy person will convey their supplications to God.[38] In medieval times, Abraham and Sarah's tomb in Hebron was a site of such a pilgrimage; one unable to make the trip himself could ask a traveling friend to do so on his behalf. Rachel's tomb south of Jerusalem, Simeon bar Yohai's on Mount Meron, and Elijah's cave near Haifa have also long been favorite sites for the barren to pray for a child. In the tenth century, a Karaite Jew railed against the custom of visiting tombs in the Holy Land to plead for pregnancy and complained that magic had become entwined with religious rites. Indeed, such pleas were often accompanied by lighting candles, burning incense, and tying scapegoats to a palm tree near the tomb.[39] Although the performance of many religious duties is often accompanied by candle lighting, incense burning and scapegoats were probably used, in that period, to exorcise evil spirits.

In the Diaspora, too, Jews continue to recite prayers at the tombs of holy men, inspired by those who enjoyed happy results after doing likewise.[40] Jacob ben Abraham Solomon wrote a book of cemetery prayers, *Ma'aneh lashon,* first printed in Hebrew in Prague, in 1615, and reprinted many times subsequently, as well as in Yiddish translation. Orthodox Jews still pray from this book today:

> May it be Your will, O God . . . that You give me seed that is desirable, worthy, good, wholesome, proper, and accepted, which will be fit to exist and to mature without any sin or guilt. Bless me and my house with offspring, so that I shall know peace in my home, and may You endow my seed with vitality, spirit, and soul from the pure and holy source . . . I beseech you, Lord of Hosts. . . . [41]

This prayer is similar to that recited by a man before joining his wife in bed after her immersion in the *mikveh.*

Childless Jewish women in Baghdad and in Morocco traditionally prayed at the tombs of holy men: their prayers in Hebrew or Judeo-Arabic were emotional supplications to God to answer the woman's deep desire and not to leave her miserably childless.[42]

A Punishment for Sins: Repentance and Good Deeds

From biblical times until our own, childless couples have asked why God would withhold the blessing of fertility. According to the Bible, infertility is a punishment for sins, especially for illicit sexual relations. Throughout the ages, Jews have developed the idea, in rabbinic commentaries, ethical texts, prayers, and tales, that sins can cause childlessness and have taught that repentance, charity, and good deeds merit the reward of children.[43]

A hasidic tale, in a collection of Hebrew folktales compiled in the nineteenth century, draws a connection between infertility and punishment, on the one hand, and fertility and reward, on the other. Once there was a wealthy, but impious, tailor who lived in Lemberg, Poland. One cold winter day, he passed on the street a poor man dressed in rags, shivering in the snow and clearly close to death. The tailor took pity on him and gave him his warm coat, remaining himself but flimsily dressed. Predictably, the rich man caught cold and was forced to take to his bed. The angels noticed he was more dead than alive and discussed what should be his fate.

"For such a good deed," said some of them, "he deserves to have a son who will be a great Torah scholar."

"His good deed may entitle him to such a son," retorted other, less charitable angels, "but how can one guilty of so many profanities father a great Torah scholar?"

Eventually, the angels compromised, rewarding him with an outstanding son, but only after he had suffered illness for many years to atone for his earlier sins. The tailor lay in bed for thirty years, and when he reached the age of seventy, he miraculously recovered and fathered a son. The boy grew up to be a great Torah scholar and a revered hasidic rabbi, but his father's name remains unknown, for it would not befit such a saintly man to be linked to a sinful father.[44]

As in the story of Abraham and Sarah, the late arrival of a son to aged parents is considered to be a gift from God.

Another legend, involving the Baal Shem Tov, touches on a similar theme. An old couple, a village bookbinder and his wife, became progressively poorer as the years passed, until one day they had no money left and could not even buy the bare necessities for honoring the Sabbath. They lacked money for candles and wine, for flour to bake the plaited loaf, and for fish for the meal. Because the husband did not want charity, he requested his wife not to accept anything from the neighbors.

That Sabbath evening, he went straight from work to the prayer house and tarried there longer than usual, not wanting others to see him going home to a dark house. When he eventually set out for home, however, he noticed that despite what he had told his wife, there was a bright light burning in the window. When he stepped inside, he found the Sabbath table laid with all the items for the blessings and with food for the Sabbath meal. He feared that his wife had succumbed to neighborly charity, but she quickly explained that this was not the case. Knowing that she had nothing to cook, she had instead put her energies into an unusually thorough housecleaning, and had been amazed to find an old sleeve, lost long ago, with fine gold and silver buttons on it. She had run with these to the goldsmith, and with the money from these had prepared a wonderful Sabbath meal.

The couple danced with joy. The Baal Shem Tov learned of their adventure, and when the Sabbath was over, he visited the couple and told them that the "hosts of heaven" had rejoiced with them, joining them in their dance. He then prophesied that they would soon have a child despite their advanced age.[45] The boy was named Israel, after Israel ben Eliezer, the Baal Shem Tov, who had brought the good tidings. The child grew up to become the Maggid of Koznitz, the holy man whom the childless villagers consulted in the previous tale and who had charged them fifty-two gulden.

The moral of these tales about childless couples reinforces the fundamental Jewish principles of repentance (as in the Gehenna tale), charity (as performed by the tailor), honoring the Sabbath (in the fashion of the bookbinder and his wife), and faith in God (like the poor villager with the bag of copper coins). These stories teach that those who observe these important aspects of Judaism may also be blessed with a child.

Natural Causes: Medical Solutions

Even in talmudic times, sages recognized that infertility could have physiological causes and was not always a moral punishment or the result of evil forces. They pointed to a husband's impotence as one cause of infertility, although they understood that such impotence was often only temporary if it resulted from undernourishment, fatigue, illness, fear of war, or even failure to empty the bladder regularly, as in the case of the students of a certain rabbi whose long lectures prevented them from relieving themselves when necessary. The sages also recognized that developmental factors in a woman could account for her barrenness, for example, if she had never menstruated. These wise men recommended various foods to increase sexual potency and desire, such as garlic, fish, and eggs.[46]

Medieval physicians believed that sterility, like other diseases, resulted from imbalances among the four bodily humors: phlegm, black bile (melancholy), yellow bile (choler), and the blood. Many remedies involved treatments intended to warm and thicken the blood, which was the medium thought to foster procreation. Maimonides, the most eminent medieval physician, believed that sperm was a product of digestion. He provided many recipes for food that was good for warming the blood and moistening the body, and he believed that such measures were favorable for sperm production and for increased virility and libido. Around the year 1190, Maimonides wrote a treatise on how to increase sexual potency—*Treatise on Cohabitation*—at the request of a Syrian sultan, the nephew of Saladin the Great of Egypt, who may have had trouble satisfying the desires of his harem. Maimonides' medical aphorisms, gleaned mainly from Greco-Roman and some Arabic sources, also included advice on this topic.[47]

Maimonides was the most influential of the many Jewish medieval physicians. Yet others, too, addressed the practical problems of increasing sexual desire, regulating body temperatures and menses, and treating diseases of the generative parts, especially in the womb, where so many complications could arise. For example, Sheshet Benveniste (c. 1131–1209), a talented contemporary of Maimonides, was a physician to the kings of Aragon. He wrote a gynecological treatise in Arabic, which (like Maimonides' work) was soon translated into Hebrew. He wrote:

> It seems to me that the nature of your wife is cold and damp and your nature, my brother, is cold and dry and here the qualities of dampness with dryness is the cause of your lack of children, because the humors must be compatible . . . and so, my brother, I will set out for you in this medical thesis the proven remedies, most of which need to be done by your wife, and a few of them by both of you together. First, in any case, her body must be cleaned each time with primula. . . . and a drink must be prepared for her. . . . with artemesia, marjoram, fennel, geranium, mint, borage, licorice . . . all soaked in white wine for a night, enough wine to cover all the ingredients, and in the morning add some clean water, cook well and then sieve. Add white whipped honey and cook some more. Add ginger, cinnamon and cloves . . . [48]

Another treatise from this period, written in Hebrew and entitled *Recollections [about] the Diseases Occurring in the Generative Organs*, describes in detail how to regulate the menses and how to treat various diseases affecting the womb. It also addresses briefly the problem of male sterility:

> When there is too little seed and no lust: The reason is a special illness in the organ or the bad humor therein. Or because of the inability of the organ [for erection] or of the two testicles and the generative organs [sic]. Or because of the bad humor which is cold and dry or because of a weakness of the kidneys . . . or weakness of the heart, the liver or the brain, or any of the peripheral organs . . . The cure is to make the opposite to the cause of the condition: if the impotence is due to a cold humor, the cure is to apply warming lotions and oils, such as millet oil . . . and the patient has to desist from cooling foods and drinks, but eat instead meat that is easily digested . . . and give him food that strengthens and warms like birds and baby doves and bird brains and meat from a one-year-old lamb, essences of cinnamon and ginger. He should eat peeled hazelnuts, almonds, pistachios, coconut, peanuts . . . [49]

Yet another medieval Hebrew text, entitled *Book on Generation*, offered remedial advice for female sterility, in the form of medicinal vaginal tampons intended to induce or regulate the menses and purify the womb.[50]

None of the remedies that assign physiological reasons for infertility are characteristically Jewish. In medieval times, however, Jewish physicians were important in advancing the science and practice of medicine in Europe, including gynecology and obstetrics, because their linguistic and intellectual skills enabled them to integrate Greco-Roman and Arabic medical knowledge. They enjoyed status in the Gentile high society, and students studied their treatises and translations at the leading medical schools, such as at Montpellier in Southern France.

There was little real progress in understanding the causes of infertility in the early modern period. Folk cures in the many remedy books popular at that time are of particular Jewish interest (as discussed later in this book), but they did not advance the scientific understanding of infertility. In 1683, Jacob Zahalon, an Italian physician and rabbi, identified five conditions causing infertility: if the husband was incapable of emitting his seed "like an arrow"; if the seed spilled out immediately; if the humors were imbalanced (too hot and dry); if there was not enough premenstrual blood to serve as nutrient for the embryo; and finally, if there was witchcraft. Zahalon offered medicinal potions for these causes. In the case of sorcery, he added the suggestion that a holy man pray for the couple.[51] In the early eighteenth century an Italian physician and rabbi, Isaac Lampronti, mentioned in his monumental encyclopedia only impotence as a cause of male infertility and developmental factors as the cause of female infertility, thereby offering no more wisdom on this topic than the Talmud.[52]

Another encyclopedia, written at this time by an Ashkenazi physician, Tobias Cohn (1652–1729), who practiced medicine in Poland and eventually became physician to the sultans in Constantinople, included a full section on gynecology and obstetrics, with a chapter on female infertility.[53] He identified the same causes of infertility as had Zahalon, but he did not include witchcraft. He pointed out that, in a very young girl, the sperm may not have reached the womb because the husband was impotent or spilled his seed early, or because the seed did not stay inside her long enough or received insufficient nourishment in the womb. However, Cohn thought that, in an older woman, the womb may have become impermeable, blocked, or too narrow. He also suggested that a woman may be infertile because she detested having sexual intercourse, "and there are many like this." He devoted a chapter to the problem of women's lack of libido in which he noted the role of the clitoris and the effects of venereal disease; in another chapter, he discussed the "suffocation" of the womb, or "hysteria" (*hystera* is the Greek word for womb), a term, very popular in medieval medicine, that Hippocrates and Soranus used in antiquity, and that referred to inexplicable female syndromes, somehow associated with the womb.[54] Cohn suggested an ancient but, in his day, still popular method of asserting which spouse was responsible for the failure of conception: each urinated on some grains, and if these grains germinated, the urine had fertilizing properties; if they did not germinate, then the person was sterile.[55] (The results of this method may have helped a wife wishing to sue for divorce on the grounds of childlessness). If the problem lay with a young woman, Cohn advised waiting until she matured, but in the case of an old woman, he had only folk remedies to offer. One of these, which he asserted had been tested, he attributed to the medieval Ashkenazi Hasid, Judah the Pious: an infusion of bugloss in wine, drunk on the night the woman undergoes her ritual immersion.

Psychological Causes: Psychotherapy

The Bible recounts that both Sarah and Rachel conceived after the birth of their husband's babies by their handmaids. Medieval rabbis likewise noticed that the adoption of a husband's child by another woman can have a positive effect on a woman's fertility, by bringing about psychosomatic changes in her physiology that enable her subsequently to conceive. On occasion, a modern-day couple who adopts a baby after being unable to conceive a child themselves finds soon after that they are no longer infertile.[56]

Since ancient times, Jews have attempted to cure barrenness through psychotherapy. Ahead of their time, talmudic rabbis recognized that one's mental state can influence bodily functioning, including conception. They maintained that a widowed or divorced woman who had no intention of remarrying would not conceive even if she were to find herself eventually back in the marital bed.[57] Moreover, they recognized that marital incompatibility could cause childlessness. One talmudic tale tells of a rabbi's role as a marital therapist when, instead of granting a divorce, he invited a couple to dine together to become better acquainted with each other.[58]

A tale from the Hasidei Ashkenaz, dating from about 1200, revealed a radical form of psychotherapy. A woman who had borne a few children, but had long since ceased to conceive, sought the advice of Judah the Pious. He recommended that her children place her in an open grave, like a corpse. As she lay there, armed men hired by the rabbi suddenly attacked the "funeral" group. The frightened children fled the scene, leaving their mother for dead. When the danger passed, she emerged from the grave, as if reborn with new life, and soon after became pregnant.[59]

Another much later (early nineteenth century) hasidic tale, centering on the advice given by a rabbi to a barren woman, also involves a psychological trauma, but of a very different nature. When the woman visited Rabbi Yisakhar Baer (d. 1843), he yelled at her, "What's all this about wanting children, you impudent hussy! Out with you!" She was so distressed by this unexpected treatment that she complained to her mother-in-law, who went herself to see the rabbi. He told her that the problem was now over and explained that there was no other way to help her daughter-in-law than to stir her "to the very depths." Indeed, the young woman conceived.[60]

In the early twentieth century, in Kurdistan, the entire community assisted a young Jewish bride who showed still no signs of pregnancy many months after her wedding. The barren girl was subjected to a ceremony involving prayers, incantations, and other rites intended to exorcise harmful spirits that might be responsible for her infertility.[61]

Sorcery: Magic

The Bible states clearly, "Suffer not a witch to live" (Exodus 22:17), and the Mishnah forbids the practice of pagan magic, but these proscriptions did not curb a real fear from antiquity to modern times that the Evil Eye, wicked demons, and nasty spells would hamper conception.[62] Jewish books of folk remedies, in contrast to medical treatises, offered advice tinged with mysticism and magic to ward off evil forces believed to be at large. Thus, Jewish incantations and amulets featured prayers and biblical verses intended to protect against evil spirits that might cause barrenness. In addition, Jews invoked demons, angels, and magic symbols, such as seals, and they employed mystical techniques to harness supernatural powers and direct them according to their needs. Such "practical kabbalah" had remedial purposes.

A talmudic fable, set in Babylon, told of a witch who cast a spell on a poor Jew, making him childless, and showed how a rabbi succeeded in exorcising it. Rabbi Joshua ben Hanania and Rabbi Eliezer ben Hyrcanus traveled through Babylon; one evening, they chanced on a Jewish home where they stopped for the night. Here the atmosphere hung heavy, for the young couple hosting them was childless, and the aging father had shut himself in his room in his sorrow, vowing not to emerge until a grandson was born. Rabbi Joshua agreed to try to help. He asked for some seeds of flax, spread them out on the table, and sprinkled some water on them. Suddenly, they began to sprout. Within a moment, there was a small growth of ripe flax on the tabletop, and the rabbi reached into the center to grab a bunch. To everyone's amazement, as he raised his hand out of the flax, he pulled out a witch by her hair. He looked her straight in the eyes and commanded: "I order you to break the spell you have cast over this man, so that he may have a child of his own." Terrified, the witch confessed that the spell was written on a charm that she had cast into the sea. The young couple's barrenness was clearly due to the witch's spell, but Rabbi Joshua did not give up. When he released the witch, she sank back into the table, and the flax withered back to a few scattered seeds. The sage went to the seaside, where he invoked the Prince of the Sea to retrieve the curse. Rabbi Joshua burned the curse, breaking the spell for ever, and within a year the long-awaited son was born.[63]

Rabbinic tradition interprets the biblical injunction against sorcery as referring only to those who invoke evil spirits to exploit them for harmful purposes and to heretics believed to consort with the devil. Because the magic performed by the rabbi in this tale, like the magic of some other rabbis in Jewish history, is beneficial, it is permissible.[64]

Tradition traces knowledge of healing magic back to King Solomon. Another talmudic legend tells of a conversation between King Solomon and Asmodeus, "king of the demons."[65] It assumes that Asmodeus studied in the "academy on high" and possessed knowledge of interest to Solomon. *The Testament of Solomon* (third century) portrays the demon as a sower of discord between husband and wife who seeks to prevent conjugal relations; the text offers advice to frustrate the demon's actions.[66] The manuscript was copied, altered, and added to in the centuries that followed. The story that unfolded provided the inspiration for a similar tale found in an eighteenth-century remedy book, in which Asmodeus revealed to Solomon the causes of a woman's barrenness and the corresponding remedies. The demon disclosed that seven spirits prevent pregnancy. These spirits cause unsatisfactory relations between the couple as well as menstrual problems. For example, one causes the wife to break into a sweat and to suffer pain in her bones when her husband desires her; another prevents her from being satisfied during sexual relations with her husband; another delays her menses by two or three months; and yet another gives her acute menstrual pains. The remedy recommended against each spirit was a specific potion concocted from animal ingredients, such as the womb of a wolf or the spleen of a bear.[67]

The Zohar warned its readers not to follow advice taken from the book that Asmodeus gave to King Solomon. However, if the Book of Zohar found it necessary to issue such a warning, we can assume that such remedies were well known in medieval Spain.[68]

Fear of sorcery was particularly rampant in the Middle Ages, among both Jews and non-Jews. *Sefer Hasidim*, an important ethical work attributed to Judah ben Samuel "the Pious" (c. 1150–1217), mentioned sorcery as a cause of infertility. This book taught that a couple who had been bewitched, so their union remained fruitless, could divorce, remarry, and both have children with new partners. Thus, the evil spell affected the couple's union, and not one or the other partner. In another instance, *Sefer Hasidim* told of a childless man who visited a sage at his deathbed. Just before the elder died, the man requested that, when the sage presented himself before God, he supplicate God to bless the barren couple with a child. The medieval text revealed faith that the sage interceded, for the evil spell was destroyed, and that same year the woman conceived. In a third case, one woman allegedly inflicted infertility on another at the bathhouse. Rather than focus on sorcery, the source implied that the barren woman did not immerse herself in the proper fashion, thus teaching that the infertility was her punishment.[69]

Since antiquity, many Jews have believed that a person desiring to harm another could do so by inflicting an evil decree, such as by means of the Evil Eye or by casting a spell. This idea has lost popularity in recent times, in the face of medical explanations of infertility, but Barukh, a Jew born in Morocco in the middle of the twentieth century, was certain that his lack of children stemmed from such a source. His first wife was very young and died after delivering a stillborn child. Her mother wanted him to marry the girl's younger sister, but he chose not to wait the many years until she would be old enough, and he soon married another woman. This second marriage proved childless, however, even though he visited doctors and rabbis and gave considerable sums to charity. Even after ten years, he refused to undergo medical treatment or to agree to divorce. He believed that his childlessness was his punishment for not satisfying his mother-in-law's request long before, and only repentance could lift the evil sentence. (We have no information about his wife's views on the matter.)[70]

Many Jewish remedy books include magic formulas for writing amulets for barrenness. Such formulas are usually ancient, copied from earlier manuscripts, and the meaning of their magical words and angel script (combinations of little circles and connecting lines) is now unknown.[71]

In talmudic times, Jews used amulets for protective purposes, if these amulets were issued by an expert and had proved useful. They were not permitted as remedies and cures but merely to protect against evil spirits.[72] Nevertheless, throughout the ages, Jews employed amulets and precious stones to promote fertility. When making an amulet, a rabbi inscribed magical forms of God's name and biblical verses (often only their initials) on parchment (and later, on paper, too), cloth, pottery, silver, or stone, to invoke God's attention. Certain inscriptions were commonly found on amulets for barren women. For example, such an amulet bore Hebrew quotations from Genesis referring to God's eventual blessing of fertility to the matriarchs, such as "No woman in your land shall miscarry or be barren" (Exodus 23:26), or "you shall not have cause to weep . . . [God] will respond . . ." (Isaiah 30:19), or simply the straightforward plea, "grant her pregnancy soon from her husband."[73]

Jews also used fertility amulets that were not inscribed, but involved some form of contagious magic that was not characteristically Jewish. For example, in talmudic times, barren women wore a special stone with protective properties. The Talmud tells that when the authentic item, which was extremely rare and valuable, was unavailable, Jews made use of another stone, which was the counterweight of a preserving stone. The Talmud, however, does not name or describe the precious stone. Medieval rabbis in France and Germany and a Polish talmudist in the sixteenth century were able to describe such a stone, which was still in use. The stone was hollow, with a smaller stone inside: the stone within a stone represented a fetus in the womb. The stone was probably aetite or eagle stone, a hollow nodule of clay-rich iron oxide with a loose nucleus.[74] Similarly, Jews in parts of the Ottoman Empire sought out a "pregnant almond" (a double nut) as a charm for fertility.[75] Ashkenazi Jews valued a "pregnant" fish—a small fish inside a large fish—and an "egg within an egg" in just the same way.[76] They hoped that the suggestive nature of the "pregnant" object was contagious, transferable to whoever possessed this rare find.

Jewish Folk Remedies

When prayers apparently remained unanswered, good deeds unrewarded, and evil spirits unexorcised, the desire for children led people to try yet other remedies. Sometimes a fumigation test was first performed to see whether the woman was capable of conceiving. If she passed the test, she went on to try all the remedies in the remedy book. Such tests and folk remedies did not usually depend on an understanding of the causes of infertility; these nostrums included animal, vegetable, or mineral ingredients boiled in wine or honeyed water, fumigations, suppositories, and ointments. Some of these tests and remedies came from the recommendations of the great physicians of medical history, such as Hippocrates, Dioscorides, Galen, and Rhazes, whereas others evolved from local folk tradition and often involved a belief in the magical transference of fertility. Thus, a woman entered the ritual bath directly after one who had just given birth, or she imbibed a potion made of placenta, pig's testicles, or mare's milk, or she even swallowed the foreskin of a recently circumcised newborn.[77] Although these remedies merely show that some desperate women would try anything in the hope of conceiving, some other remedies, involving mandrakes, red stones, hare's stomach, and willow leaves, developed Jewish significance in imaginative ways.

Mandragora. The Bible (Genesis 30:14–16) documents the most ancient folk cure for barrenness. However, it is not clear how Rachel used the *duda'im*, usually translated as mandragora or mandrake, to help her relations with Jacob bear fruit. The Hebrew word *duda'im* derives from "love." The ancient Greeks called the plant a "love-apple," using the mandrake apple, soaked in wine, as a love potion. They also believed that it helped barren women to conceive.

Josephus Flavius (37–100 C.E.) carefully described the routine for harvesting the mandrake plant, which was greatly valued in his time for casting out devils: when a dog tied to the plant with a rope tried to run away, the tug uprooted the plant and the dog died, presumably from the invisible powers in the plant.[78] An authority today on plants of the Bible, Nissim Krispil, has pointed out that Reuben, who brought Rachel the *duda'im*, may have used a donkey to extract the plant in this way, because the biblical phrase "Issachar is a strong-boned ass (*ḥamor garem*)" (Genesis 49:14) may be read instead as "Issachar's [birth] was caused (*garam*) by a donkey," if a donkey helped to procure the fertility potion that led to his conception.[79]

A medieval recipe for a fertility cure made use of only the seeds of the plant. Sheshet Benveniste, mentioned already, recommended soaking these seeds in white wine. He assured his readers that many women had profited from his recipe, including one fifty-year-old woman who conceived after taking this medicine.[80] This remedy therefore fell into the desirable category of "tried and proved." Physicians were not the only people to recommend *duda'im*, for curing sterility: Bahya ben Asher, the thirteenth-century preacher, kabbalist, and biblical exegete, was probably more responsible than anyone else for the popular use of this cure among Jews in subsequent centuries. He mentioned this remedy in his readable commentary on Exodus. This commentary was frequently reprinted and quoted, influencing Jews worldwide.[81]

A fifteenth-century illustrated Hebrew pharmacopoeia, from Italy, also recommended the mandrake plant for curing infertility. It depicted a small, leafy plant with two apples sticking up vertically and a long and disproportionally large root in the shape of a man.[82] Earlier medieval artists had already stressed the real human likeness of the mandrake root, which has features resembling legs, body, hands, and head.

The French historian, Basnage, who wrote almost three hundred years ago, had clearly never set eyes on this plant, which grows wild in the Middle East. An illustration of the plant, resembling an outsize banana tree, accompanied his text:

> Once, at the time of the wheat harvest, Reuben came across some *duda'im* in the field, and brought them to his mother Leah ... (Genesis 30:14). Several interpreters, ours in particular ... have translated the term as mandrakes, which are, so it is told, a sort of fruit whose seeds render women fertile; and these are, so they claim, what Rachel needed. [Rachel] was very angry at being barren and craved to eat of this plant, so she decided to cede to Leah her conjugal privileges (those that women want for themselves and do not give up easily) in return for some of this plant. Other learned interpreters consider the mandrake hallucinatory and say that this plant resembles a shrubby tree and is pleasing to the eye, and its fruit has an exquisite taste. Reuben found this plant, which could not have been common, was charmed by its beauty and the goodness of its fruit, and brought it to his mother who used it as we have seen. It seems that the *duda'im* were not mandrakes, nor flowers like the lily of the valley or the violet, but a delicate and fragrant fruit, full of sugar.[83]

In the nineteenth century, Jews in Morocco placed the mandrake root on a small fire, and the barren woman bent over it, thus enabling the smoke to enter her private parts. These Jews referred to the apples as "eggs of the witch" because they induce hallucinations and insanity. Also in the nineteenth century, Sephardic women in Jerusalem either ate these apples or tied the roots to their bodies as a charm. Some who ate the apples became insane for three days subsequently. In 1878, a Jerusalem newspaper advertised a sale of mandrakes with roots in human forms, "a remedy for barrenness." Several popular remedy books compiled by Sephardic Jews at that time included advice and anecdotal evidence that *duda'im* cured barrenness.[84]

The discussion of the true identity of the biblical *duda'im* and how they were used continues today. Mandrakes are native to Mediterranean countries, but not to Mesopotamia, where Jacob and his wives lived, so it is possible that Rachel's *duda'im* were not, in fact, mandrakes. Perhaps she used the heady smell of the jasmine flower as an aphrodisiac.[85] Laboratory tests have revealed that mandrake roots, leaves, and fruit have only negligible quantities of estrogen, about the same amount found in tomatoes, barley, and yeast. However, the plant has both narcotic and sedative properties, and it may have served its purpose by relaxing the person who used it.

Rubies and Red Stones. Jews used reddish gems, especially ruby, for many centuries as charms for pregnancy, associating them with Reuben's role in helping Rachel to conceive. Of the twelve precious stones on the breastplate of the high priest, representing the twelve tribes of Israel, Reuben's stone was red.[86] Since antiquity, Jews and non-Jews alike have believed that precious stones have wondrous properties, even magic powers, and have valued them for remedial purposes.[87]

In medieval times, Jews were the major importers and dealers in gems and were fully aware of all their possible uses. Bahya ben Asher's commentary on the high priest's breastplate proposed that the red stone representing Reuben grew in certain places in the sea—apparently coral—and explained its accepted use in promoting fertility by a method of word association. He pointed out that the Hebrew words for red (*odem*) and for man (*adam*) have the same letters, signaling the effect of the former (the red stone) on the latter (to bring about the birth of a man).[88] A fourteenth-century Ashkenazi manuscript, *Sefer gematriot*, similarly discussed the properties of the precious stones in the breastplate and noted that Reuben's stone, a carnelian or ruby, consumed with food and drink, enhances fertility, like Reuben's *duda'im*.[89] Bahya ben Asher, who was writing in Spain, and the Germanic author of the Ashkenazi manuscript probably both knew of an older text on the medical use of gemstones.

In the eighteenth and nineteenth centuries, remedy books continued to recommend red gems to promote childbearing, although these texts did not acknowledge reasons or sources. Jewish folk recipes suggested a fertility potion of ruby powder mixed with wine or, alternatively, that the barren woman wear a ruby as a charm. A remedy book used among Jews in Syria repeated the advice of *Sefer gematriot*, but did not mention this source.[90] The Galician rabbi Avraham Itzhak Sperling (1851–1921) included "the charm of gems" in his study of many Jewish laws and customs and offered the remedy of *Sefer gematriot*. However, Sperling gave his source as an eighteenth-century anthology of aggadic material compiled by a Sephardic rabbi in Izmir.[91] In contrast, two remedy books published in Izmir, in the late nineteenth century, quoted Bahya ben Asher's wisdom concerning the red stone, also without naming this source.[92]

In Izmir, Turkey, in the late nineteenth and early twentieth centuries, a ring with a red stone was a treasured family heirloom, passed on by a parent to a young bride in the hope of ensuring her fertility.[93] Amuletic rings made of carnelian some-

times bore the inscription "Joseph is a fruitful bough . . . " (Genesis 49:22), a verse that
the Talmud had recommended as an incantation against the Evil Eye. In some hasidic
communities, barren women still borrow reddish stones to wear in the hope of conception. Success stories accompany such stones, giving hope and strength to each
woman who borrows one. She returns it to the rabbi's wife when birth is imminent.[94]

Potions. An ancient treatise on the laws of female purity, *Tosefta atikta*, warned against
using unclean ingredients in remedies for barrenness, an apparent indication of the
use of such remedies. This text considered the wife of Manoah, in the Book of Judges,
who suffered from barrenness before she eventually gave birth to Samson. It taught
that God blessed the woman with fertility for her pious avoidance of a (presumably)
well-known "unclean" potion made of burnt fox skin. A footnote added to this text,
in Poland in 1890, justified the use of the stomach of a hare (*be-keiva arnevet*) in fertility potions by the fact that the Hebrew phrase is numerically equivalent (according to *gematria*) to that for conceiving and bearing a child (*tazri'a ve-yalda*).[95] Such a
rationale suggests that a potion using the stomach of the hare was commonplace.

Since ancient times, many peoples have thought the hare rich in magical
powers.[96] A medieval Hebrew adaptation of a second-century Greek obstetric text
included the stomach of a hare as an ingredient in a vaginal pessary for remedying barrenness, with the author's specification that it had proved successful.[97] Sheshet
Benveniste assured his readers that "many doctors have agreed that the stomach of a
hare steeped in wine and drunk or kneaded with some butter [into a pessary] and
placed in the womb" would enable a woman to conceive immediately.[98]

The exact remedy forbidden in the *Tosefta atikta* (using burnt fox skin)
was actually recommended in a popular remedy book by a wonderworking rabbi
(*baal shem*), Eliahu ben Moshe Luntz (seventeenth century), which was first published
in Eastern Europe in 1720.[99] The stomach of the hare was an ingredient in a fertility potion in yet another well-read remedy book by a Lithuanian contemporary,
Zekhariah ben Jacob Simner, which was also first published in Eastern Europe, a few
years later. Simner took care to recommend maintaining cleanliness in preparing a
dose for both husband and wife to drink after the ritual bath and for three consecu-
tive nights before having sexual relations:

> Take the stomach of a hare, clean it well of faeces, and take care that
> it does not touch the ground. Burn it on a new unused metal utensil
> until it turns into ash. Lay the metal [utensil] on the coals [to cool]
> and then crush the ash to a fine [powder] and drink [it] in [a cup of]
> still water. . . . then she will conceive.[100]

A Hebrew remedy book, used especially by Sephardic Jews, recommended
this ingredient for a cure for barrenness and justified its use by pointing out the *gematria* of the Hebrew words, but this book wrongly attributed this calculation to the
well-respected *Pirkei de-rabbi Eliezer* (eighth century).[101]

Herbs, grasses, and especially the willow and the citron used in the ritual of
the Feast of Tabernacles (Sukkot) also were used in cures for barrenness. Ancient rites
to induce rainfall and to renew the fertility of the land may have led to the use of the
willow and citron in the Sukkot ritual at the end of summer. A book of medicine

drawn from the practical Kabbalah that flourished in Jerusalem from the sixteenth century to modern times attributed a fertility remedy consisting of a dish of meat roasted on willow branches to the famous kabbalist Isaac ben Solomon Luria, "The Ari," (d. 1573).[102] In the late nineteenth century, an Eastern European rabbi told of a person whose wife drank an infusion of willow leaves and subsequently had children. He pointed out that in *gematria*, the Hebrew word for willow (*aravah*) is numerically equivalent to that for male seed (*zera*). A Sephardic rabbi from Morocco reported that the drink was tried and had proved successful. Another plant used at Sukkot is the citron: until the early twentieth century, Jewish women in Alsace bit off its stem in the hope of conception in the coming months.[103]

Childlessness has always been one of the greatest afflictions that can befall a Jew. The active search for causes of infertility and remedies has intensified in the twentieth century, however, and our generation has witnessed important scientific discoveries disclosing many medical causes of infertility as well as revolutionary techniques for overcoming them and enabling conception. Israel has become one of the world's centers for infertility research, with many infertility clinics available to help Jews have the children they desire. The search for new methods of helping people become parents continues, and new forms of treatment, now "tried and proved" in scientific ways, raise hopes for those who have not conceived naturally.

Identification of the medical problem and subsequent fertility treatment can be long and difficult, and sometimes doctors admit they cannot help. Some people may choose to have a family using modern methods of combining a donor's egg with a husband's sperm or a donor's sperm with a wife's egg, or by adopting a child. These options solve the problem of how to become a parent, but they can cause other emotional problems, and raise legal and, sometimes, religious issues as well.

As many people have discovered, modern medicine does not hold all the answers. A couple may decide to abandon the effort to become parents, and (like the second-century scholar Ben Azzai, who chose to study and not to have children) find other ways of fulfilling themselves. Today, as Rabbi Michael Gold points out, prayer, repentance, and good deeds do not solve the problem of infertility, but these traditional behaviors can keep a person's faith alive and provide strength to pursue the dream of having a family or to make an alternative decision.[104] Some observant Jewish women in traditional communities also maintain faith in traditional fertility amulets that they know have helped others, or they consult community faith healers (usually Orthodox Jews) whose popularity never dims. In Western countries, psychotherapists (not usually the rabbi) have also helped childless couples to find strength to discover a solution, in different ways. Although many psychotherapists are Jewish, their methods of building up a person's spiritual strength and approaching the problem of childlessness are not often based on their Jewish education.

With the advance of Western civilization, we have also witnessed an important shift in popular attitudes, away from the prejudice and stigma against those who cannot have children to a gentler and more sympathetic concern for their suffering. Although some people may appear insensitive if they are ignorant of a couple's efforts to conceive or of their loss of fertility, relatives, friends, counselors, and medical staff who are aware of the couple's problem do sympathize. The pain and suffering of infertility can be shared. Jewish literature is replete with tales of pain and suffering; this is part of our heritage. As we have seen, some tales relate the experiences and emotions of the childless. When a tale ends sadly, narrator and listener cry together and share their distress. Often, however, Jews find happy endings to tell each other, to strengthen the soul and try to heal the pain.

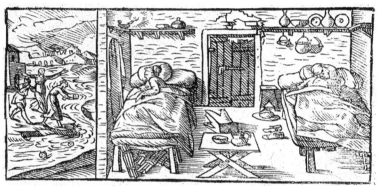

Plate 5. *Husband and Wife Sleep in Separate Beds to Avoid Conception.* Venice Haggadah, 1609.
Woodcut. Jewish National University Library, Jerusalem.

Chapter Three

Contraception and Abortion

When a woman knows that pregnancy is likely to be life-threatening, she may take contraceptive precautions or, failing this, seek an abortion. This is the case among Jews, for Jews have always valued the preservation of existing life more than potential life. Some Jews have considered contraception and abortion in other circumstances, too, such as during the worst periods of anti-Semitic persecutions or during war or famine. In addition, some Jews have delayed having children to pursue religious studies or alternative intellectual goals. Furthermore, prospective parents fearing an overabundance of daughters[1] or worrying that their baby would grow up to a life of poor quality have attempted to avoid childbirth. In addition, harlots, adulterers, and those in dire financial straits have sometimes wished to avoid having babies. Because such behavior threatens the moral fabric of Jewish society, birth control and abortion have generated much Jewish legal debate, especially in modern times, in light of improved medical techniques. However, Jews, like non-Jews, have always considered the prevention of conception preferable to abortion. In addition, today both prenatal diagnosis of various disorders and genetic counseling for carriers of inherited syndromes have created new issues for Jewish medical ethics. The halakhic controversies on these topics are not the focus of this study:[2] here we will examine instead situations in which Jews have sought to prevent childbirth and the methods used to reach their goal.

ABSTINENCE

Jewish tradition has always recognized the importance of sexual relations for marital happiness and has discouraged couples from abstaining from this aspect of marriage.

The Mishnah lists sexual relations as one of a husband's duties toward his wife. A husband's failure to fulfill this duty can be grounds for divorce.[3] Jewish society has considered a spouse, whether husband or wife, "rebellious" if he or she insists on abstaining from the marital duty of making love. The decision not to have more children can be a reason for such rebelliousness. A scholar in talmudic times, Shimon ben Azzai (early second century), set a precedent by giving priority to his Torah studies.[4] Contemporary and later rabbis condemned him for abstaining from his procreative duty, but these later rabbis did not know whether he married and abstained from marital relations or whether, like King Hezekiah, he had avoided the wedding canopy altogether.

Sometimes both partners agree to abstain from sexual relations to prevent conception. Talmudic tales teach, however, that, even when conditions are terrible, it is not good to abstain from sexual relations and the possibility of procreation. The first tale tells of the difficult times in Egypt before the Exodus; the second tells of the despondency following the destruction of the Second Temple in Jerusalem. In the first tale, when Pharaoh decreed the tossing into the river of all Israelite newborn sons, one couple (Amram and his wife Jochebed) feared for the baby they had conceived three months previously. Amram saw no future for the Israelites and begged his men to divorce their wives, just as he had divorced his beloved Jochebed. However, in the tale, their daughter, Miriam, reproached him: "Your order is harder than Pharaoh's, for he decreed against male children only, but what you ask precludes the birth of both sons and daughters. Pharaoh is wicked, but as you might be able to outwit him, there is a doubt whether the Israelites will obey his ruling. You, however, are pious and your people will certainly fulfill your request. Your decision," she continued, "will prevent the birth of children both in this world and in the World to Come. You are therefore even more severe than Pharaoh." Amram listened and hastened to withdraw his plea to his fellow men. His son, Moses, was born a few months later, laid in a wicker basket among the river reeds, and, as is well known, survived.[5]

The other talmudic tale is set in the rubble of the Second Temple, in the heavily anti-Semitic atmosphere of the Roman victory against the Jews; the sages thought of banning marriage to prevent childbirth, but they did not do so for they recognized this would mean an end to the Jewish people.[6] However bleak the future appeared, and history is not short of periods when Jews lived under oppression, when they were massacred or forced to convert, Jews continued to have children.

Orthodox Jewish couples do not have sexual relations during the wife's "unclean" period (during menstruation and before ritual purification), and therefore they abstain for some twelve to fourteen days each month. Although Jewish tradition sees sexual relations as a man's duty toward his wife, these relations are considered to be a woman's pleasure, and she can choose to forgo this pleasure at any time. However, Maimonides and the later Shulḥan Arukh warned couples against abstaining from marital relations during the permitted time, unless they had already fulfilled the commandment to procreate.[7]

In antiquity, Jews were not certain at what point in the monthly cycle a woman conceived, but by the Middle Ages, they recognized that a woman may conceive at any time between her immersion and the onset of her subsequent menstrual period. Nevertheless, some Orthodox women have discreetly delayed their purification by a few days, hoping to avoid pregnancy by having sexual relations only in the latter half of their menstrual cycle.[8]

Although Jewish men have often wedded before they reach the age of twenty, some have postponed marriage to delay parenthood. Although the Talmud recommends marrying young, it also advocates first building a house, planting a vineyard, and then marrying—in other words, first establishing the means to provide a home for a wife and family. Responsa from the fourteenth century until modern times concerning the necessity to coerce a man into marriage after a certain age show that, in the past, some men have postponed marriage because they could not find a suitable bride or because they could not afford a wife and family. However, in most cases the rabbis agreed that a court should not force a man into marrying.[9]

A talmudic tale about King Hezekiah instructs that Jews should not prevent procreation because of expected undesirable qualities in the children. The sages told that he chose not to marry because he foresaw the wickedness of his offspring. Isaiah supposedly rebuked him: "The secrets of God are none of your business. You have to perform your obligation, to do what is pleasing to God" (*B. Berakhot* 10a). Nevertheless, since talmudic times, Jews have encouraged the practice of eugenics in their effort to avoid hereditary diseases. They have checked for undesirable symptoms in the family of a future bride for fear of what her children might inherit. However, the aim of Jewish eugenics has not been concern for the quality of life of a particular individual, but rather for the long-term strength and purity of the Jewish people.[10] The moral of the tale is that procreation is an act of faith in God, and no person may pass judgment on whether another's life is worth living.

CONTRACEPTION

Jews have often had recourse to contraception rather than having to abstain from the act of love. However, rabbis have found some of the available methods for avoiding pregnancy more acceptable than others.

Coitus Interruptus

The Book of Genesis tells the story of Er and Onan. Er, the first-born of Judah, married Tamar but "was displeasing to the Lord, and the Lord took his life" (Genesis 38:7). The rabbis of the talmudic period reasoned that although Er enjoyed conjugal relations, he ensured that his exceedingly beautiful wife would not conceive, and therefore God condemned him to death for taking this precaution. When Er died, Onan, his brother, was forced into a levirate marriage with Tamar, but he knew that the child she conceived would not count as his, and he let his seed go to waste [lit. "spoil on the ground"] whenever he joined with his brother's wife. God did not approve of this behavior either and took his life, too.[11] From these two cases, the sages deduced that unnatural sexual intercourse is sinful, and "Whoever emits semen in vain deserves death" (*B. Niddah* 13b). Ever since, rabbis have argued over whether the contraceptive intention or the deviant and unnatural nature of the sexual act was in fact hateful to God.[12]

In medieval times, Maimonides clearly forbade coitus interruptus, the Hasidei Ashkenaz declared that spilling seed in vain delays the coming of the Messiah, and the Zohar was adamant that the destruction of generative seed is a sin "lower than the lowest, worse than murder, that does not admit repentance."[13] The message for Jews concerning this practice was clear.

Male Sterilization

Since talmudic times, Jews have associated sterilization with the biblical proscription against castration. They have assumed that the proscription applies to men only, because women were never castrated. The ancient Assyrians and Persians sometimes castrated slaves, and in the Roman era, eunuchs achieved positions of status as political advisors. In Moslem lands, too, the ruling gentry valued the service of eunuchs, especially in their harems. In the face of all these local customs, Jews were vehement in their condemnation of castration.[14]

Castration was also practiced during the Middle Ages, by some zealous Christians desiring to prevent sexual sins. Zealous Jews of medieval Germany, the Hasidei Ashkenaz, warned their people against this practice. Judah the Pious insisted that a Jewish man who misbehaved with women should not render himself sterile.

Castration is no longer relevant today. Instead, the availability of male sterilization by vasectomy is now the issue. Although doctors perform this operation for men who want this form of contraception, Orthodox rabbis consider it a serious offense, and many Jews who no longer adhere to tradition still recoil at the thought.[15]

The "Cup of Roots"

In talmudic times, Jews knew of a remedy for jaundice or anemia that caused temporary—and in large doses, permanent—sterility. This "cup of roots" was a mixture of gum arabic, alum, and garden crocus roots powdered and mixed with wine.[16]

The Talmud relates that a woman named Judith had suffered so much in childbirth that she never wanted to become pregnant again. She was surely not the first woman to feel that way, nor by any means the last, but she was determined. She disguised herself well and went to consult her husband, Rabbi Hiyya. She asked him only one question, whether women are commanded to propagate the race, and received the negative answer she had hoped for. The rabbi stated that the duty was strictly a man's. Judith went home and drank a sterilizing potion to avoid future conception. When the sage discovered what his wife had done, he was greatly upset. Nevertheless, her action set a precedent for women to use an oral contraceptive, which is considered acceptable in Orthodox communities today usually only when conception is likely to cause a woman serious health hazards, or when, like Judith, a woman has helped her husband to fulfill his procreative duty, at least minimally, and has suffered severely in the process.[17]

The talmudic sages were fully aware of how such potions could be abused for hedonistic reasons. They suggested that Er may have given Tamar a dose of the "cup" as a sterilizing potion, so she would not lose her beauty to pregnancy.[18] They spun a similar tale about Lamech, son of Cain, who kept two wives in the corrupt years before the Great Flood and who, like Er, also perished for his sins by divine punishment: the sages said that Lamech gave one of his women the contraceptive "cup of roots" to preserve her beauty.[19]

As Jews left the Middle East to settle in all corners of the world, the ingredients of the talmudic potions were often unavailable, and women made use of alternative, local recipes or those recommended in the pharmacopoeia of Jewish physicians. For example, a medieval Hebrew textbook of gynecology asserted that drinking an infusion of acacia would cause permanent sterility and that this recipe had been "tried and proved."[20] Sheshet Benveniste, the Jewish physician in Spain whose advice on infertility is quoted in Chapter 2, prescribed a drink of an infusion made of the leaves, flowers, and apples of another plant, *shalzir*, for permanent sterilization.[21]

In contrast to the medieval Hasidei Ashkenaz, who forbade male steriliza-tion even in cases of sexual deviancy, an early fourteenth-century talmudist, Yom Tov Ishbili, allowed a man to drink a contraceptive potion "in order to rid himself of his lusts and lewd thoughts," provided he had already fulfilled his procreative duty. Ishbili said he knew of great men who had treated themselves in this way.[22]

Disregarding (or unaware of) Isaiah's condemnation of King Hezekiah, a Jewish woman in sixteenth-century Poland, whose children did not "walk in an upright path," consumed a contraceptive "cup of roots" to avoid bearing any more wayward offspring. Rabbis in seventeenth-century Poland permitted a woman with childbearing difficulties to swallow this potion.[23] Jewish physicians continued to pre-scribe a sterilizing potion in eighteenth-century Italy, when the need arose.[24] How-ever, in the nineteenth century, three rabbis in Germany and Poland voiced hesitations about the safety of the "cup." The exact nature of the potion "must have been for-gotten in the course of time." As recently as 1946, a woman complained to the rab-binic court of Petah Tikva, in the Holy Land, that the "cup of roots" she had drunk had proved ineffective, and she asked for an alternative method of contraception. The rabbi who answered her question suggested that she seek a more "tried and proved" potion from a "more expert" physician.[25]

The modern contraceptive pill has replaced the talmudic "cup of roots." Worried about the loosening of morals in Jewish society, Orthodox rabbis continue to maintain that women should take this pill only if conception would be dangerous for them.

Contraceptive Tampon

The Talmud often mentions another type of precaution against preg-nancy, an absorbent tampon, *mokh*, and assumes readers' familiarity with the item. The Talmud does not describe what it was made of or exactly how it was used.[26] However, Soranus, the Alexandrian physician who lived in the early second century, gave a detailed description of what must have been the talmudic *mokh*: it was a piece of fine wool, steeped in a cooling, clogging liquid that would not allow semen to pass through the female orifice.[27]

The Talmud points to several situations when this contraceptive was used. Girls married before the onset of menstruation, who were less than twelve years old, required such a tampon to prevent the real danger of pregnancy in their immature bodies. Pregnant women also employed a *mokh*, perhaps to protect against physical damage or infection occurring from conjugal relations. However, some people feared that a woman could conceive a second baby while pregnant with the first, and there-fore gravid women may have used a *mokh* in the hope of preventing the formation of a new fetus that could endanger the first. In addition, nursing mothers favored such a tampon, for fear that a new fetus would harm lactation and pose a threat to the nursling. By taking this precaution against conception, a mother gave her nursing child the best possible nourishment for the first twenty-four months. The Talmud reveals that harlots and rape victims were two more categories of women who used a *mokh* to prevent conception.[28]

The *mokh* may not have been used beyond the talmudic period, or it may not have been effective, because post-talmudic rabbis mentioned that harlots sometimes sought abortion and, moreover, discussed the possibility of abortion for an adulterous woman (as discussed later). Its notable absence from remedy books implies that perhaps the post-talmudic rabbinic discussion of whether the tampon may or must be used, and whether its use should be precoital or postcoital, was theoretical and did not reflect popular practice. In the Middle Ages, the Hebrew version of Soranus' treatise, the *Book on Generation*, entirely omitted his paragraph about contraceptives and used the word *mokh* to refer to a vaginal suppository, concocted by a pharmacist or midwife, to induce menses and promote fertility or to encourage the expulsion of a retained placenta.[29] A book of remedies, the *Book of Medical Experiences*, attributed to Abraham ibn Ezra (1089–1164), offered a recipe for a contraceptive suppository (*p'tilah*, not *mokh*) of mint leaves, for insertion before coitus or even during menstruation.[30] None of the Jewish remedy books consulted in this study revealed directions for making a contraceptive *mokh*.

Other Methods

Although both the Bible and the Talmud warn against the practice of magic, many folk remedies for avoiding conception were clearly magical.[31] For example, a chapter in the *Book of Medical Experiences* entitled "On the Prevention of Pregnancy" advised that a woman hang on herself the heart of a hare to prevent conception.[32] This text, which offered other magical recommendations, has been attributed to Abraham ibn Ezra, although a man as erudite as he, in Jewish matters as well as in medicine, is unlikely to have recommended the amuletic use of a hare to a rabbi's wife who needed to avoid childbearing for medical reasons. Perhaps Abraham ibn Ezra included all known treatments for the sake of comprehensiveness.

A fifteenth-century remedy book in Yiddish recommended use of the heart of a mouse. Hayyim Vital (1542–1620), a mystic and physician who drew on medical treatises that he had read as well as on advice received from other doctors, reported six possible contraceptive methods. One of these methods required that a woman hang on herself the skin or hair of a hare. Whereas Vital frequently reported having tried out his remedies, he did not note his experience in this regard.[33] In addition, an eighteenth-century remedy book from Eastern Europe opted using the heart or the foot of a hare or the heart of a mouse.[34] In the early twentieth century, too, Jewish women in Egypt desiring to avoid conception hung the foot of a hare around their necks. The principle of contagious magic is probably behind these amuletic proposals, for both animals flee when humans approach.

Such remedies clearly do not originate within the Jewish community and, in view of their magical nature, should have had no place there; however, their inclusion in Jewish remedy books suggests that some people wanted to prevent pregnancy and no more reliable methods were known. Raphael Patai has studied the magical potions used among Jews in different parts of the world and has pointed out similarities with other cultures.[35] These remedies are not of any particular Jewish interest other than to reveal that, through the ages, Jews have attempted to prevent conception in ways not sanctioned by the rabbis.

A special form of Jewish magic was performed by some Jewish mystics. Their texts of practical Kabbalah sometimes offered magical incantations and instructions for making amulets to prevent pregnancy. Two nineteenth-century remedy books included formulas for this purpose. One of these was composed by a Sephardic Jew, Avraham Hamoi, and the formula included the letters of the Divine Name. The other remedy book was used by Yemenite Jews and recorded an amuletic formula for contraception with esoteric kabbalistic angel characters.[36] Whereas Jews under the influence of the Enlightenment in the West ceased to practice magic, such charms were in use until the middle of the twentieth century in many parts of Eastern Europe, North Africa, and in the Eastern Jewish communities.

Aletta Jacobs (1854–1929) was the first of several Jewish women to advocate and teach birth control methods publicly. She studied medicine at a Dutch university, opened a women's clinic in Amsterdam, and helped to develop a contraceptive diaphragm. She was especially concerned with helping poor women free themselves from the burden of childbearing. Women's desire for a reliable form of contraception was such that, in 1916, when a birth control clinic opened in the Jewish neighborhood of Brownsville in Brooklyn, there was a long queue of those seeking advice, even though dispensing information about contraception was illegal. In the early decades of the twentieth century, the law did not deter Emma Goldman in the United States, or Rose Witcop in England, from openly dispensing and publishing birth control information.[37]

Many Orthodox Jews today maintain the traditional view that only women may use contraception, and only for medical reasons. Outside Orthodox communities, however, most young Jewish couples, like non-Jews, use contraceptives to plan the size and spacing of their family. Their choice of method is likely to depend on medical considerations and not on Jewish tradition.

ABORTION

Much of the Jewish legal discussion about abortion serves the purpose of upholding and reinforcing the ethics and morals of Jewish society. It is based on little material in ancient or medieval Jewish rabbinic sources. Most of the responsa date from the seventeenth century and later, with an almost exponential increase in written replies to questions on this subject in the twentieth century, since abortion became relatively safe to perform in the early months of pregnancy. Some of these are responses of rabbis to real, individual cases. For example, a pregnant woman suffered terribly and wanted to miscarry. Another was remorseful about having conceived through adultery and asked for an abortion. An epileptic woman feared her baby would be born with the same disorder and wanted her pregnancy terminated. A woman with terminal cancer was told that her health was deteriorating more rapidly on account of her pregnancy, but she refused to have her fetus destroyed. A Gentile demanded that a Jewish physician perform an abortion. Jews have considered the possibility of abortion in light of the tragic effects of maternal rubella and of thalidomide on a growing fetus. More recently, the ability to diagnose genetic syndromes and disorders in early pregnancy has precipitated yet more questions about the ethics of abortion. Fully aware that the decisions reached in all these situations set precedents for future cases, rabbis have taken great care when issuing their rulings. Because each case of permitted abortion has wider implications for society, rabbis have set down clearly their reasoning for each particular decision.

To Save a Mother's Life

The Mishnah rules that a fetus endangering its mother's life must be removed, because her life has priority over that of the unborn child: "If a woman is in hard travail [and her life cannot otherwise be saved], one cuts up the child within her womb and extracts it member by member, because her life comes before that of [the child]. But if the greater part [or the head] was delivered, one may not touch it, for one may not set aside one person's life for the sake of another" (*Oholot* 7:6). This ruling is almost two thousand years old. However, this embryotomy in advanced pregnancy (discussed in Chapter 9) is not the same as an abortion induced in the first trimester.

The Talmud and Maimonides regarded an unborn baby that endangers a woman's life as an aggressor intent on killing and taught that, in such a situation, the baby may be destroyed, by drug or by hand, but (in the spirit of the Mishnah) only if its head has not yet been delivered.[38]

Practical advice for the birth attendant in this situation was offered in medieval times. A fourteenth-century Jewish philosopher, Meir Aldabi, gave several recipes that he had found for inducing abortion in a woman who suffered terribly and wanted to miscarry. He explained how to concoct a few potions, materials for fumigation, and a vaginal suppository.[39] A compendium of midwifery, dating from the same period, recommended an abortifacient for a young girl or a woman with a deformity of the genitalia, for whom delivery of a full-term infant would be fatal.[40]

In the seventeenth century, rabbis recognized extreme mental anguish as a life-threatening condition. This mental anguish included suicidal tendencies and hysterical behavior that could damage others.[41] Nowadays, women who have suffered schizophrenia or postnatal psychosis also are categorized as having a life-threatening condition.

After Adultery

A Jewish physician, Asaph Judaeus (c. seventh century), followed Hippocrates in condemning abortion, but in marked contrast to the Greek, Asaph limited his condemnation to abortion of a fetus conceived by harlotry. This limitation left room for permitting abortion when a woman's life was endangered by pregnancy.[42] Many Jewish students qualifying as physicians pronounce Asaph's oath to this day.

The medical ethics against aborting a child conceived through promiscuity were unambiguous, but in the seventeenth century a woman's great distress may have moved a Jewish physician to send her to a rabbi for a second opinion. There is documentation of such an instance in which a woman was pregnant as the result of adultery; the remorseful woman sought permission for an abortion from Yair Bacharach (1638–1702), a rabbi who headed the Jewish community of Worms, Germany. Although the rabbi maintained that no clear prohibition against this practice existed in Jewish law, he said that the illegitimate status of the embryo did not change his opinion that abortion is morally wrong. He warned that rabbinic sanctioning of abortion in such a case would open the gates to immorality and debauchery.[43]

In contrast, fairly recently, Rabbi Benzion Ouziel (d. 1953), Sephardic Chief Rabbi of Israel, permitted abortion in the case of a woman pregnant from adultery, to prevent her disgrace. Unlike Bacharach, Ouziel based his decision on the illegitimate status of the baby. The child of such an illegitimate union is a bastard (*mamzer*); Orthodox Jewish society stigmatizes such a child, banning eventual marriage to another Jew of legitimate birth. To avoid such a curse, Ouziel permitted the woman to abort her fetus. He declined, however, to grant the same permission to an unwed mother who wanted her pregnancy terminated, for her child would not classify as a *mamzer*.[44]

After Rape

The Bible tells the story of Dinah, the daughter of Leah and Jacob, who was out visiting one day when Shechem, the son of Hamor the Hivite, saw her, desired her, and raped her. Jacob was greatly distressed over this act, and two of his sons, Dinah's brothers, were so furious that they decided to take revenge. Shechem declared he had fallen in love with Dinah and asked her father for permission to marry her, at any price. Jacob set his condition for his daughter's sake, but within a few days the angry brothers had killed Shechem, and Dinah remained defiled, without a husband.[45]

Dinah's predicament has been embellished over the centuries into a full-fledged folktale with a happy ending. This story tells that Dinah conceived from Shechem and that her brothers intended to kill her, too, to safeguard the honor and good name of the Israelite women. However, Jacob determined to ensure the lives of both his daughter and her expected child. He made Dinah a gold protective amulet, inscribed with the Holy Name, and sent her to the wilderness, where her brothers would not find her. A baby girl was born in the shade of a thorn bush, and Dinah put her father's amulet around the infant's neck. That same day, Michael the archangel, disguised as an eagle, flew down and snatched the baby away. Dinah returned childless to her father's home, while the angel carried the baby to Egypt, to Potiphar and his wife, who were barren and had prayed for a child. They named her Asenath. Years later, when Joseph was in Egypt, he saw Asenath and recognized the amulet that she was wearing as the one his father had made. He married her, returning her to the Israelite family and enabling her to reunite with her mother.[46] The tale conveniently removed the unwanted baby and permitted mother and daughter to live happily ever after, but that is not what happens in real life when a woman is raped.

Postcoital contraception and abortion after rape were neither available nor discussed until modern times. The talmudic sages discussed whether a raped woman would try to prevent conception using a *mokh* postcoitally; the talmudic conclusion was that one cannot assume that this practice prevented conception.[47] In the late nineteenth century, a suction device to remove semen straight after the incident gave some rape victims hope of preventing an unwanted pregnancy. In 1891, Rabbi Yehudah L. Perilman of Minsk said that a woman may destroy seed implanted within her illegally, against her will, especially if the rapist were not Jewish. The destruction of seed had to be done by a woman, however, because of the prohibition incumbent on men not to destroy male seed.[48] In contrast, in the last twenty years, the former Chief Rabbi of England, Rabbi I. Jakobovits, an authority on Jewish medical ethics, has taken a severe stance against the abortion of a fetus conceived through rape, because he believes that every fetus has a right to be born, and society must assume the burden of its care.[49]

Abortifacients

A rape victim and a woman who wanted as soon as possible to rid herself of evidence of her adultery were probably not concerned with the ethics of abortion. In talmudic times, these women may have taken the extra precaution of rising quickly after sexual intercourse and twisting and shaking themselves violently to spill out the seed.[50] They may also have tried abortifacients in the days and weeks that followed impregnation, rather than wait until pregnancy advanced sufficiently for a surgical embryotomy that could kill mother as well as baby. Since ancient times, Jewish women have attempted to induce abortion by resorting to emetics, vaginal astringents, irritants, fumigation, strong smells, weight lifting, and magical methods. Medieval and later remedy books usually suggested several abortifacients, attesting to the fact that they often did not work. Jews were familiar with remedies for expelling a dead fetus from a mother's womb and for hastening a reluctant birth, and they may have applied this knowledge to induce abortion: remedy books sometimes warned that a particularly powerful remedy would expel the fetus "dead or alive."

Abortifacients were not unknown in talmudic times. The Talmud mentions an abortifacient drug that Cleopatra allegedly administered to her pregnant slaves.[51] A magical manuscript, *The Sword of Moses*, dating from this period, told how to deploy black magic for terminating pregnancy.[52] In addition, educated Jews were familiar with the Greek writings of Dioscorides (first century) and Soranus, who both provided numerous recipes for abortifacients, although these writers considered avoiding conception preferable to destroying a fetus.[53]

Medieval Jewish medical writers provided instructions and recipes for abortifacients, with ingredients expected to kill the fetus and induce its expulsion. The popular *Book of Medical Experiences* included a chapter on how to terminate pregnancy. It offered several recommendations, such as a sniff of arum, a suppository of opopanax root or of colocynth and oxgall, or alternatively fumigation with the smoke of burning horse or pigeon dung or with steam from satureia herb.[54] Another medieval manuscript recommended similar ingredients for inducing abortion, but of a fetus presumed to be dead.[55] Sheshet Benveniste advised instead a potion made of powdered lodestone mixed with artemisia or rue water.[56] A Judeo-Arabic pharmacopoeia, also dating from the Middle Ages, reported that a dose of blue licorice helps to expel a fetus.[57]

Medical manuscripts authored or compiled by Jews did not always stipulate that these "remedies" were to be limited to therapeutic cases, such as when a woman's life is endangered by continuation of pregnancy or when the fetus has died in the womb. Yet a thirteenth-century medieval source included a warning together with a prescription for abortion. The anonymous writer commented that a physician must know how to guard himself against any evil that may occur from such a forbidden practice, because certain licentious women desire to abort their illegitimate fruit, with the permission of some leading scholars. This author stressed that he himself would have nothing to do with this, in the absence of danger to the mother, and sharply criticized women physicians, quacks, and surgeons who were not medically trained but offered their services for financial gain among Jews, just as among Gentiles.[58]

Two Yiddish remedy books, one dating from the fifteenth century, and another from a century or two later, recommended eating horseradish on an empty stomach.[59] A sixteenth-century manuscript, written in cursive Ashkenazi calligraphy, suggested seven different recipes for abortion, including the suppositories of opopanax or colocynth (attributed to Greek sages) referred to in the *Book of Medical Experiences* and fumigation with smoking pig's dung. Aristotle was the alleged source for a recipe involving boiled *etrog* (citron) leaves.[60]

Judah Ayash (d. 1760), a famous rabbi of Algiers, noted that women "prepare medicines and potions, known among them, in order to abort the fetus."[61] These remedies could be found in books of home remedies, in Hebrew, Yiddish, Judeo-Arabic, or Aramaic and included fumigations, drinking potions, and magical methods often involving a kabbalistic incantation. A popular eighteenth-century remedy book provided a recipe in Aramaic for expelling a fetus that died in the womb; the author added that this potion would successfully expel a live fetus, "with the help of God," if its birth presented a great danger to the mother.[62] Distraught women used such home remedies well into the twentieth century.[63]

It is unlikely that the documentation of all these abortifacients was solely for the sake of comprehensiveness or that these remedies were used only by heathens and harlots. It also seems unlikely that Jews used such recipes only for the purpose of saving a woman's life. Midwives certainly knew how to try to expel a dead fetus or a retained placenta, and they may have resorted occasionally to this knowledge in a discreet attempt to aid a woman determined to terminate her pregnancy.

However, we can guess that the popular remedies described previously were unlikely to result in abortion and, until recent times, surgical intervention was the only sure method. In the past, surgical abortion could well have killed the mother as well as her fetus, and therefore, a Jewish surgeon or midwife would probably not have consented to this procedure. Asaph Judaeus was not the only Jewish physician to proclaim an oath against performing abortion. A *Marrano* physician, Amatus Lusitanus (1511–1568), also vowed not to help a woman bring about an abortion.[64] In addition, a seventeenth-century Italian physician and rabbi, Jacob Zahalon

(1630–1693), who was particularly concerned with the ethics of medical practice, repeated this same warning in a prayer he composed for physicians to recite: "[Let me not be enticed] to perform an abortion on a pregnant woman."[65] In the early twentieth century, Emma Goldman, who was a qualified midwife, saw the desperate circumstances of working-class women with unwanted pregnancies, but she refused to perform abortions because they were too dangerous.[66]

Twentieth-Century Issues

In modern times, as in the past, some Jewish women have sought abortion of an unwanted conception. However, only in recent times has help become available for women in the early months of pregnancy, in a relatively safe and reliable manner.

During the Holocaust, especially, many women sought abortion. Some feared Nazi experiments on pregnant women, and others sought to terminate pregnancy because they had lost any hope for a better future. For example, Dr. Adina Blady Szwajger treated starving children in a Polish hospital where the only way that she could reduce their suffering was to give them lethal doses of morphine. Her husband was taken to Auschwitz. When Dr. Szwajger discovered that she was pregnant, she arranged for an abortion for herself, although she had no anesthetic, and helped three of her friends in the same way, because she was convinced that "children had no right to be born" in those terrible times. In 1942, a rabbi allowed Jewish women in the Kovno ghetto to undergo abortion when the Nazis decreed that every pregnant Jewish woman must be killed.[67]

Although some who witnessed the Holocaust believe strongly that it is deeply wrong to destroy potential life, Dr. Henry Morgentaler, an Auschwitz survivor, became a gynecologist, opened abortion clinics in Canada in the 1960s, and challenged local laws that restricted women's access to abortion. Dr. Morgentaler had witnessed the distress of women coerced into giving birth or having abortions against their will during the Second World War, and he strongly believed in giving women the freedom to choose whether to bring a child into the world.[68]

Advances in modern medicine have led to new choices and new problems in Jewish medical ethics. For example, although disabilities were common in the past (the Talmud describes infants born with physical disorders), the question of abortion of a handicapped fetus is recent, with no precedents in classic Jewish sources, because only in recent times have tests been able to determine certain disorders reliably before birth.

Rabbis have distinguished between an abortion for the mother's health and one performed on account of the child's expected quality of life. They have been sympathetic and willing to take into consideration the risk to a mother's mental health, her severe anguish over the birth of a child with a genetic syndrome or disability, and her request for compassion. In contrast, rabbis have not been willing to consider aborting a fetus whose potential was unknown. However, now that diagnostic testing of the unborn fetus can produce reliable information concerning some severe disabilities, some rabbis have reviewed their attitudes to therapeutic abortion in these special cases.[69] Although rabbis are concerned to safeguard the standards of

Jewish medical ethics, their views may not concern non-Orthodox Jewish parents who discover that their fetus is multiply handicapped. Their decision regarding abortion is their own personal choice.

In 1972, the American Jewish Congress issued the following statement: "Restrictive or prohibitive abortion laws violate the right of a woman to choose whether to bear a child, her right of privacy and her liberty in matters pertaining to marriage, family and sex. . . . Those who find abortion unacceptable as a matter of religious conviction or conscience are free to hold and live by their beliefs, but should not seek to impose such beliefs, by government actions, on others. . . ."[70]

Although safer and more reliable than ever before, abortion remains an emotional issue not only for Orthodox Jews, Holocaust survivors, and expectant parents who discover that their unborn child will be handicapped, but also for many other people faced with an unwanted pregnancy.

Part II
Pregnancy

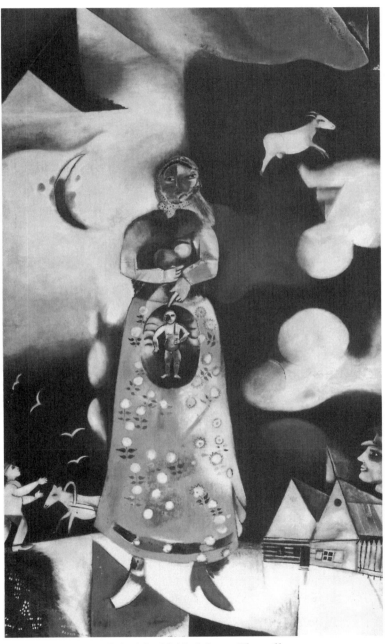

Plate 6. *Maternité*. 1912–1913, Marc Chagall.
Oil on canvas, 194 × cm. Stedelijk Museum, Amsterdam.
Copyright: ADAGP, Paris.

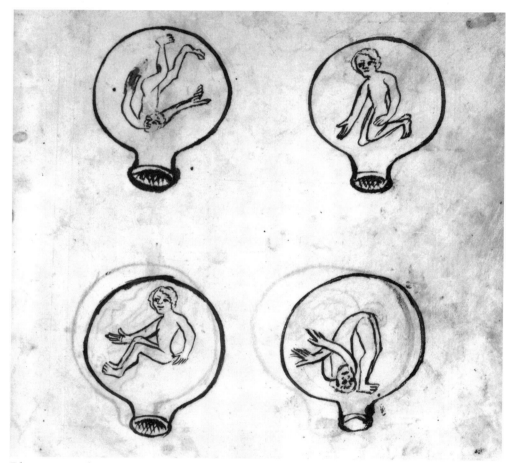

Plate 7. Fetal positions, obstetrical manuscript. Spain, fourteenth century.
Copyright: Cliché Bibliothèque Nationale de France, Paris. Ms Heb. 1120
f.70r.

Chapter Four

The Formation of the Embryo

Until recently, our understanding of embryology was speculative. Jews have pondered the creation of the embryo and how it acquires its soul, the essence that gives a baby vitality, breath, and eventually wisdom. They have been fascinated by the physical and psychological influences on conception. Nowadays, molecular biologists are revealing the minute details of the formation of an embryo, but understanding the nature of the soul appears still to be beyond our grasp. The influences on conception are also topics of ongoing scientific research, to help those who have difficulty in conceiving and those who miscarry, and to understand and prevent congenital disorders.

CONCEPTION

Jews have always believed that there are three partners in the creation of new life—God, father, and mother, and they have formulated theories about how each partner contributes to conception.

God's Role

Time and again, the Bible repeats God's primary role in enabling conception.[1] Job formulated the earliest theory of embryology: "...You [God] fashioned me like clay ... poured me out like milk, congealed me like cheese; You clothed me with skin and flesh, and wove me of bones and sinews" (Job 10:10). Extending this insight, the talmudic sages depicted God as the catalyst causing the interaction of the male white substance with the female substance, which they thought was red. They imagined that a woman's womb was full of standing blood (which flowed out during menstruation in the absence of conception), and when a drop of white seed entered the womb, if it were God's will, the blood congealed and took form, like a drop of rennet falling into a bowl of milk.[2]

Talmudic rabbis reasoned that the father supplied the baby's bones, sinews, nails, brain, and even the white in the eye, in his drop of "white substance," whereas the skin, flesh, hair, blood, and the black of the eye developed from the mother's "red substance." God gave the baby its soul, breath, sight, hearing, speech, and understanding, as well as the ability to walk, and physical beauty. Thus, God supplied the soul to the physical embryonic matter but reclaimed it when the person died.[3]

The sages imagined that God created all human souls at the time of the creation of the universe. God chose one of these to enter each human conception and dispatched it with angel messengers to enter the embryo in the mother's womb.[4]

In the post-talmudic period and the Middle Ages, Jewish philosophers and mystics continued to ponder God's role in conception. They wondered about the source of the soul and its descent into the baby. For example, Sa'adia Gaon (882–942), a Babylonian philosopher, did not accept the idea of preexistent souls and argued instead that God creates the soul "simultaneously with the completion of the bodily form of the human being."[5] Maimonides (1135–1204) followed Gaon on this point, but other medieval philosophers, such as Bahya ibn Paquda (c. 1050–c. 1150), did not.[6]

Bahya and other Jewish philosophers in medieval Spain, such as Solomon ibn Gabirol (c. 1021–c. 1057),[7] Isaac ibn Ghayyat (1038–1089),[8] and Shem Tov Falaquera (c. 1225–1295),[9] contemplated, in poetry and discourses, the divine origin of the human soul. These philosophers believed that God is the Creator, enabler of conception and birth, the source of breath and wisdom, but not of evil inclinations, for which each person himself must take responsibility.

The Jewish mystics, too, accepted the talmudic idea of the primordial origin of all human souls. They proposed that, because the soul returns to its source when a person dies, God could choose it again for a new conceptus, and therefore any soul could have several visitations on earth. Some kabbalists imagined the divine source of human souls as a tree on which each soul blooms. A river carries the souls downward from this source to the celestial paradise, the location of the storehouse of souls, where the souls await their calling to descend further to the earthly world.[10] Some mystics imagined the supernal storehouse in the form of a curtain woven of all the souls that God created, which hangs before the Throne of Glory on high.[11]

In the Zohar, Moses de Leon (1240–1305) depicted each soul as both male and female, created out of the womb of the feminine element of God. According to this view, when a couple unite in love to procreate, their thoughts rise up and reach the celestial paradise, where they unite, and here the baby is conceived, in the divine realm. God determines the nature of the soul; for example, that it will be strong and wise and not meek and dim, and assigns its gender as it descends the levels of the divine world. God entrusts it to angelic messengers, who are instructed where to deposit it on earth. These angelic messengers give the soul its good and evil inclinations. However, the Zohar warns that when a couple unite with impure thoughts, God is absent from the union and has no share in the conception, so the result is certainly wicked.[12]

Isaac Luria (1534–1572), "The Ari," one of the most influential and original thinkers among Jewish mystics, proposed that human souls are in fact sparks of Adam's soul, scattered after his first sin, which seek through every reincarnation to return to their original structure. He believed that when this happens, the final redemption will take place. The original souls that fell from Adam may undergo fission to produce sparks of new souls. Luria thought that biblical and talmudic personalities were reincarnations of the souls of Adam, of Eve and the serpent, and of Cain and Abel.[13]

Hasidic stories tell of the unusual origins of the souls of some wonderworking rabbis that account for the outstanding personalities of these men. For example, one tale relates the special circumstances of the birth of Israel ben Eliezer, the Baal Shem Tov. Toward the end of the seventeenth century, times were bad, with many anti-Semitic massacres. The Prophet Elijah noticed the plight of the Jews and pleaded with God to send down an innocent soul to sweeten their lives, but it was not easy to influence God. Nevertheless, eventually God noticed a pious Jew and his wife who had endured slavery, separation, and many other hardships for seventeen long years and decided to grant Elijah's plea. God called on an innocent soul to become the son of this couple's reunion in their old age. Their son was named Israel ben Eliezer.[14]

Since the late twelfth century, kabbalists have argued about how many times a soul may be reborn into a new body; some said three times, others proposed that the wicked may go on and on transmigrating for one thousand generations. When a child showed unusual qualities but then died, some kabbalists found comfort in the belief that the child was a reincarnation of an illustrious person who was making a visitation on earth. Similarly, some kabbalists rationalized that a soul of one sex may enter a body of the opposite sex.[15]

When does the soul enter the baby's body? Just as opinions have varied about the nature of the source of the soul, so Jews have also differed in their thoughts about the timing of ensoulment. Some, such as the compiler of the Mishnah, believed that the soul entered at the time of conception.[16] Others, such as the author of the Zohar, believed that the soul—the *nefesh* (the source of human vitality)—entered the body at the moment of birth, and the two other components, *ruah* and *neshamah*, the anima and the spirit, took form later in life, when the intellect had matured.[17] Yet other Jews thought that the soul entered the baby's body after birth, when the baby was named, assuming a connection between a soul and its given name. Thus, when an infant was named after a deceased relative, the soul of the departed could leave its resting place in Heaven and return to earth in the body of the infant. This thought probably convinced Judah the Pious, in Germany in the early thirteenth century, to rule in his will that none of his descendants should be given either his name or his father's name.[18] Isaac Luria believed that if a father of an unborn child died before the baby was born, the baby would receive the father's soul and should therefore be given his name. Jews who believed in such transmigration thought that the soul carried with it a certain character and fate passed down from one reincarnation to the next, a way of explaining the inheritance of characteristics.[19]

A hasidic tale about Rabbi Solomon Halevi of Karlin (1738–1792) reveals the belief that the soul enters the baby's body at birth. This man allegedly had the extraordinary gift of seeing the destinies of the souls of all men. One day, two people came to ask him for help. One came for a rich man who lay dying, and the other came for a woman in the poorhouse who had been in labor for days without being able to give birth. The Hasid saw that the soul of the rich man was destined for the poor woman's unborn baby and understood that the child could not be born until the man had died. As it happened, news of the successful delivery of a baby boy soon followed word of the man's death. The rabbi believed that the baby had inherited the rich man's soul and put aside some of the dead man's legacy for the boy's upbringing. As the child grew, however, he began behaving as though he were the wealthy man's heir, much to the distress of the biological sons of the departed person. Only the rabbi understood and regretted his ability to perceive the destinies of souls.[20]

Such folktales show that mystical ideas about the origins of the soul and the descent of the soul into the baby's body offered plausible and comforting explanations for some of the problems of childbearing.[21]

Since the seventeenth century, Jewish rationalist philosophers have no longer sought the origin of souls, nor are they concerned with ensoulment; instead, they have studied the Cartesian mind-body dichotomy, thought about whether the soul may be immortal, and attempted to understand human consciousness. Discussions about when the soul enters the fetus have arisen, marginally, in the context of Jewish medical ethics, when rabbis have questioned the legality of abortion, with the conclusion that the timing of ensoulment is irrelevant to the case.[22]

The Parents' Role

Aristotle (384–322 B.C.E.), who used the same cheese simile as Job in his treatise *On the Generation of Animals*, believed that male seed coagulated the blood in the womb, which was a passive medium and not female seed. Before him, Hippocrates (460–377 B.C.E.) had postulated that the fetus formed from the combination of male seed and the blood in the womb, or female seed. These two differing ancient Greek theories strongly influenced Jewish ideas about how each parent contributed to the creation of a baby, and therefore it is important to mention them.[23]

The idea that the male seed molds blood in the womb to form the embryo appears in the *Wisdom of Solomon*, written in Greek by an Alexandrian Jew, perhaps in the third century B.C.E.[24] Later, during the talmudic period, Jews followed the Hippocratic theory that each parent contributes specific elements to the baby's formation.

In medieval times, however, the Aristotelian theory dominated. Maimonides, the most brilliant of medieval physicians, studied closely the Greek school of rational thinkers, as well as the Talmud and Arabic medicine. Like his Arabic contemporaries, Maimonides maintained that the male seed contained the power to guide the development of the fetus, and the woman provided nourishment for the embryo. He proposed that semen contained the procreating and growth energy, the forces that gave shape, quality, and structure to the fetus.[25] Maimonides postulated that semen contained various procreating and developmental forces that caused a woman to conceive, and these male forces gave shape and quality to the fetus. Maimonides knew, from his own surgical practice, that women have two ovaries and ducts where their "seed" ripens, but he did not speculate on whether the ovaries participated in the formation of the fetus.[26]

Maimonides was not the only medieval Jewish physician to take an interest in how conception occurs, nor was he the only philosopher to focus on the particular problem of what constitutes female seed.[27] The discussion centered on the biblical word *tazri'a*, meaning literally "[a woman] seminates" or "she gives forth seed."[28] In Maimonides' day, many physicians and philosophers believed that women seminated the premenstrual "blood of the uterus," and female seed was a passive medium molded into fetal form by the forces in male seed. For example, Abraham ibn Ezra (1089–1164), Shem Tov Falaquera (mentioned previously), and Bahya ben Asher (c. 1260–1340), thought of woman's seed (premenstrual blood) as a nurturing medium, as earth acts on grain to make it grow.[29] However, certain Hebrew medical manuscripts from the twelfth century and later supported the earlier rabbinic position that female seed is an active force contributing to embryonic formation.[30] Levi ben Gershom (1288–1344) offered yet another idea: he proposed that female seed prepared the premenstrual blood for the formative action of the male seed.[31]

Nahmanides (1194–1270), who was a rabbi, philosopher, and physician, discussed "the well-known controversy about the reproductive process" in his biblical commentary. He imagined that women had "eggs" like the eggs [testicles] of a man, but these were not generative. He believed that female seed was the blood in the womb that united with the male sperm to form a baby.[32] The Aristotelian influence is clear in *The Holy Letter*, which scholars have attributed to Nahmanides. Here the author depicts the seed of woman as the natural substance given form by the seed of man, according to God's design.[33]

One more medieval physician worthy of mention is Simon ben Tzemah Duran (1361–1444), who repeated the Aristotelian view that the fetus formed from the action of male seed on the red matter. Duran proposed a new idea, however, that the biblical word for female semination, *tazri'a*, in fact referred to female orgasm, which he thought had no role in the act of conception, but was for pleasure alone.[34]

Nahmanides, Bahya, and Duran admitted that women had eggs and drew parallels with hens' eggs, which can either be fertilized by a rooster and hatch or remain cold on the ground. The problem of how conception occurred remained philosophical, however.

Only centuries later, in 1672, Regnier de Graaf discovered the follicles on the surface of the ovary and reasoned that the small lumps were generative. He guessed that one of these follicles could make its way to the womb to become the beginning of an embryo, and he realized that the comparison of female seed with a hen's egg was probably correct. Five years later, in 1677, Antonie van Leeuwenhoek observed human spermatozoa under his homemade microscope. Jacob Emden (1697–1776), a German rabbi and kabbalist, was unusually well-read in the sciences and could understand Dutch, the language of de Graaf and Leeuwenhoek, and Latin, the language of scientific publications. Emden reported the discovery of the cluster of eggs in the woman's ovary and explained that one of these eggs constituted the substance of the fetus. The egg closest to the uterus absorbed the sperm, he said, which had a warm vapor containing the spirit of life and the finite form of the embryo. The action of the sperm, he explained, is "like leaven in the dough." Nourished by the egg, the sperm used its procreating and growth power to invest the egg with life and movement. This then moved to a more spacious area to grow into the fetus.[35]

Elijah Pinhas ben Meir (c. 1742–1821), another kabbalist with a keen interest in science, also wrote about embryology, in his encyclopedic *Sefer ha-brit*. About three days after a woman receives her husband's seed, he explained, one of her eggs travels through a duct (the fallopian tube) to the womb. He was delighted that these facts matched the talmudic guidance to pray for absorption of the seed in the first three days. He pointed out that the husk of the egg forms the placenta and the fetus abides in the placenta like the chick in its egg. This, too, supported the talmudic imagery of a fetus in the womb "like a nut in a cup of water." He reported that one or two sperm enter the female ovum, absorb its moisture, and grow. He also referred to an ongoing controversy in the scientific world between those who believed that all human features lie in wait in the egg and those who thought that they all lie in a homunculus in the sperm. He concluded: "Only God knows the truth in this matter!"[36]

The female ovum was actually identified under a microscope only in 1827, by Karl Ernst von Baer. Since then, biologists studying the newly formed cells of a fertilized egg have observed that its chromosomes—the microscopic, threadlike part of the cell that carries hereditary information in the form of genes—derive equally from both parents. Biologists have discovered that, while the mother and father contribute equally to the genetic makeup of the embryo, the mother makes, in addition, an extra contribution to the formation of the fetus through the placenta. Thus, the subtle differences between the paternal and maternal contributions are now analyzed at a molecular level.

Parental Experiences During Conception

Jews have believed that parental experiences at the time of conception may influence the formation of the baby and have sometimes exploited these beliefs to encourage morality.

The Bible tells that Jacob placed striated wooden sticks near the drinking trough of Laban's sheep and goats so the animals would bear speckled and spotted young.[37] (Jacob had struck a deal with Laban, his uncle and father-in-law, with whom his relations had soured, that Jacob would leave the area and take only the speckled and spotted flock. He therefore wanted to increase the number of these animals in the flock.) Jacob may have believed that what mothers saw at the time of conception affected the color of the babies, and therefore he placed the striated wooden sticks in the ewe's field of vision. Only a few biblical commentators (notably, Rashi in the eleventh century and Nahmanides in the thirteenth) attributed the abundance of speckled and spotted newborns to divine intervention in Jacob's favor.[38] Thus, many Jews, from antiquity to modern times (as discussed later), have believed that what a mother sees before or during conception affects the baby she conceives.

A popular story, told in various versions during the talmudic period, illustrates this belief. When the King of Arabia (some say an Ethiopian, or a Moor) saw the fair skin of his newborn son, he suspected his wife of adultery. Before he took any drastic steps against her, however, he consulted Rabbi Akiva, who was known for his great wisdom. Is it possible, the King asked, that he and his wife, whose skins are dark as the night, could engender such a fair baby? The rabbi first asked about the color of the statues that decorated the royal bedroom. He then explained that the mother must have looked at the white statues when conceiving, and their coloring influenced the child's complexion.[39]

Rabbis taught that a woman's experiences on her way home from the ritual bath may affect the child conceived later that evening. The Talmud recounts that vain Rabbi Yohanan chose to sit at dusk at the gates of the *mikveh* in the hope that women would look at his phenomenal beauty and would beget children as handsome as he. His intent was not to incite adulterous thoughts, but merely to convey a pleasant image to the embryo.[40] Along the same lines, a legend about Rabbi Yishmael, the high priest, attributes his exceptional beauty to the angel Gabriel who, disguised as his father, accompanied his mother home from the ritual bath.[41]

Conversely, rabbis in the late nineteenth and early twentieth centuries warned women not to look at anything unpleasant on their way home, but to look first at the sky, and then to look down only if they were sure to look at a pleasant scene. Before reaching home, if they came across an unclean sight, such as a dog, a donkey, or a camel, they were to return to the bath house to purify themselves again. Traditional Jews in Eastern Europe, the Ottoman Empire, and North Africa observed this advice until recently. There were tales of pious women who returned several times to the ritual bath for immersion before they eventually reached home.[42] In Djerba, Jews attributed the wisdom of a certain rabbi to his mother's having returned fourteen times on one night.[43]

The talmudic sages also taught that impure thoughts, unnatural coital positions, drunkenness, or lewdness during the marital act could influence the formation of a baby conceived in that act.[44] Thus, the Talmud warns that if parents are on bad terms, their baby may grow into an ill-tempered child. If their conduct is improper, the baby may be handicapped. Moreover, sinful coupling results in rebellious and problematic offspring. However, the sages knew that the negative need not win out; many illegitimate children are bright because of love and joy in their parents' union.[45] In medieval times, the Zohar warned that demons become aroused by impure thoughts and give birth to evil; later, kabbalists warned of the dangers of demonic offspring, as discussed later in this chapter.

Unlike the talmudic sages and medieval mystics, Asaph Judaeus (c. seventh century) was a physician, who had studied Greek as well as Eastern medicine, and he, too, believed that certain factors at the time of conception affected a child. In his *Book of Medicine*, Asaph stated that the humor dominating the sperm at the time of conception conveyed a potential for illness to the embryo. For example, in the early hours of the day or night, the sanguine humor was dominant, whereas at midday and midnight, red bile was dominant; he reasoned that sperm from blood-filled organs was warm and wet and gave a healthy character to the conception, whereas sperm under the influence of red bile was likely to transmit ill humor to the fetus.[46]

A tenth-century midrash elaborated on the biblical story of Isaac's conception, by explaining that God made Isaac to resemble Abraham, to silence any gossip of questionable paternity that could have arisen from Sarah's pregnancy so late in life. The midrash told that God commands an angel to shape a fetus to be like his father, so everybody should see who the father is.[47] Similarly, God could direct this angel to shape the baby of an adulteress to resemble the object of her thoughts, a warning to women to be faithful to their husbands.

Although angelic intervention may have accounted for the inheritance of parental characteristics in medieval times, these rabbinic ideas formed a guide to righteous behavior and were hardly embryological insights. A passing glance of a handsome rabbi or the couple's coital position are not now considered significant in influencing an unborn child, but a woman's overall psychological peace or mental turmoil undoubtedly affects the child she bears.

Unusual Conception

Virgin Pregnancy

A satire about Jeremiah, thought to have originated in the East in the gaonic period (after the rise of Islam), relates how conception could occur even without physical contact between man and woman. This story tells that in the days of Zedekiah, Jeremiah the prophet once went to the bath house and found everyone there masturbating. As soon as he noticed this, he wanted to run away, but the men caught him and would not let go. They dunked him and beat him and said that, because of what he witnessed, they would not release him until he had done the same. Jeremiah pleaded with them to let go of him and swore that he would never tell anyone what he had seen. The men argued, however, that just as Zedekiah, who had seen Nebuchadnezzar eating a live rabbit, swore that he would not tell and later canceled his oath, so too might Jeremiah. The sinners then threatened the prophet with sodomy. Immediately, he did as he was told and cursed his days. Afterward, he repented and fasted, immersed himself, and purified himself. Later, Jeremiah's daughter came to the bath house, and his seed, which had not putrefied in the water, entered her and she conceived. After seven months, she bore a son. He was born with the gift of speech, but his mother was ashamed of him, afraid that people would say that the daughter of Jeremiah had conceived her son in harlotry. The baby told her, "Mother, do not be ashamed, I am Ben Sira [ben zera, "son of seed"]."[48]

A similar tale about the conception of the savior Saoshyans from the seed of Zoroaster implies a Persian influence to this story. However, the Talmud may have provided the inspiration in its theoretical discussion of whether a virgin who finds herself pregnant may marry a high priest, although the sages concluded that a virgin cannot be impregnated in the bath.[49] Many manuscripts have told the story of Ben Sira's conception, often abridged to omit the pornographic details of the original.

Unnatural pregnancy from conception without sexual contact is a popular motif in mythology all over the world, not only among Jews. Jewish folktales tell of pregnancy conceived from a snake's lust, an idea that originated in talmudic insinuations concerning Cain's conception.[50] Similar folktales, collected and transcribed in recent years, reveal that Jews have also assumed that a woman could become pregnant from swallowing something, without engaging in sexual intercourse; there are tales of offspring begotten from magic apples, a suspicious bone, and a powder made of ground skulls.[51] These fantasies thrived among Jews who believed strongly in the supernatural and did not know how the body worked. Such stories were not so extraordinary in the past, when there was far more mystery about the creation of new life.

In recent times, rabbis have referred to the story of Ben Sira's conception when seeking halakhic acceptance for artificial insemination, because both in the story and in the modern medical procedure, conception occurs without sexual intercourse.[52]

Demon Babies

Another form of unnatural conception involves spirits and demons, also part of God's world. Since talmudic times, Jewish legends have told of demon conceptions: Adam had relations with Lilith, a female spirit; Eve bore Cain, not from Adam, but from Samael, an archangel, chief of the demons, who disguised himself as the snake in the Garden of Eden; Lilith coupled with Cain and produced numerous spirits and demons; and when Cain killed Abel, Adam separated from Eve, and two female spirits came and made merry with him, begetting spirits and demons that roamed the world, while Eve also produced demonic offspring.[53]

Through the ages, many Jews believed that temptresses from the netherworld provoked men to masturbate or have nocturnal emissions that could result in demonic offspring. In seventh-century Babylon, Jewish bills of divorce against Lilith and her escorts were written in Aramaic on pottery bowls, to annul weddings between mortal men and demonic wives who tricked them into matrimony.[54] In thirteenth-century Spain, the Zohar told that Adam begot spirits and demons against his will, through "spontaneous emission of seed."[55] The same text warned that when a man has erotic dreams, female spirits play with him, become aroused, and bear demons called the Plagues of Mankind. These demons look like men, but have no hair on their heads. In a similar manner, male spirits sport with women and impregnate them, so they give birth to spirits, all of them Plagues of Mankind.[56]

The sixteenth-century Polish kabbalist, Naphtali ben Jacob Bacharach, lectured at length on how to perform the act of love in holiness. He warned specifically of the danger posed by Lilith, who hid in the bed linen, waiting to snatch the "sparks" of semen inevitably lost during love making. The kabbalist imagined that Lilith fashioned these into demons and spirits and advised that, during sexual intercourse, a man should direct his heart to God and should utter an incantation to keep her away: "You [who are] wrapped in velvet [Lilith], who comes incidentally, stay away, stay away. You will not be of help and you will result in nothing good, not from your hand and not from your bond. Go back, go back to the tumultuous sea; its waves call you. I hold on to God, wrap myself into the King's holiness." The husband was then instructed to pull the sheets over the couple's heads for one hour.[57]

Prayers and incantations to disown and nullify the influence of children conceived through inappropriate sexual arousal were popular in Eastern Europe in the seventeenth century, and rabbis discussed whether demonic intercourse constituted adultery.[58]

A cautionary tale dating from the early eighteenth century warned married men not to masturbate or have sexual relations with prostitutes. In the tale, a beautiful female demon seduced a married Jewish man in his little stone house on the main street of Poznan, Poland. She bore him several children, but, in due course, his lawful wife discovered the infidelity and consulted her rabbi. He summoned the husband, who confessed his guilt, and the rabbi wrote a powerful amulet to expel the demon. Just before the man died, the demon visited him with a final request, that he leave her and her children the cellar of the house. The cellar door remained locked for many years. Eventually, the man's lawful widow and children died, and someone unknowingly bought the house. The new owner forced open the cellar and, fifteen minutes later, was found dead, for no apparent reason. Then havoc began, as the demons took over the house, claiming it as theirs, throwing dust in the food of the new occupants, causing their lamps to topple, and making their lives so unbearable that they abandoned the house. The new owners of the house consulted the wonderworking rabbi, Rabbi Joel Baal Shem of Zamosc (d. 1703). Invoking holy names, the rabbi adjured the demons to reveal their claim on the house. The demons told him that they had inherited the cellar from their human father. The Baal Shem promptly took the demons to court, where they could be heard but not seen. The court ruled in favor of the humans and banished the demons to the forests and deserts where they belonged.[59]

STAGES OF FETAL DEVELOPMENT

In talmudic times, Jews noticed the maturational stages of an embryo and, like other peoples, formulated theories about what influences its growth. Some of these theories were significant in Jewish life. For example, the view, widely held by Jews and non-Jews alike, that a baby born after only eight months of gestation was not viable dictated the management of the baby's delivery on the Sabbath. In addition, a rabbi who knew the variations in gestation periods could refute an accusation that a woman had conceived adulterously.

The talmudic semantics for the various stages of fetal development reveal the contemporary understanding of embryology. Thus, the Talmud depicts both men and women as having "seed," which develops into the "fruit of the belly." As discussed earlier in this chapter, the womb was thought of as a nourishing soil in which the implanted seed matured into a human fruit. The talmudic sages thought that a woman's menstrual flow ceased with conception because the blood passed instead to her breasts, where it turned into milk for the baby, hence the swelling of the breasts in early pregnancy.[60] For the first six weeks of fetal life, the formless embryo was called a *golem*, the material that God molds and infuses with vitality.

In the seventh week of gestation, a "textured amnion" began to take shape, having form and tissues: talmudic sages described the "textured amnion" as having eyes and nostrils like "drippings of a fly," a mouth like "a stretched hair," and a male member the size of a lentil or a female organ like the slit on a barley grain.[61] The sages discussed the ancient Greek theory that a male embryo was fully fashioned by the forty-first day, whereas a female was fully fashioned only by the eighty-first day, and they reported an experiment that confirmed this theory. Queen Cleopatra's servants, whom she had sentenced to death, were inseminated a month or two before death, and the embryos were examined at postmortem surgery. Although some sages believed the reported results, most did not.[62] Two thousand years ago, Jews did not dissect human bodies to obtain scientific knowledge; they gained their knowledge from studying miscarriages.

The Talmud refers to a baby more than three months in the womb as an embryo or fetus; in later pregnancy, it is "one that is [to be] born." A baby that is viable, meaning a child who will survive when born, was "one whose months [of pregnancy] have been completed." The text compared an embryo to a nut floating in a bowl of water or, in advanced pregnancy, to a folded writing tablet. In advanced pregnancy, the baby's hands rest on its temples, its elbows on its legs, its heels against its buttocks, its head between its knees, its mouth closed, and its navel open. The rabbis assumed that it ate and drank what its mother consumed, but it produced no excrement, for that would surely kill the mother.[63]

The Gestation Period

The talmudic sages observed that the normal duration of pregnancy was 271 to 273 days (nine months) from conception (the first coitus after the last menstrual period): curiously, the numerical value for the letters in the Hebrew word for pregnancy, *herayon*, is 271. Sometimes a pregnancy is unusually short or unusually long. Thus, the Talmud tells that the minimum period of pregnancy for a viable baby is 212 days from conception (seven months), although a baby born after six and a half months could survive, and, at the other end of the spectrum, a twelve-month pregnancy was possible.[64]

The Talmud proposes two normal gestation periods for human embryos that yield viable babies: one at seven months and the other at nine months. A baby born after eight months was therefore either a seven-month fetus born one month late, after the completion of its natural gestation period and thus expected to survive, or a premature nine-month baby who would certainly die. A premature baby was identifiable by poor development of the hair and nails. This concept of viability came from Hippocrates, who reported that a baby born in the eighth month was more likely to die than one born in the seventh or ninth month of pregnancy.[65] One rabbi justified this idea by pointing out that the Greek letter *zeta*, which has the numerical value of seven, means "thou shalt live," whereas *eta*, which has the numerical value of eight, means "mischance" or "destruction."[66]

The nonviability of an eight-month fetus has had practical implications for Jews because the Talmud permits desecration of the Sabbath (for example, by cutting the umbilical cord and heating the room) to receive a seven-month and a nine-month fetus, but not for an eight-month baby, who is treated, the Talmud says, "like a stone."[67]

The Talmud cites the strange case of Rabbi Hiyya's twin sons, who were born three months apart; one was mature at the beginning of seven months, the other was mature only at the end of nine months.[68] Were the two babies really twins, or was one conceived long after the other, the medical term for which is "superfetation"? Although the ancient Greeks believed that superfetation was possible, Jewish sages in talmudic times apparently did not.[69] Again, for Jews, this point was not merely theoretical; the possibility that a second conception could harm the first or could itself prove nonviable may have been the reason for pregnant women to use a contraceptive tampon during marital relations.[70]

How influential was this talmudic embryology? Throughout the ages, rabbis have often referred back to this important Jewish source to solve a particular problem. Like so much talmudic material, these ideas have provided fertile ground for tales and legends. There are stories of unusually long gestations, which sometimes cast doubt on a woman's faithfulness to her husband, and of unusually short pregnancies, such as that of Leah, whose sons were reputedly born after seven months; Moses was born after six months and the prophets after seven months, and some told tales of twins born a couple of months apart.[71]

One story, dating from the fifteenth century, tells of a young woman who gave birth eleven months after her husband had left for a distant city to further his studies. The incident created a local scandal. The young husband, from Enns, Austria, was named Shlumiel, a Yiddish name that depicts a bungler whose enterprises invariably go awry. The matter was discussed in the rabbinic court, whose elderly members were persuaded by the wife's obvious piety and who researched Jewish sources for enlightenment on the problem. The members of the court succeeded in stifling suspicions when they announced that such a long pregnancy, although rare, had in fact occurred before.[72]

Obstetrical texts documented the viability of a seven-month baby and the nonviability of an eight-month baby until the late eighteenth century, and this concept was evident in prayer books that included one prayer for safe delivery for the seventh month of pregnancy and another for the ninth month. Meir Aldabi, a Jewish philosopher in early fourteenth-century Spain, offered an astrological explanation for the two different gestation periods. He explained that while Saturn (a planet characterized by its relative immobility, being cold and dry) dominates the sperm at the time of conception, Jupiter (warm and wet) encourages the shaping and forming of the embryo, and in the following months, Mars, the Sun, Venus, and Mercury enable the development of all the organs; the moon gives the baby strength in the seventh month, and if it is not born then, the ruling of Saturn in the eighth month can cause its weakness and death; if the pregnancy continues into the ninth month, however, Jupiter's positive power gives the baby strength for a successful full-term delivery.[73] A Hebrew medical manuscript dating from the same period repeated that Saturn, the planet associated with weakness and death, rules in the eighth month of pregnancy.[74]

Astrology was one way of rationalizing the problem of the two gestation periods and the nonviability of a baby born in the eighth month, but a century later, Solomon ben Simon Duran (c. 1400–1467), a rabbi of Algiers who was well-read in medicine and philosophy, gave the effect of the planets as only one of three possible reasons. He believed that viability also depended on the balance of the humors (following Greco-Roman ideas and Asaph Judaeus). He also extrapolated his father's crisis theory of illness to offer a third reason: this theory stated that a crisis on the seventh day of an illness is a sign of the patient's strong constitution and a crisis on the ninth reveals a little weakness, but a crisis on the eighth day shows great weakness.[75]

Until the seventeenth century, Jewish physicians favored the astrological rationalization of the gestation periods, which had no Jewish relevance, over an alternative proposal by Sa'adia Gaon based purely on talmudic conjecture that, in the last trimester of pregnancy, the embryo moved from the middle chamber in the womb to the highest. He suggested that, in contrast to the seventh and ninth months, in the eighth month the [birth canal] opening was too narrow for safe delivery.[76]

References in the post-talmudic literature to twins born months apart show that some Jews believed that superfetation was possible. Although not a medical text, the thirteenth-century *Sefer Hasidim* taught that a woman could conceive from two men in the first forty days from the end of her last menstrual period, but not after this time.[77] In the late sixteenth century, a rabbi wrote that he witnessed in Rome the stoning of a Roman Catholic woman who had given birth twice in a four-month interval: she had confessed that her second child was conceived adulterously in the fifth month of her first pregnancy. Another rabbi, in early eighteenth-century Egypt, reported the case of a woman who gave birth shortly after her husband had left the country and then delivered another baby a few months later. Absolving her of adultery, the rabbi assumed that she had become pregnant the second time while her husband was still living with her.[78] Medical literature also offered some cases; for example, *Marrano* physicians Rodrigo de Castro (c. 1550–1627) and Isaac Cardoso (1604–1681) discussed superfetation in learned Latin treatises.[79]

We now know that superfetation cannot occur because ovulation ceases at the onset of pregnancy, and women rarely conceive twins by two different men, a phenomenon called superfecundation.

It appears that, although historically Jews took an interest in embryology, they did not make any significant contributions to the advance of this science until modern times. One reason was the prohibition against desecration of the dead, out of respect for them. Thus, Jews did not undertake dissection to further scientific knowledge, except when it could save life in the future. As the Enlightenment spread among Jews, many chose to abandon Jewish law in their pursuit of academic goals. Robert Remak (1815–1865), at the University of Berlin, was one of the first Jewish physicians to obtain a university post in modern times and was one of a few Jews to carry out pioneering work in embryology in the nineteenth century. Remak identified three different layers of the embryo. Since then, countless Jews have contributed to the understanding of the development of the fetus, especially in the field of molecular biology.

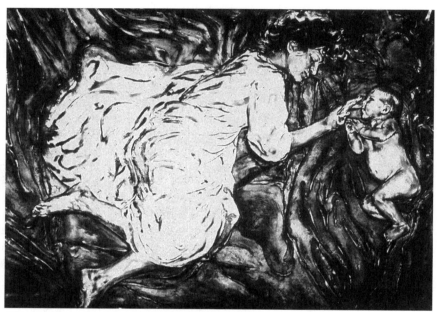

Plate 8. *Awakening I*. 1986, Ruth Weisberg.
Lithograph. Courtesy of the artist.

Chapter Five

The Experiences of Pregnancy

In their concern for fine offspring, Jews have provided guidelines for all aspects of behavior during pregnancy, including intellectual stimulation, diet, and marital relations. Expectant parents naturally are anxious for the baby to be well formed and to develop healthily in the womb. Nowadays, prenatal clinics offer diagnostic tests to check on the fetus, but in the past, Jews sought forecasts and omens to reduce this anxiety.

ACKNOWLEDGING PREGNANCY

Pregnancy Tests

It is sometimes important to find out as soon as possible whether a woman has conceived. Although this knowledge may be a joy to the prospective parents, traditionally Jews are often wary of sharing it with others until after the birth.

A woman usually guesses that she is pregnant when she has missed a menstrual period, feels nauseated, and suffers swollen and painful breasts. Some women only notice one or two of these signs, and on occasion, a woman may not realize for some months that she has conceived. In the past, it was sometimes difficult to notice the first pregnancy of a very young woman, but usually, pregnancy was identified by the end of the first trimester.[1] Waistlines were hidden behind an apron or a loose dress, but sooner or later, others noticed a neighbor's failure to make her monthly visit to the ritual bath, or they noticed a woman's heavy gait and knew that she had conceived.[2]

The Talmud gives criteria for the early identification of pregnancy: menses cease and convert to breast milk, and a woman experiences heaviness of head and limbs.[3] Knowledge of the time of conception was sometimes important to determine an expected child's paternity, to determine inheritance rights. For example, when a husband died or left home for an extended period and his wife later found that she was pregnant, it was necessary to establish the identity of the father before aspersions were cast on her virtue and the infant denied paternal dues.

The oldest remedy books contained advice on how to test for pregnancy.[4] A method used in ancient Egypt required a sample of the woman's urine, which was sprinkled on cereal seeds in the earth. If the grain failed to grow, the urine lacked life-giving elements, signifying that the woman had not conceived, whereas sprouting grain confirmed pregnancy.[5] Passed on from one generation to the next, this test survived into the late nineteenth century.[6] (It was actually used more often as a test of barrenness, applied to both husband and wife, to see which one was responsible for the couple's childlessness.[7]

An astrological handbook, attributed to Abraham ibn Ezra (1092–1167), reveals that Jewish astrologers were sometimes asked to confirm a woman's pregnancy by studying the configuration of the stars and planets in the night sky.[8]

A medieval Hebrew fable, written down by Berekhiah Ha-nakdan (c. 1200), tells of a pregnancy test from a blood sample. The fable relates that a physician once drew some blood from a sick man for analysis, to see whether the patient had a chance of recovery. The doctor asked the man to keep the blood sample in a safe place for three days and promised to return then to make his diagnosis. Fearing the sample might spill, the sick man gave it to his daughter for safekeeping. She placed it out of harm's way, underneath her cupboard. Unfortunately, a cat upset the dish, and the dismayed girl was at a loss about what to do. Innocently, she decided to replenish it with her own blood. The physician returned on the promised day and examined the blood. He grew angry and shouted at the sick man: "So, you are pregnant! Never has there been such a thing and never shall there be, that a male should bear a child! I do not wonder that you are sick! Your wickedness and your sins have brought about this unheard-of phenomenon." With that, the physician departed. The bewildered father called his daughter for an explanation. Tearfully, she told the truth: that his blood had spilt and she had added hers to the dish. The sick man thus learnt that his daughter, whom he had regarded as extremely chaste, was pregnant.[9] Berekhiah did not say whether the father ever rose from his sick bed after such devastating news.

Celebrating Pregnancy

Celebrating pregnancy has never been part of Jewish ritual, but rather is a recent custom, practiced only in some Jewish communities. Ethnographers have observed that Ashkenazi Jews have taken care that a woman's gravid state should not be noticeable for as long as possible, whereas in the early twentieth century, Sephardic and some Kurdistani Jews celebrated the prospect of a first birth with a ceremonial preparation of the layette for the newborn.

Ashkenazi Jews in the shtetl believed that proud talk when a pregnancy was barely established would invite catastrophe. Like other Jews, they feared the Evil Eye, expecting it to do harm when their affairs were prospering. Moreover, hasidic rabbis taught that a man who discovered a new way in which to serve God should keep it secret for nine months, as though he were pregnant with it, and inform others of it only at the end of that time, like a birth.[10] Ashkenazi Jews today usually buy nothing for an expected baby until after the birth.[11]

In contrast, Sephardic Jews have often celebrated a first pregnancy. This celebration has been named *kortadura de fashadura* (in Judeo-Spanish) or *tekti'a el-g'daouère* (in Judeo-Arabic), meaning "the cutting of the swaddling clothes." The ceremonial cutting of a cloth to make the baby's first costume, which is the same for a girl or a boy, is an old Sephardic custom still continued by some Jews in Istanbul. When a Jewish woman reaches the fifth month of her first pregnancy, her family invites all her female relatives and in-laws, as well as friends and neighbors. Liqueurs and chocolates, tea, cakes, and sugared almonds are set out on the best china, on hand-embroidered tablecloths. The cloth is of excellent quality and traditionally comes from the expectant woman's dowry. A relative who is herself a mother and whose own parents are still alive (a good omen for long life) receives the honor of making the first cut in the cloth. At the moment of the cut, the pregnant woman throws white sugared almonds on the cloth, to symbolize the sweet and prosperous future she wishes for her child.[12]

Sephardic Jews in Algeria and Morocco celebrated the cutting of the first layette when a woman was in the last trimester of her first pregnancy. The pregnant woman's parents provided lengths of cloth on a copper tray covered with a silk scarf. In Algeria, the person who made the first cut was similarly a woman whose parents were still alive and who clearly lived in a happy home. In Morocco, the midwife cut the cloth into swaddling clothes in the presence of women friends and relatives who offered their good wishes and shared tea and cakes.[13] Apparently, this was a very festive occasion, for in 1904 the rabbi of Sefrou decreed against the ostentation displayed at these celebrations.[14] When conception followed a period of barrenness that had been cured by a pilgrimage to the tomb of a famous rabbi, the pregnant woman returned to the tomb for a celebration of cakes and arrack, and she distributed charity to yeshivah students and the poor. By the middle of the twentieth century, a few Jewish families still continued these traditions, fearing bad luck if, by abandoning them, they omitted the blessings and good wishes for the future child.

In the Holy Land, during the last decades of the Ottoman Empire, Sephardic Jews prepared baby clothes during the last months of a woman's pregnancy, but there appears to be no record of a celebration or ceremony. In one account, women sewed the layette from old pieces of cloth, with the most effort put into the baby's bonnet, the only item that would be visible above layers of swaddling and blanketing. Women decorated the bonnet with colored ribbons and a little sprig of rue against the Evil Eye.[15]

Jewish women in Amadiya, Kurdistan, in the early twentieth century, also celebrated a first pregnancy. When a young woman was certain that she had conceived, she went to her father's house, where her mother and female relatives sewed clothes for the expected baby. They bestowed the honor of making the sheets for the cradle on an old woman who had delivered many babies. The women invited musicians, sang and danced, and offered the mother-to-be tidbits of advice about childbearing. In the evening, they prepared a feast for the men in the husband's house. These Jews may have learned this custom of celebrating "the joy of pregnancy" (known as *parḥiya semaḥa*) from their local neighbors, because elsewhere in Kurdistan, Jews kept the first pregnancy secret as long as possible.[16]

Jews in Yemen and Aden prepared clothes for the newborn in the seventh month of a woman's pregnancy, but without ceremony. It was customary to conceal pregnancy from the public eye for as long as possible, and each woman sewed what she would need for her own baby.[17] When a woman realized that she was pregnant, she shared her knowledge with her mother: "Oh mother, we have sown a generation." This expression received the standard reply: "Oh daughter, the tidings will come at the hour of birth."[18]

Although, in recent years, Sephardic and Kurdistani Jews have refrained from making preparations for an unborn child, increasing numbers of Western Jewish women are celebrating events in the life cycle that are unique to women. Unlike the Bat Mitzvah at puberty and the wedding, which both mark a change in status, no Jewish ritual marks the new role of becoming a mother. Some women have sought to create a new ceremony, in the style of a Jewish ritual, to express their feelings of spirituality and Jewish identity at this milestone in their lives.[19] For example, one woman chose Rosh Hodesh, the first day of the new moon (a day when women have abstained from heavy work), as a good time for a pregnancy ritual at home. In this ceremony, she recited benedictions over candles and had a plaited loaf (hallah) and sweet wine as well as special blessings for the occasion, just as in other Jewish celebrations. She also incorporated symbolism into the celebration, with motifs of fertility and birth.[20] Another woman opted for a ritual performed in synagogue. She desired a ceremony in which she could publicly affirm her performance of the duty to procreate and acknowledge God's partnership in conception. Here she undertook, like Manoah's wife, not to do anything that could harm the growing fetus and received the *mi-shebeirakh* blessing, that God should hear her prayers.[21]

These ceremonies reflect the fact that, for most Jewish women outside the Orthodox tradition, childbearing is no longer a foregone conclusion, but is now a particular stage in life, reached after conscious decision making. In such a ceremony, a woman acknowledges her responsibility for creating a new life, prepares herself to accept her new role, and commits herself to fulfilling it within the framework of Judaism, just as she may have done at her wedding or at her Bat Mitzvah when she was twelve years old. Although these new ceremonies may have some common aims, they differ greatly in their performance and are not a formalized part of Jewish ritual. As each woman chooses the ideas, blessings, and rituals of her celebration, she endows the occasion with her own personal spiritual significance.

EXPERIENCES INSIDE THE WOMB

Once a woman is pregnant, Judaism considers her fetus part of her body, just as her limbs are part of her body.[22] Jews have always recognized that a fetus is much more than a mere limb, however. Some have thought that an unborn baby is capable of emotions and intellectual activity and that elements of its adult personality are evident even before birth. Some have also believed that the fetus is capable of self-expression and can influence the mother's behavior.

Spiritual Life of the Embryo

Talmudic sages were interested not only in the physical characteristics of the developing fetus, but also in its spiritual existence. They imagined that, at the beginning of time, God created all the divine sparks that give babies their uniqueness and essence of human being, and an angel delivered these to the mothers' wombs when needed.[23] The sages pictured the spiritual experiences of the embryo before birth, and the medieval mystics later embellished this imagery.[24] For example, a midrash tells that when husband and wife engage in the act of love, God calls on an angel to bring up the husband's seed. God then calls on another angel to fetch a soul for this seed. God decides whether the soul will be strong or weak, tall or short, male or female, foolish or wise, rich or poor, but not, of course, whether it will be pious or wicked. However, this soul prefers the holy and pure upper world where it has resided until chosen and pleads with God not to force it into the evil-smelling droplet. God ignores these protests and places it in the seed, and the angel delivers it to the wife's womb where it will grow into a baby. God assigns two angels to guard the seed lest it fall out.

The tale continues. A light burning above the head of the fetus in the womb enables it to see from one end of the world to the other. In the morning, one angel shows the baby the Garden of Eden where the righteous sit in glory, and in the evening they visit Gehenna, where the wicked are punished and beaten with rods of fire. On this trip, the baby learns that soon it will leave the womb. It learns, too, that if it grows into a righteous adult, its soul will live forever in the Garden of Eden and not in Gehenna. The angel shows the baby its path in life and eventual burial place and then locks the opening of the womb.

When the time comes for the baby's birth, again the little soul, who has become accustomed to life in the womb, protests the change. The soul's fate is to enter the womb against its will and to emerge against its will. As the infant emerges, the angel hits it under the nose (making the little mark above the upper lip) and extinguishes the light that burned above its head, to make the infant forget everything it saw. When the baby is born, it cries instantly for the world that it has just left.[25]

In the zoharic version of this tale, when the parents are pious people, four angels—Michael, Gabriel, Nuriel, and Raphael—accompany the soul on its descent from the supernal world to the baby's body. Gabriel, the angel of the good inclination, teaches the baby the entire Torah and seventy languages. However, when the parents are sinful and unworthy, the guardian angels in the womb are from the Other Side—Anger, Destruction, Depravity, and Wrath—ruled by Samael, the angel of the evil inclination, who wipes out all the baby's prenatal knowledge at birth.[26]

The Hasidim, too, have perpetuated this legend. Keen to develop the idea of God's participation in a baby's formation, they teach that divine guidance of embryonic life sets the pattern for a person's existence in this world. Thus, the baby's prenatal knowledge of Torah, the Garden of Eden, and Gehenna dictates the soul's yearning for divine light. The moral of the tale is that a life of piety, righteousness, prayer, faith, learning, humility, and charity enables the soul to retrieve all the prenatal knowledge given to it by God and thereby restore the divine light.[27]

This legend inspired Itzik Manger's (1901–1969) delightful story, *The Book of Paradise*, first published in Yiddish, in Warsaw in 1939 and eventually translated into Hebrew, English, and some other European languages.[28]

This picture of prenatal activity has provided an existential basis for the birth of a Jewish baby and a rationale for a person's Jewish lifestyle. Its popularity throughout the ages reflects, on the one hand, nostalgia for the coziness and security of life in the womb and, on the other hand, acceptance of a lifelong responsibility to maintain the purity of one's soul through righteous behavior.

Maternal Experiences Affecting the Baby

Like other peoples, Jews have believed that a pregnant mother's experiences and events in her vicinity may influence her baby's characteristics and personality. Jews have been liberal with advice concerning her diet and cravings for special foods as well as her spiritual and intellectual well-being.

Since ancient times, a woman's diet during pregnancy has been of utmost importance. The Book of Judges relates that an angel warned Manoah's wife not to drink wine or eat impure foods when pregnant.[29] Centuries later, the Talmud detailed a diet for pregnant women: some meat and wine, in moderation (to ensure the baby's robust constitution), eggs (for the baby's eyesight), and fish (for gracefulness), as well as fresh vegetables and fruit, celery, or parsley (for brilliance), coriander (to make the baby plump), and citron (for fragrance). The same text warns pregnant women against eating mustard (lest the child become gluttonous or intemperate), cress (for fear of bleary-eyed offspring), fish brine (which could also affect the baby's eyes), intoxicating liquor (which could cause the child's eventual ungainliness), and clay (causing ugliness). During pregnancy some women indeed crave clay, soot, or ashes, a syndrome known as pica.[30]

In contrast to the Talmud, a medieval treatise on pregnancy warned that expectant mothers should not eat celery or parsley, lest the baby develop boils or blisters, and they should refrain from consuming spicy foods, which cause bleeding.[31]

Although fashions have changed over the years concerning which foods are healthiest, the principle that a pregnant woman's cravings must be satisfied, lest the fetus be harmed, has remained remarkably stable throughout the ages. Jews have believed that an expectant mother should eat anything she craves, even a tiny morsel if it is the Day of Atonement, the holy day when Jews fast. A talmudic anecdote relates that on such an occasion a rabbi advised whispering in a pregnant woman's ear to remind her that it was the Day of Atonement. Her craving immediately disappeared, and the son whom she bore became a great rabbi. However, another woman with similar cravings who ignored the rabbi's whisper gave birth to a wicked, selfish son. This homily serves several purposes: to remind one that God rewards the virtuous woman; to teach that the fetus causes the mother's craving; and to signify that the baby's character expresses itself in the womb.[32]

In medieval times, Maimonides and Meir Aldabi both adopted the existing Greco-Roman theory that sickness, nausea, and cravings of normal early pregnancy are due to an imbalance in bodily humors (in particular, the predominance of an unfavorable cold humor). They elaborated that women who suffer in this way harbored "bad liquids" in the folds of the stomach at the time of conception, from their failure to release premenstrual blood; when these liquids penetrate the stomach, a woman craves sour and pungent things, even soot or ashes, and she eliminates these unpleasant juices by vomiting. Maimonides and Meir Aldabi observed that the growth of the fetus reduces the effects of these liquids.[33]

A Hebrew version of Soranus' treatise on obstetrics, dating from the fourteenth century, recommended astringent potions to counteract the abundance of humors that cause pregnant women to crave pottery shards and ashes. This text advised a one-day fast if the cravings persist beyond the first few months, with minimal food intake on the next few days; it allowed a little draft of water, followed by wine. Doctors today do not approve of this advice, because the lack of fluids can endanger the fetus. The medieval text went on to counsel expectant mothers to listen to some music and do some pleasant reading.[34]

A few centuries later, the physicians Abraham Zacuto Lusitanus (1575–1642) and Tobias Cohn (1652–1729) offered several potions (such as a mint or cinnamon infusion) for coping with pica, other cravings, vomiting, and other first-trimester discomforts, which they list as asthma, hoarseness, loosening of the bowels, stomachache, toothache, headache, and dizziness.[35]

In her memoirs, Gluckel of Hameln (1645–1724) cited her own experience to warn women that it can be dangerous to ignore a craving during pregnancy. She had borne thirteen children and was also a successful businesswoman. She admitted laughing at those who thought they would suffer harm by not indulging a craving during pregnancy. Many times when she was pregnant she noticed some nice fruit in the market that she fancied but did not buy, for it was too expensive, and she suffered no ill effects. However, on the last day of one of her pregnancies, she saw some medlars (a small brown apple-like fruit), which she had wanted to eat, but had not done so. The baby was born with brown spots on his head and body, refused to suckle, and appeared as though "his soul had departed." When there was no improvement after three days, Gluckel remembered the medlars and asked that some be obtained for her. When the medlars arrived, she squeezed some of the juice into the baby's mouth. He drank it eagerly and then accepted his mother's breast. By the eighth day, the day of circumcision, he was perfectly well. She warned young pregnant women that if at any time they fancy a fruit or anything tasty, they should sample it and ignore "their own silly heads which say, 'Ay, it cannot harm you!' . . . For it can, God forbid, be a matter of life and death to them, as well as to the unborn child, as I found to my cost."[36]

Rabbis and midwives have warned of dire consequences, such as miscarriage, birthmarks, or handicap, if such cravings are not fulfilled. However, this attitude is not characteristically Jewish. Such fears have been common worldwide, among the Jews of North Africa,[37] Eastern Europe,[38] the Ottoman Empire,[39] Persia, Iraq, and Kurdistan,[40] as well as among many other peoples.[41] In the early twentieth century, Yemenite and Kurdistani Jews believed that refusing a pregnant woman's gastronomic whims caused birthmarks and even blindness: a popular proverb advised "give her to eat lest the baby be born with one eye."[42]

An elderly Jewish woman, Ghitta Sternberg, recently recalled that, during her first pregnancy in Canada, where she had moved from her Rumanian shtetl, she mentioned to a friend that she would like to have a kvosnetze, the pickled sweet apple she had loved in her home village. To her utter amazement, her friend went to great trouble to obtain this special apple, which was surely unknown in Canada.[43] The reason for the friend's efforts was her fear that if a craving were not satisfied, the pregnant woman risked miscarrying. When discussing this subject, an Israeli woman told of her craving for a guava when she was last pregnant. She dismissed her desire for this fruit as extravagant, because it was out of season, but she was not surprised when her son was born with a guava-shaped birthmark. Such stories are less common today, but were widespread a generation ago.

Jews have taught that it is not only food that affects the baby: the Talmud tells of the mother of Joshua ben Hananyah (first to second century C.E.), who visited every house of study in her city when she was pregnant and begged scholars to pray for her baby, that he should grow up to be wise and learned. After the birth, she resumed these visits, carrying the infant in the cradle, so from his earliest experiences he would learn to love the atmosphere of study. He eventually fulfilled her hopes, by serving in the Temple in Jerusalem before its destruction and becoming a man of great wisdom.[44]

Almost two millennia later, Ghitta Sternberg's mother had the same idea when she listened to music in her shtetl in the hope that her future child would grow up with musical talent. Behind her house was a little park, where a local military band gave Sunday concerts. When she was pregnant, she deliberately sat on her back porch to listen to the music. (In the shtetl, the opportunity for listening to music was otherwise limited to weddings, occasional concerts, and scratchy gramophone records, amplified with a wooden horn.) Ghitta joked that her mother's efforts worked, because her own musical talents are just about at the level of the shtetl military band.[45]

A recommendation from an early twentieth-century remedy book advises pregnant women to immerse themselves in the *mikveh* in their ninth month, to erase evil influences on the baby.[46] A simple immersion could wash away some of a woman's fears for her baby, and she could hope that her prayers at the ritual bath might attract God's favor and the blessing of an easy and safe delivery. The many prayers for the well-being of a pregnant woman and her fetus are discussed in the next chapter.

Nowadays cravings are no longer blamed for miscarriage, handicaps, or birthmarks, although pregnant women are encouraged to maintain a healthy diet. They may also take the advice offered in the fourteenth century and listen to music or read a pleasant book for relaxation.

MARITAL RELATIONS DURING PREGNANCY

Sexual Relations

Jewish sources provide comprehensive guidance for all realms of human behavior, including marital relations during pregnancy. The importance of sexual enjoyment during pregnancy among Jews is in marked contrast to the practices of other peoples, such as the early and medieval Christians, some African tribes, and some in New Guinea, who encourage sexual relations for procreation only. At the beginning of the Christian era, the Stoic school preached strict control of one's passions, but only the Essenes, a Jewish sect living near the Dead Sea at that time, limited sexual relations to begetting children and therefore refrained from this activity during pregnancy.[47] This was the only exception to Jewish approval of making love during pregnancy.

Although the Talmud warns that sexual relations may harm pregnancy in the first few weeks, it claims these relations are especially beneficial in the last trimester. The warning stems from the theory that the baby rises in the woman's belly as pregnancy progresses; in the first trimester, the fetus resides in the lowest chamber of the womb, but it moves to the middle chamber for the next trimester and spends the last three months in the highest chamber. It then turns over to exit head first into the world outside. Thus, the talmudic sages thought that when the fetus was in the lowest chamber, deep penetration by the husband could harm both the mother and her embryo. The sages feared that, in the middle trimester, the vitalizing semen could possibly benefit the baby, but the intrusion could cause the mother to miscarry. They reasoned that when the baby was in the highest chamber, physical damage from sexual relations was less likely; during the last trimester, both mother and baby could benefit from the life-giving powers of the semen and the invigorating exercise of the act of love.[48]

Medieval rabbis pointed out that sexual relations during pregnancy were clearly not for procreation, but were mainly for a woman's pleasure and, in the last trimester, for the baby's strength, too. Moreover, it has been considered a mitzvah for a husband to give his pregnant wife pleasure in this way.[49] However, real life has often been far from the Jewish ideal that sexual relations are primarily for a wife's pleasure, over and above a husband's gratification. Recognizing the force of male libido, rabbis made allowances for a husband to satisfy his needs, even if his wife had shown no desire to make love.[50] Maimonides, for example, considered that marital sex for the relief of a husband's physical pressures was physically and morally healthy, although he warned against excess.[51] His contemporary, Abraham ben David of Posquières (c. 1125–1198), encouraged a husband to have sexual relations with his wife if by doing so he avoided "thoughts of sin." He stressed, however, that it was better for a man to desire his pregnant wife for the benefits to her and their baby than for his own personal gratification.[52]

The physiological and hormonal changes that occur during pregnancy cause some women to lack libido; they feel too tired, they suffer physically, or they fear miscarriage. Conversely, some women do not enjoy sexual relations and use pregnancy as an excuse for abstaining. Pregnancy may also affect a husband's physical interest in his wife; some men find the pregnant body unattractive or frightening, or they fear they may harm the baby. One 21-year-old woman who became pregnant within six months of her marriage said recently: "Our [sexual] relations are as they were before I conceived, only now I am often too tired . . . but I have to think of him!" Another woman, married less than two years, who had a one-year-old toddler and who was eight months' pregnant with twins, said that, until the sixth month of her current pregnancy, sexual relations were normal, but since then she just had not been interested. She commented that her husband sometimes expressed his annoyance, but suddenly added: "He's a man!" These two women were fully aware of their husbands' needs and paid tribute to the age-old impression that a man's sexual drive is immensely powerful. Jews have called it the evil inclination (*yetzer ha-ra*), believing that if it dominates a man's actions, he will become wicked. At the same time, they have acknowledged that God created this inclination for a purpose: it is the force that leads men to marry and have children, to build homes, and to earn a living. Jews have considered it one of the driving forces of life that men must learn to control.[53]

In all their statements about sexual relations during pregnancy, rabbis have advised expectant parents according to their ideas of what is respectable and moral.

The overall intention has always been to encourage couples to be considerate of each others' needs and comfort.

Companionship and Support

Marital relations are, of course, not only sexual. The traditional Jewish marriage contract obliges the husband to "cherish, honor, support, and maintain" his wife; happy companionship is also a purpose of marriage. Most women enjoy support from their husbands during pregnancy. In communities where daily physical chores have clearly been a woman's role, a husband's help during pregnancy and birth has been mainly spiritual, expressed through his prayers. Today, Orthodox Jewish husbands still help in this way (and in other ways, too), whereas among the non-Orthodox, any extra help is more likely to be physical, with a husband's shopping, cleaning, or washing dishes, to reduce his wife's exertions.

Two Israeli fathers felt the need to help others learn from their experiences of pregnancy and wrote a tongue-in-cheek guide for prospective fathers. It began with a useful list of instructions on how to treat a pregnant wife: do not nag her but do spoil her; show interest and inform yourself about childbearing; promise her all she desires; do not be infantile or jealous; do not allow her to exert herself; do not complain; keep healthy; let her choose the baby's name; go on holiday (without her!); find new hobbies; and, finally, when you hear her inevitably remonstrate "have you forgotten that I am pregnant?", answer amicably "have you forgotten who *made* you pregnant?"—but in case she has a surprising retort to that, it is better to kiss her and stroke her hair. The two men went on to say that pregnancy is the only time a father is able to enjoy his baby, because after the birth the baby falls in love with its mother, the grandmother takes over the house, and everyone forgets the father until the next pregnancy. While recommending that a husband be supportive to his pregnant wife, these authors advised that he should sometimes escape from this burden, and they warned of the rejection (real or imagined) that they could experience after birth.[54] Here again, the main issue is the mutual consideration of each person's needs and comfort, and not the particular details.

Pregnant Beauty

Despite the traditional importance of having children and the subjectivity of beauty, Jews have perceived childbearing as detrimental to a woman's beauty. Midrashic elaborations of biblical stories tell that pregnancy disfigures and detracts from a woman's grace. For example, according to midrash, Lamech and Er took contraceptive precautions for the sake of preserving the beauty of their wives.[55]

Physical beauty is a distinction that women seek and that Jewish men (like all others) appreciate, although they are wary of it. Ever since ancient times, women have enhanced their beauty by ornamenting themselves, using cosmetics, and wearing fine clothes.[56] Nevertheless, an ancient Jewish proverb, still a rabbinic favorite, warns: "Grace is deceptive, beauty is illusory" (Proverbs 31:30). An Orthodox Jewish woman dresses with propriety and does not wear her hair loose in public or expose bare arms or legs. She dons her fine clothes, which are modest, on the Sabbath and festivals, and for other celebrations, but never presents herself as a sex object.[57]

There are many ways of appreciating a woman's beauty. Yet the expressions of this beauty in art—sculpture, painting, and poetry—have sought perfection mainly in physical characteristics. Throughout the ages, Jewish art avoided pregnant women as subjects. Only at the beginning of the twentieth century did the artistic freedom sought by the Impressionists enable a few Jewish artists to look at pregnant women and perceive their beauty. Marc Chagall captured it wonderfully in a sketch and a painting done between 1912 and 1913: he perceived the beauty of the swollen belly in the vitality of what is inside it and did not pay attention to the stretch marks on the outside.[58] A pregnant woman reflects, and sometimes also radiates, that vitality. Sculptures of pregnant women by Israeli artists are a reminder, but not a revival, of the ancient Canaanite fertility goddesses. These artists are not worshiping the enlarged abdomen, but are instead proclaiming the inner richness of the fertile female body. For example, Meira Grossinger has worked in wood and clay to reveal the inner softness of a pregnant woman's emotions. The distended bellies of her figures represent woman's spiritual fullness.[59]

Although since the Song of Songs Jewish poets have sought a woman's beauty in her physical characteristics, they have described spiritual beauty in the supernal world and in God's relationship with humankind. One exception is seen in the words of a Jewish poet of the Salonika Academy who lived in the sixteenth century. In a love song, David Onkinerah noticed more than what is skin deep: he noticed an inner light and joy in the radiant eyes of his lover.[60] Nevertheless, throughout the ages, the ideal woman of a male poet's dreams has been physically beautiful. She was not, and is still not, a pregnant woman.

One can seek beauty in a woman's inner vitality (like Chagall), in the radiance of her eyes (like Onkinerah), in her warmth, loving kindness, and consideration for others, and in the inner peace that a pregnant woman sometimes gains from the life inside her. The inner, spiritual beauty is difficult to define and perhaps equally difficult to attain, but it is definitely recognizable. To use the language of Jewish mystics, spiritual beauty perhaps represents a pure soul untainted by the evil of this world, and such a quality can be perceived in some people.

FORECASTS AND OMENS

Expectant parents often fear the uncertain outcome of pregnancy; one way of coping with these fears is to seek predictions. Nowadays, ultrasound scanning, blood tests, and other highly specialized techniques can assure expectant parents that their baby is developing normally, but until these methods became available, people forecasted a baby's future by interpreting dreams, the stars, or certain events.

Dreams

Some expectant parents remember their dreams more during pregnancy than at other times. Many have vivid dreams, some clearly arising from fears associated with childbearing. Since biblical times, some Jews have noted their dreams and have learned from the messages they sometimes seem to bear.

Since antiquity, Jews have interpreted dreams as indicators of events of the day or as visions of the future. They have believed in dreams as vehicles of communication of supernatural forces; angels could convey God's messages to the dreamer, demons could disturb one's sleep with their antics, and sometimes, a dream could carry a message directly from God.

Philo Judaeus (d. circa 50 C.E.) wrote five books on dreams and their interpretation; Jews, like other ancient peoples, took this subject seriously. There was some criticism, notably in the apocryphal Wisdom of Ben Sira, but the Talmud includes many pages of dream interpretations as well as instructions for neutralizing nightmares. Jews interpreted dreams of the proverbial vineyard and olive trees, as well as dreams about certain birds, as prediction or confirmation of pregnancy. According to the Talmud, a man who dreams of a vine laden with fruit should expect his wife not to miscarry, a dream of an olive tree portends many sons, and a dream of a cock indicates the birth of a son.[61]

Throughout the ages, Jews have continued to interpret dreams. Thus, in the tenth century, Sa'adia Gaon's interpretations in Babylonia followed the Talmud closely. He confirmed the significance of dreaming of a vineyard; the wife of the dreamer would surely conceive. One who dreamed of many trees would have many sons, but one who dreamed of being surrounded by many trees would father many children who would die. Gaon repeated that dreaming of a cock indicated the birth of a son. In the thirteenth century, Hasidei Ashkenaz in Germany also paid great attention to the study of dreams: a dream of sleeping under or inside trees was an omen that the dreamer would have children; a dream of apple trees growing in one's home was an omen that a wise son would be born, as well as a silly son; a dream of trees that never bore fruit indicated that the dreamer's unborn sons would be wicked; a dream of eating white sugar told that a son would be born or that the dreamer would become wealthy; a dream of passing blood in one's urine indicated that the dreamer's wife would miscarry; a dream of hunting an eagle foretold the birth of a son, whereas a raven or a crow indicated the imminent birth of a baby of either sex, and a hen in hand foretold the birth of a daughter.[62] When a man dreamed of carrying a bird in his bosom, a child would be born to him. If the bird flew away, however, disaster would follow. If a man dreamed of a woman giving birth, someone near him would die.

In 1515, Solomon Almoli, a Spanish Jew who eventually settled in Constantinople, published a manual for understanding dreams based on these earlier sources and including the foregoing interpretations. It became a popular Jewish dream dictionary, especially among Yiddish-speaking Jews.[63] A Yemenite dream dictionary bound into a manuscript of prayers, supplications, and verses of Torah seemed to have culled at least some of its interpretations from local Arabic sources, although it was written by a Jew and contained Jewish concepts. The only two items relevant to our topic reveal that if a Yemenite Jew dreamed that he saw an ox gored, he would surely have a wise son, whereas if he dreamed that his beard grew, he would be blessed with a daughter.[64]

The traditional Jewish means of preventing the misfortunes predicted in dreams are fasting (sometimes even on the Sabbath), praying, repenting, giving to charity, or "improving" the nightmare in a dawn ritual. The sad dreamer should gather together three loving friends and announce: "I have seen a good dream" (even though it was a nightmare). These friends then respond in unison seven times: "Good it is and good may it be," followed by a series of biblical verses including the words "turn," "redeem," and "peace." In addition to these traditional measures, Almoli suggested abrogating the omen by acting out the dream, thereby fulfilling the dream harmlessly.[65]

In the early seventeenth century, the kabbalist Hayyim Vital recorded his dreams. His first son had died in infancy, but his wife had conceived again three years later, and when she was in her seventh month of pregnancy, Vital dreamed that he was at the grave of a sage. While he circled the tomb with others, a man offered him a jewel bright as the sun and said: "First they gave you a burning light, but the oil was consumed and the light went out. But now they are giving you a precious jewel which needs no oil and will not go out." At that moment, Vital awoke. He understood that the light that had gone out was his dead son, and the jewel in his dream was the expected baby. He could relax, for his dream had predicted that the baby would live. When the boy was born, Vital named him after the sage whose tomb he had visited in his dream.[66]

Almost two hundred years ago, Nahman of Bratslav (1772–1810) drew on his dreams for several of his wonderful tales. He advised that if one wanted a dream to come true, one should write it down and note the time and place. Several hasidic rabbis followed this advice. One tale of dream interpretation has survived from Nahman's era: a woman who had lost several babies in early infancy reported a vivid dream on the night before she gave birth to yet another child whom she feared would soon die. She dreamed that she was led into a great hall, where old men wearing crowns and white robes sat at a long table listening to a boy who headed the meeting. She noticed that the boy was her last son, Moshe, who had survived the longest of her children, but had died when he was seven. She wanted to run up to him and embrace him, but he warned her not to touch him and blessed her for a safe delivery. A hasidic rabbi interpreted the dream as a warning: if she wanted her next child to survive into adulthood, her soul would have to stay on earth and not wander about in the heavenly palace.[67] It is not clear from this mystical interpretation what the poor woman should have done to prevent the death of her next child. Perhaps he meant that she should stop yearning for her children whose souls are in heaven and should compose herself to care for the baby for whom she had received a blessing in her dream.

Expectant parents today sometimes have adulterous dreams. Moroccan Jews liked to say that dreams about an unfaithful husband foretold the arrival of a baby girl, and those about an unfaithful wife were a sign of a baby boy.[68] Pregnant women have commonly dreamed of giving birth or that their baby is already born. Traditional Jewish women often dream while pregnant of the circumcision ritual.

Other Means of Prediction

The midrash teaches that a woman may guess her baby's future from sensations of the fetus in her womb. In addition to the homily described previously, which suggested that the wisdom and holiness of her offspring depended on whether the embryo caused her to eat on the Day of Atonement, legend tells that Jochebed, mother of Moses, sensed during pregnancy that her baby was destined for great things, whereas the kicking in Rebekah's womb warned her that one of her twins would be wicked.[69] Legend also tells that King David composed songs when still in his mother's womb.[70]

In view of the preference for boys, it is hardly surprising that women interpreted a good complexion, being good at housework, and lively kicks from the womb as evidence that a son had been conceived. In ancient and medieval times, people thought that the right testicle and the right side of the uterus were warmer, being nearer the liver than the left, and this warmth favored male conception; therefore, a fuller and firmer right breast presaged a boy.[71]

Since late antiquity and until the eighteenth century, some expectant parents consulted Jewish astrologers for information about their child. A medieval manuscript, in Judeo-Arabic, showed that someone had asked the astrologer whether a woman would miscarry. The astrologer studied the stars and planets and foretold an increased incidence of miscarriages. A Hebrew astrological handbook attributed to Abraham ibn Ezra asked questions concerning not only the sex but also the life span of the expected baby, but gave no answers. (Maimonides was alone in rejecting astrology of this sort during his era.)[72]

Since antiquity and until recent times, some Jews resorted to the practice of divination to predict the future. In the fifteenth century, some German Jews used a Bible to forecast the outcome of pregnancy from the verse at the beginning of the page or touched by the thumb when the book was opened at random.[73]

Remedy books often offered several methods of determining the sex of an unborn child. A popular test required drops of a pregnant woman's breast milk; if the drops sank in water, a girl would be born, but if they floated, the baby was a boy.[74] A rabbi in fifteenth-century Constantinople used this method postnatally to determine maternity when two mothers suspected that their newborns (one boy and one girl) had been interchanged.[75]

Jews sometimes made use of *gematria*, a Jewish method of practical Kabbalah, for predicting the sex of a baby. For example, one Jewish remedy book from Damacus suggested adding the numerical values of the parents' names and the month of expected delivery and dividing by nine: if the remainder were 1, 2, 3, 4, or 7, the baby would be female; otherwise, it would be male. The same book also offered another way of performing the calculation. Perhaps one of the two variables, if not both, would produce the correct result.[76]

In a Russian Jewish family in the late nineteenth century, pregnant women used the lemon-like *etrog* (after Sukkot) to make predictions. Whoever succeeded in biting off the nipple-shaped end of the fruit would give birth to a boy. In addition, the difficulty with which this end came off foretold the eventual difficulty of giving birth.[77]

Although some Jews have reasoned that one cannot make predictions about a baby while it is still in the womb, the variety of predictive methods nevertheless confirms the extent of parental desire to seek knowledge of unborn offspring. The variety of methods, however, attests to their unreliability.[78]

Modern Diagnostic Testing

Today, women seek predictions much as their ancestors did, but the results they can obtain are more accurate than ever before. Answers to parental questions about fetal health come now from doctors and scientists with highly specialized skills, equipment, and laboratories, rather than from astrologers, rabbis, or even midwives.

Special tests in the first trimester of pregnancy enable early identification of congenital syndromes that are more common among Ashkenazi Jews than among other peoples.[79] For example, the Tay–Sachs syndrome, which is caused by a genetic enzyme attacking the brain and nerves and results in the death of the child usually within five years of birth; Gaucher disease, which is caused by an enzyme deficiency that results in organ damage, bone weakening, and even death; Niemann–Pick disease, yet another enzyme deficiency, which causes metabolic disorder and degeneration resulting in death in early childhood; and mucolipidosis 4, which is a disorder of the central nervous system that causes partial or complete blindness and mental retardation. When a test confirms such a fetal abnormality or another severe disorder, abortion is often possible.

As seen in Chapter 3, in ultra–Orthodox Jewish communities, however, women may consider abortion of such a fetus only when a doctor warns of a danger to maternal health. Problems sometimes arise when a woman consults her rabbi about the medical diagnosis and the rabbi's opinion contradicts the doctor's advice. For example, in Israel one woman lost her baby when she started premature labor on Shabbat and her rabbi told her not to worry and wait until after Shabbat to go to the hospital.[80]

Other diagnostic tests, such as ultrasound examinations and amniocentesis, are outside the scope of this book; although these tests are important, they have no particular Jewish significance. Even with the most sophisticated tests, however, doctors are still a long way from being able to predict much of what can go wrong in the formation of new life. When the result of one test invalidates one specific fear, other fears can take its place in the mind of any anxious expectant parent.

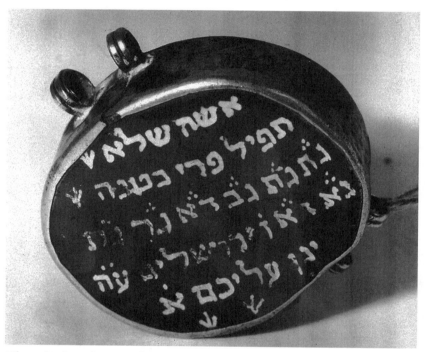

Plate 9. Amulet pendant, inscription: "For a woman not to lose the fruit of her womb," followed by letters with magical significance. Kuba, Dagestan, twentieth century. Grishashvili Museum of the History and Ethnography of Tbilisi, Georgia. Photo: Beth Hatefutsoth Photo Archive.

Chapter Six

Pregnancy Loss

Pregnancy has always carried risks, and Jews, like other peoples, have been careful to take precautions to avoid tragedy. Such precautions have depended on perceptions of the causes of pregnancy loss. In the past, these perceptions were often colored by beliefs in divine retribution and demonic mischief, but today one usually looks for physiological and environmental causes.

Although most pregnant women today give birth to healthy babies, one pregnancy in five still ends in misfortune, often in the first trimester, but sometimes later in pregnancy, involving considerable trauma. One way of coming to terms with such a difficult experience is to seek to understand why it happened; another way is to acknowledge one's mourning the misfortune.

MISCARRIAGE

The Hebrew word for an aborted fetus "who never saw the light" (Job 3:16) is a *nefel*, something that has fallen or dropped out.

In talmudic times, the sages took an interest in the nature of miscarriage, in the context of the Jewish laws regarding female impurity. They ruled that a woman remains ritually impure for a shorter period if her uterine discharge is merely menstruation and not a birth. Thus, a woman who aborted a sac of liquid or unidentifiable matter counted her days of impurity as if she had not conceived, but one who aborted a fetus whose limbs were formed purified herself as after giving birth.[1] The talmudic rabbis likened the shape of an aborted fetus to a fish, a beast, a bird, a serpent, and even to Lilith, who, they imagined, had a human face but a body with wings.[2]

Causes

Jews have realized that miscarriage may have numerous causes. The Bible portrays full-term pregnancy as God's reward to the righteous and pregnancy loss (like barrenness) as a divine punishment. This distinction is clear from God's promise to Moses on Mount Sinai, "No woman in your land shall miscarry" (Exodus 23:26), among those who obey the commandments. Later, Hosea, the Israelite prophet, begged God to punish his iniquitous people: "Give them a womb that miscarries" (Hosea 9:14).

Since antiquity, Jews have marveled at the divine favor that enables a pregnant woman to stand without the fetus' falling out. The talmudic rabbis taught that

God decides when the womb shall open and reasoned that a baby could fall out prematurely if God's goodwill were withdrawn for some reason. For example, a woman's immorality or any feelings of hatred, even groundless hatred, in her household could provide such a reason.[3]

The Bible and the Talmud also blame pregnancy failure on physical and emotional trauma, as well as on evil winds and spirits. Thus, a physical blow, a great fright, the strong smell of burned meat, a south wind, and even cut-off fingernails or toenails (associated with witchcraft in many cultures) were believed in ancient times to be causes of miscarriage.[4] Legend tells that, when Joseph made himself known to his brothers, Judah's outcry and the ensuing tumult caused the women in Egypt to give birth prematurely. Moreover, when Esther heard of Mordecai's mourning for the plight of the Jewish people, she, too, was most upset and miscarried.[5] The Book of Kings relates that Elisha threw salt into a spring near Jericho to neutralize its harmful effects.[6] The pollution in the water, perceived as the cause of miscarriage and infant death, may have been demonic rather than toxic, because throwing salt is an ancient protection against evil spirits.

Incantations and stories inscribed on Jewish amulets from post-talmudic Palestine and medieval North Africa tell of demonic forces that could kill a fetus in the womb. Similarly, a remedy book first published in Eastern Europe in the early eighteenth century tells that Samael, the evil demon, was slighted by the archangel Michael and was therefore bent on harming the growing fetus.[7]

As mentioned in the previous chapter, the Talmud assumes that sexual intercourse can occasion miscarriage, but in a specific way: a woman could abort a compressed, flattened, and lifeless fetus if she conceived a second fetus that pressed on the first.[8] In addition, Jews feared that unfulfilled cravings could induce miscarriage or handicap.

Medieval physicians recognized illness, an abscess in the womb, and a woman's excessive leanness, obesity, or deformity as causes of miscarriage.[9] In the twelfth century, Maimonides elaborated that a woman could miscarry as a result of exertion or steambathing. He said that "excessive anointing of her head with oil" could induce a coughing fit that could expel the fetus. His contemporary in Germany, Judah the Pious, warned that the tendency to miscarry could be hereditary.[10]

In the early fourteenth century, Meir Aldabi accepted the popular medical theory that the planets influence maternal health and the growing fetus. He noted that Saturn could induce pregnancy loss in the eighth month. In the late sixteenth century, Hayyim Vital accepted and quoted from this thesis.[11]

Today there are still women who consider miscarriage as punishment for some misdemeanor or as the result of an emotion, especially if the doctor cannot explain why it happened.[12] Doctors usually limit their investigation of pregnancy loss to physiological and biochemical analysis.

A "Wind Egg" or False Pregnancy

Since antiquity, some women have displayed all the symptoms of pregnancy only to discover some months later that they had not actually conceived.

False pregnancies were common when confirmation of pregnancy was not entirely objective.

A metaphor in the Bible, describing Isaiah's futile efforts, recognizes the phenomenon of false pregnancy: "We were with child, we writhed—It is as though we had given birth to wind" (Isaiah 26:18). Some centuries later, the Talmud mentions the case of a woman who gave birth to a lifeless "wind egg."[13] Another source dating from the talmudic period tells of a winged spirit who impregnated beautiful women, causing them to become pregnant and then to give birth to wind.[14]

The ancient Greeks described a uterine growth, a *mola*: a woman would think she had conceived, and her belly would swell, but at the time of birth nothing would come out. Eventually, she would become dangerously ill with dysentery and would abort the *mola* as a fleshy lump. The most influential obstetrical treatises, namely Soranus' in the second century, and that of ibn Sina (also known as Avicenna) in the early eleventh century, repeated this observation. Thus, *The Book on Generation*, a Hebrew version of Soranus' text, instructed midwives on the management of a false pregnancy caused by a *mola*, and in the seventeenth century, Abraham Zacuto Lusitanus, a Jewish physician of *Marrano* birth, defined the signs, causes, and treatment of a *mola* and documented his own case studies.[15]

In the early eighteenth century, another physician, Tobias Cohn, noted the possibility of a pregnancy ending in the delivery of mere air, or of a meaty, formless lump, after a woman had shown all the usual signs of a developing fetus. He believed that this could result from the effect of a woman's imagination on her menstrual blood, in the absence of male seed. He warned Jewish women against looking at strange sights, which could affect menstrual blood or the fetus, and noted that such weird conceptions were more common in other nations.[16]

Tales of birth pangs that suddenly stopped, producing nothing but air, survived into the twentieth century. In 1987, an Iraqi Jew reported that a woman who felt a baby kick inside her, but who gave birth only to gases, thought that she had been impregnated by evil spirits. Iraqi Jews called this phenomenon a "pregnancy of the devils," reminiscent of the winged spirit of the talmudic period. In contrast to the medical descriptions of this phenomenon, the Iraqi tales document the deep disappointment of a woman who learned that she had no baby.[17] These tales are not stories for entertainment, nor do they teach a moral lesson; they are for healing purposes only. They have grown out of true experiences and have been handed down from generation to generation as a form of medicine for coping with the pain of false pregnancy.

PRECAUTIONS

Jews have encouraged a lifestyle of righteous behavior and prayer at all times in life, including during pregnancy. Thus, piety, donations to charity, and repentance have been especially important to Jews who interpret miscarriage as a punishment for sins. However, when a righteous woman repeatedly miscarries, and neither her own prayers nor anyone else's seem to help, she may look for other methods of avoiding such misfortune.

Prayers

A Man's Prayers for his Wife's Pregnancy

The Talmud's instructions to men on how to pray for the growth and delivery of a healthy baby reveal fears associated with the safe outcome of pregnancy: between the fortieth day after conception and the third month of pregnancy, the expectant husband prayed that the fetus would not miscarry; throughout the second trimester, he prayed that the baby would not be stillborn; and during the last three months, he prayed for a safe delivery.[18]

In talmudic times, a man whose wife was pregnant could have formulated his petition for the well-being of his wife and fetus during his daily recitation of benedictions at the synagogue. However, pregnancy was a concern not only of the father, but also of the community as a whole, and the priests prayed for the pregnant women of the community when they fasted on Thursdays.[19]

Jews standardized prayers for recitation during pregnancy only many centuries later. From the sixteenth century onward, these prayers assumed the style of prayers for other occasions in Jewish life. Thus, prayers for pregnancy came to resemble those recited during immersion in the ritual bath, during illness, or while visiting the cemetery.

In the seventeenth century, Ashkenazi rabbis recommended that a husband recite a special prayer when his wife began her seventh month of pregnancy, and when she entered her ninth month, he needed to take a reckoning of his deeds, to repent, and to give to charity—Jews have customarily given to charity in the general hope of receiving God's protection. The composition of the two different prayers was in recognition of the two gestation periods of human embryos referred to in the Talmud (see Chapter 4). The prayer for the seventh month, but not for the ninth, included the hope that the baby not be born on the Sabbath (to avoid profaning the Sabbath if the baby were born in the eighth month).[20]

A century later, a Sephardic rabbi from Jerusalem, Hayyim Yosef David Azulai (1724–1806), also published prayers for a husband to recite during his wife's pregnancy. He, too, formulated two versions, one for the third month and the other for the ninth.[21] The former prayer specifically addressed the fear of pregnancy loss, whereas the latter was for a safe and easy delivery.

Azulai's contemporary, Eliezer ben Itzhak Papo (Rabbi of Silistra, Bulgaria, d.1824) composed a prayer for a husband to recite at some time during his wife's pregnancy that addressed all the fears of expectant parents. It expressed the hope that the mother would not miscarry, that "no sickness or blemish affect the mother or the child," and that the baby "be complete in all his limbs and senses." The prayer also placed the pregnancy in the context of a Jew's reason for living: the husband supplicates God to enable the birth of a healthy child as well as the blessing of old age for him and his wife so they can both "rejoice with our offspring when we see them doing Your will, as is Your wish. We will complete the perfection of the soul in this transmigration." This mystical prayer closed with the request that God accept the prayer, for the sake of the patriarchs, as well as Moses, Aaron, Joseph, and David.[22]

Today an Orthodox Jew who wants to pray for his pregnant wife recites one of these classic prayers.

A Woman's Prayers for Safe Pregnancy

From the sixteenth century onward, some Jews actively encouraged women to pray themselves, in the vernacular if they could not read Hebrew. For example, in 1596, Moses ben Hanokh Yerushalmi published *Brantspiegel*, a handbook in Yiddish for every aspect of women's lives, including guidance for a pregnant woman. He advised a pregnant woman to think about God and to marvel at how God gave her strength to carry and nurture the baby in her womb. He instructed her to pray daily, "with her whole heart," not to have any unkosher cravings that could lead her to eat what is forbidden, not to miscarry, and to have easy delivery of a healthy baby.[23]

In the eighteenth and nineteenth centuries, many European Jewish women owned their own prayer books instructing them in the laws of ritual purification and containing prayers for recital during ritual immersion, as well as lengthy prayers for use in childbearing. Some of these books were printed, but sometimes a woman owned a handwritten and beautifully bound volume, specially made for her own use. One tiny exemplar from Mannheim, 1733, bound in red velvet with a silver buckle, includes supplications that the baby not be disturbed by demons and that the woman not miscarry; these prayers were written in German and Yiddish using Hebrew calligraphy. Italian Jewish women used similar prayer books, written in Hebrew and Italian.[24]

Women who did not own such a book could obtain a handwritten prayer from their rabbi or circumciser.[25] A woman who could not read, like many living in Moslem and Eastern countries, kept the written prayer with her throughout pregnancy, as an amulet, or recited a prayer she had learned orally.

A book of supplications for women, printed in Vilna in 1910, contains a special prayer in Yiddish for a woman fearing miscarriage. It calls on God to accept her prayer, just as Hannah had her prayer accepted in biblical times, and to allow her pregnancy to reach full term. She prays that the baby be born healthy and grow up to become a pious Jew, "for the glory of Israel."[26]

Today, Orthodox pregnant women continue to pray for a safe and healthy pregnancy in the manner of their foremothers. However, a few Jewish women have continued the tradition of innovating prayers that was started by Hannah in the Bible, by composing their own prayers. One such modern prayer, full of religious fervor, asks for the baby's well-being, for the child to enter a world free from destruction, insanity, and warfare, and for the mother's well-being, in relation both to her expected child and to her husband.[27]

Other Prayers for a Pregnant Woman

The existence of prayers for others to recite for a pregnant woman shows that pregnancy was not the sole concern of a husband and wife, but of others, too. A prayer, written by Fanny Neuda (1819–1894), for a mother to recite for her pregnant daughter gives evidence of the strong bond between the two women:

Wake, Oh God, over the feeble fruit, that she bears under her heart, that it should develop to a healthy and a strong being, and ripen in time and reach the world well kept and well nourished. Save my daughter from every evil, which sometimes affects her condition. Wake over her . . . that mother and child may come out safely from the dangerous act [of birth], and guard them from evil results.[28]

A Jewish woman in Morocco in the first half of the twentieth century prayed for her pregnant daughter, in Judeo-Arabic, in the synagogue on the Sabbath morning, when the Torah scroll was open. She expressed her hope that, for the sake of the holy books, her daughter would give birth without distress to a healthy son.[29]

Since the eighteenth century, and probably earlier, women who have lost several pregnancies have asked a rabbi to pray for them in the hope that his prayers will have more effect than theirs or those of their husbands. Sometimes, a yeshivah student studied and prayed for a pregnant woman. Jews rewarded the *Wieberlamden*, as they were commonly known in Germany, with a few coins.[30]

Certain prayers are for a sister to recite, or anyone else, such as in-laws or close friends, who cares for the well-being of the expectant mother. Jacob ben Abraham Solomon (c. 1600) of Prague composed such a prayer for reciting in the cemetery. He pleaded for God's mercy for a woman suffering from her pregnancy, that she should not miscarry, that she should give birth as easily as a hen lays her egg, and, looking ahead, that the child should grow up to a life of Torah, to marry, and to perform good deeds. Millions of Jews fearful for their pregnant women have recited this prayer in central and eastern Europe since its first publication in a prayer book, *Ma'aneh lashon*, in the early seventeenth century. A Yiddish version and bilingual versions (Hebrew and Yiddish, Hebrew and German) soon followed. The book is still in print, and Orthodox women recite this prayer today.[31]

Magical Remedies

Confronting the risks of pregnancy, Jewish women have resorted to magical customs, in addition to conventional prayers and donations to charity. Since the earliest days of Jewish history, women have used amulets, magic stones, incantations, and protective bindings in the hope of safeguarding their pregnancy.

Jewish amulets for protecting pregnancy from misfortune bear a supplication, or more generally, God's name or permutations of its letters, with relevant biblical verses or an acrostic of the verses. Extant examples from post-talmudic Palestine have revealed invocations to helpful angels to protect pregnancy, as well as efforts to bind or expel some harmful spirits. One such amulet bears Psalm 116:6 ("The Lord protects the simple; I was brought low, and He saved me") to protect against premature delivery. Another amulet invokes the help of the rod of Moses, the ring of Solomon, and possibly the shield of David in expelling an evil spirit. An amulet preserved in the Cairo *Geniza*, dating from medieval times, invokes names of God to protect against "any of those seven spirits that enter into the entrails of women and spoil their offspring" and to ensure that she should not abort her fetus.[32]

A medieval Judeo-Arabic text on the magical use of psalms recommended an amulet inscribed with Psalm 1 to protect against miscarriage, advice repeated in a widely circulated medieval guide to the protective use of psalms. The latter also recommended the writing of Psalm 128 ("... Your wife shall be as a fruitful vine ...") on kosher parchment, which a pregnant woman could carry on herself at all times.[33]

A kabbalistic manuscript compiled in Damascus in the mid–sixteenth century, *Shoshan yesod olam*, offered seven formulas for the preparation of amulets for protection of pregnancy, including magical names for God, angelic invocations, formulas against evil spirits, magic squares, the seal of Solomon, and the shield of David (*Magen David*). A popular book, *Toldot Adam*, published in Eastern Europe in the early eighteenth century, drew from these formulas in the "tried" advice it gave for protecting against pregnancy loss. Furthermore, it specified that only a God-fearing *mekubbal* (a man trained in Kabbalah) over forty years old should inscribe such amulets. Many Yiddish-speaking Jews as well as Jews in the Ottoman Empire used this book. Amulets for protection against pregnancy loss used by Persian Jews before emigrating to Israel bear similar magical formulas.[34]

Jews invoked God's name in incantations and over potions for protecting pregnancy, not only on amulets. For example, a prescription dating from the talmudic era against miscarriage—even if a woman bleeds vaginally—entailed whispering the unspoken name of God before drinking from a cup of wine, every day for a week. *Toldot Adam* offered a protective incantation invoking angels for a pregnant woman to recite whenever she leaves her home.[35]

Kabbalistic elements were also featured in a remedy book from Yemen, written in Hebrew in the nineteenth century, but certainly copied from earlier sources. For an amulet for a pregnant woman, the book instructed the scribe to write the names of the angels Michael, Gabriel, Shamriel, and Raphael, who guard the baby in the womb, followed by these adjurations: "By the power of the angels, by their strength, their holiness, and their purity, may they guard, protect, help and cause to fructify the fetus in its mother's womb [the woman's name is inserted here] ... that it should not be moved by anything bad, not by demons or harmful elements and not by an evil spirit. I adjure you, Lilith and your escorts, I adjure you, by the power of ..." the tetragrammaton and a series of other names for God, "... check on the fetus in its mother's womb [the woman's name is again inserted here] that it should not be moved by anything bad ..." After some further exhortations, the text finished with some angel script (magical signs) and a magic square.[36] A Yemenite Jewish woman rolled up the parchment bearing this inscription and wore it in an amulet case on her necklace until her pregnancy reached full term.

An Ashkenazi Hebrew manuscript recommended use of an amulet in a different way for protection against a future miscarriage: the names of three angels—Starbiel, Gastrakhiel, and Sandalphon—were written in Hebrew on kosher parchment and put in a grave together with the last aborted fetus.[37]

Some Jews used coins amuletically for protecting pregnancy. For example, in the Romanian shtetls in the early twentieth century, women fearing miscarriage wore a necklace on which hung a coin bought from a *tzaddik* (a saintly man) who, by blessing it, divested it with magic powers.[38]

Some Jewish women fearing miscarriage have carried what the Talmud refers to as *even t'kuma*, a "stone of preservation."[39] In medieval times, aetites, also known as eagle stones (described in Chapter 2) and red stones such as carnelians, chalcedony, or rubies were valued as preservation stones. We have already seen that Jews made use of red stones in the hope of promoting fertility; they used them in a similar manner to protect against miscarriage and, as discussed in Chapter 8, for easing delivery. A law issued by the Jewish community of Cracow in 1615 or 1616 forbade the wearing of precious stones except by pregnant women, who could wear one on a ring, for its protective powers. In the late nineteenth century, pregnant Jewish women in Poland, Russia, Dagestan, Syria, and the Holy Land carried a red stone as protection against miscarriage.[40] For example, a stone preserved in a museum in Tbilisi, Georgia, that dates from the early twentieth century, has a Hebrew inscription on it, in white ink, "for a woman not to lose the fruit of her womb," followed by some letters with magical significance. The stone is mounted in a silver frame with two loops for hanging on a necklace. A small oval carnelian, from Iraq but now in a museum in Jerusalem, has a *Magen David* and psalms inscribed on it in white ink and may have served a similar purpose.[41]

Another method of safeguarding pregnancy, not uniquely Jewish yet common among Jews in the past, is the use of a protective binding. The ancient practice of supporting a bulging belly with a form of binding continued through the Middle Ages and into the twentieth century. The soft, silk bindings used in medieval times were replaced in eighteenth- and nineteenth-century Europe with complicated whalebone or leather structures adjusted to the extended belly by a system of laces.[42]

Often, a pregnant woman's binder was not merely a physical support, but it assumed therapeutic significance through magical properties. Ethnographers have recorded this practice in the late nineteenth and early twentieth centuries in Jewish communities in different parts of the world. For example, in Salonika and Tunisia, pregnant women bound their bellies with a string that had been measured seven times around the grave of a renowned rabbi, to absorb his holiness. In Kurdistan, Jewish women made a magical binding against the Evil Eye by weaving together threads of five different colors—red, yellow, green, black, and white—while whispering the names of five notorious demons. The women wore the braid diagonally across the body, shoulder to hip, to shield the developing baby from harm. In Georgia, Jewish women rented a special leather belt decorated with amulets to protect pregnancy.[43] Jewish women in North Africa, the Middle East, and Kurdistan often attached a padlock to their protective binding, to give it additional magical retentive power.[44]

Two protective customs practiced by Orthodox Jewish women in Israel today may be hundreds of years old. In the first instance, a charm used to prevent miscarriage is made by winding scarlet embroidery twine seven times around the tomb of Rachel, the matriarch, near Bethlehem.[45] The second custom applies to a woman who conceives after several miscarriages: she ties a Torah binder around her belly in the hope that the binder will protect the growing embryo to full term. Sometimes this is done only in the last months of pregnancy, if the woman fears premature birth.[46]

In the past, when Jewish women despaired of repeated pregnancy loss, they resorted to other magical protective methods of no particular Jewish interest, in the hope of eventually delivering a healthy baby. For example, they swallowed milk of a pregnant animal in potions for preventing miscarriage, hoping for the magical transference of gravidity.[47] Today, physicians know that a hormone found in a pregnant animal may help to maintain a human pregnancy. As almost every Hebrew remedy book consulted in this study includes such potions against miscarriage, a woman was apparently prepared to do almost anything when conventional Jewish advice (such as prayer and repentance) for protecting against miscarriage failed, if she believed that it would help her predicament.

Today, many women with high-risk pregnancies accept medical treatment without knowing the source or nature of the medicine or exactly how it works. However, they have faith in the doctor who has prescribed it. Such faith stems from a belief that a doctor only prescribes a remedy of proven value. Thus, Jews have had faith in rabbis, midwives, and healers who have prescribed remedies that had proved effective for others. Some Orthodox women today have faith in the Bible or a prayer book that they put under their pillow for protective purposes; some have an amulet especially made by a *mekubbal*, and some hasidic women borrow a "tried and proved" marble-sized, reddish stone to wear on a necklace throughout pregnancy.[48]

MOURNING PREGNANCY LOSS

In the past, pregnancy loss was a well-recognized reality. Jews composed prayers in the hope of forestalling this loss, and midwives and mothers discussed remedies and exchanged charms. Today, however, miscarriage and stillbirth are hardly topics of conversation among the newly pregnant, or of prayer outside Orthodox communities, and such misfortune can be unexpected and traumatic.

Much of the social behavior surrounding pregnancy loss is a matter of custom, not law; some customs may ease the pain, the shock, the frustration, and the feelings of guilt and helplessness, whereas others may not. Judaism allows a certain freedom of behavior for bereaved parents in the special case of pregnancy loss. Thus, there is no prescribed ritual mourning for pregnancy loss, and customs regarding the circumcising, naming, and burial of a miscarried or stillborn child, which all affect the mourning process, have varied from place to place.

Jewish tradition regarding ritual mourning has biblical origins, although the applicable laws were formulated in talmudic times and have changed little through the ages. The aims of the talmudic sages in formulating these laws were to maintain "the dignity of the departed" as well as "the dignity of the living" and to ease the grief of the bereaved by sharing their sorrow.[49] In the case of miscarriage and stillbirth, under these laws, the lost baby had never seen the light of day and had been no more than a part of the mother's body, so no ritual was needed to maintain the dignity of the departed, although nothing prevents this from being done by those who so desire.

Formal Jewish mourning involves parents' staying at home for seven days in full mourning, visited by extended family and friends. After the first week, modified mourning continues until the end of the first month after the bereavement, and more limited mourning continues until the anniversary of the death. From then on, Jews mark each anniversary (*Yahrzeit*) with a prayer. This ritual facilitates the expression of feelings about loss and provides a framework for community support. In the past, it was apparently not the custom for Jews who lost a pregnancy to observe this ritual.

In the Middle Ages, many Jews living in Arab lands were familiar with an ancient Arab proverb asserting that a miscarrying woman would be quick in conceiving again.[50] For centuries, Moroccan Jews consoled themselves in another way, saying that it was better to lose a baby and receive condolences (and hope for another baby that would survive) than to have no hope of ever becoming pregnant.[51] However, as the years passed and misfortune followed misfortune, a woman may have had little comfort from such proffered consolation. As we saw in Chapter 2, such a woman, who was unable to provide her husband with live offspring, faced the added fear and pain caused by her husband's seeking another woman to bear him a child, in addition to the fear accompanying each new conception and the pain of each lost pregnancy.

In the past, the loss of a baby was certainly more common than in modern times, but this does not necessarily mean that parents suffered less than today. We wonder today why the talmudic sages did not mourn such a loss. Did they not feel a sense of loss? Or did they just decide not to express it? Did their wives feel the same way they did, or did they mourn quietly and longer? Today, we know that the sense of loss may be more severe and protracted for a woman who has lost her fetus than for the bereaved father, and women often express their emotions differently from men. Only in recent years have some bereaved parents discussed openly their need to mourn pregnancy loss, and there is no reason not to observe the mourning ritual, if one wants to.

Another recent phenomenon is that parents may want to mourn a special form of loss, which follows their decision to abort a fetus diagnosed as severely handicapped.

The New York section of the National Council of Jewish Women has pioneered a Pregnancy Loss Support Program for miscarriage, stillbirth, and newborn death, and in Israel, Yad Elisha does this work from Jerusalem. Nowadays, those who have experienced pregnancy loss assert a need for support groups in Jewish communities. The more than thirty books on pregnancy loss and infant death published between 1982 and 1996 reveal recent social recognition of the difficulty of coping with this loss. These books share experiences and offer coping strategies. They suggest ways of dealing with fear of repeated loss when conceiving again and ways to face family and community after tragedy. They also endorse the emotions that men and women experience and discuss the different ways that people grieve.[52]

Although some Jewish couples have found that observing the mourning ritual helped them to recover from their loss, in recent years, a few have searched for other ways of coping with these experiences. In 1984, Hope Kellman and David Carlen wrote their own prayer, in the style of a Jewish prayer, to form part of a collection of poetry, thoughts, and Jewish blessings, to express their feelings of love and grief for their lost baby. The prayer was part of a ceremony created to give Jewish meaning to the experience of pregnancy loss. The authors envisaged that bereaved parents would recite such a prayer privately, or during a ceremony of passage, soon after the event, and at the time when, had the pregnancy continued to term, the baby would have been born.[53]

Another couple, Penina and Steve Adelman, felt the need for social recognition of their mourning when, after a long period of infertility, they lost their first pregnancy. They desired the support of their family and community, which would have been forthcoming in the Jewish mourning ritual. Thus, they developed a ceremony for grieving pregnancy loss or infertility, based on the story of Hannah.[54] As with other Jewish rituals, a specific time was set aside for their ceremony, in this case Rosh Hodesh Tammuz (New Moon, June/July), and the ceremony included Torah study (they chose the story of Hannah) and group participation. The Adelmans created a ceremony with spirituality, Jewish meaning, and group solace for the pain of loss that the couple had suffered.

In contrast, Merle Feld, the wife of a Liberal rabbi, did not appreciate the condolences offered by others. She wanted to be alone with God and with her husband, to mourn privately. She expressed her distress in a poem entitled "Healing After a Miscarriage":

> *Nothing helps. I taste ashes*
> *in my mouth. My eyes are flat,*
> *dead. I want no platitudes,*
> *no stupid shallow comfort.*
> *I hate all pregnant women,*
> *all new mothers, all soft babies.*
> *The space I'd made inside myself*
> *where I'd moved over*
> *to give my beloved room to grow—*
> *now there's a tight angry*
> *bitter knot of hatred there instead.*
> *What is my supplication?*
> *Stupid people and new mothers,*
> *leave me alone.*
> *Deliver me, Lord,*
> *of this bitter afterbirth.*
> *Open my heart*
> *to my husband-lover-friend*
> *that we may comfort each other.*
> *Open my womb that it may yet bear*
> *living fruit.[55]*

Ritual mourning of pregnancy loss may help some people to cope with their misfortune, but not all. Because mourning pregnancy loss is not part of Jewish tradition, how each person handles mourning of pregnancy loss remains a matter of personal choice.

Part III

Birthing

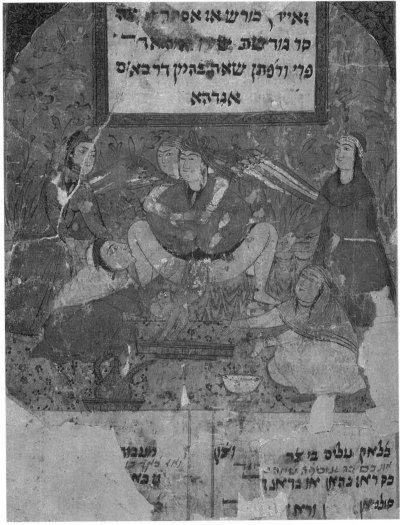

Plate 10. Queen Esther gives birth to Cyrus. *Ardashir nama.* Judeo–Persian manuscript, late seventeenth or early eighteenth century.
Jewish Theological Seminary, New York, Ms. 40919 f.154r.

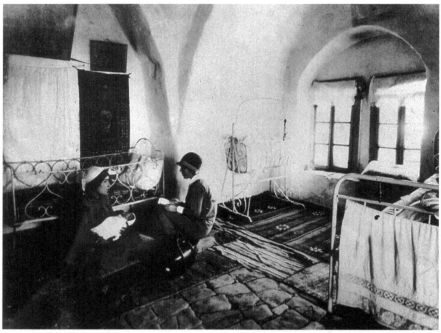

Plate 11. Hadassah nurse visiting lying-in woman in her home, Jerusalem, 1930.
Hadassah Medical Organization Archive, New York.
Photo courtesy of Beth Hatefutsoth Photo Archive.

Chapter Seven

Midwives

Jewish midwives have traditionally offered emotional support, physical help, expertise, and even spiritual guidance to their clients. Since talmudic times, Jews valued midwives' skills highly and were reluctant to trust a non-Jew with the dangerous task of bringing their newborn infants into the world. Jewish communities therefore often secured their own midwifery service, so even the poorest women could give birth with professional assistance. The role and status of the community midwife changed with the transfer of childbirth to the hospital maternity ward, however, and it is still changing today.

A MIDWIFE'S FUNCTIONS

Physical and Emotional Support

Since antiquity, Jewish women have expected assistance in birthing. The Book of Genesis tells that a midwife encouraged and comforted Rachel, whereas another delivered Tamar's twins and established which one was the first-born. Before the Exodus from Egypt, Pharaoh called on two midwives, Shiphrah and Puah, to deliver the Israelite women. Helpful women attended Phinehas' wife and comforted her with talk of a son.[1] Thus, experienced and friendly women offered sympathy and comfort as well as professional expertise. Midwives of that period may have supported the back of the laboring woman and allowed her to lean on them as she squatted. They tried to assuage her fears and assure her that God would answer her prayers and help her just as God had helped other women in their time of need.

The Bible tells that Pharaoh instructed Shiphrah and Puah to kill the infant sons of the Hebrew women. Fearing God more than the wicked ruler, the two midwives disobeyed, alleging that the Israelite women were so vigorous that they had been delivered of their infants before the midwives had time to reach them. Rabbinic tradition favors the idea that these two names indicate the midwives' functions and that the women who helped the Israelites were, in fact, Jochebed, the mother of Moses, and her daughter, Miriam, or possibly her daughter-in-law Elisheva. In Jewish lore, Jochebed and her daughter are the most righteous of women, each having the ideal personality for midwifery.[2]

The talmudic sages proposed that the name Shiphrah derived from a Hebrew verb for cleaning or swaddling a baby, or for being fruitful. Similarly, the name Puah may have come from the Hebrew verb meaning to cry out because a midwife tried to calm the cries of the woman in labor by uttering encouragement, a prayer, or an incantation in her ear.[3] A fourteenth-century biblical commentator suggested that Shiphrah earned her name from the Hebrew word for a tube, *shforferet*, "since it is the custom of midwives, when the child is stillborn, to insert a tube of reed into its bowels, blowing into it and thus reviving the child."[4]

Josephus Flavius (first century C.E.) suggested that Shiphrah and Puah may have been Egyptian midwives whom Pharaoh trusted to carry out his instructions. In recent times, scholars have proposed that these women may have headed a caste system of midwives, and their names may have derived from ancient Egyptian and Ugaritic names for "fair one" and "girl," and not from Hebrew terms.[5]

A Jewish midwife is a "wise woman" in the Mishnah (second century), implying greater knowledge and skill than other women. In the talmudic period, midwives knew how to use oil to lubricate the baby's passage, where to press during delivery to prevent tearing of the mother's tissues, and how to prevent the umbilical cord from strangling the baby.[6]

The Ideal Midwife

By the Middle Ages, wisdom was not the only requirement for a Jewish midwife. The fourteenth-century Hebrew version of Soranus' treatise on gynecology recommended: "A woman suitable to be a midwife is God-fearing, respectable, learned, wise, intelligent, clean, innocent, strong, skillful, and patient, who is accustomed to working with womanly affairs and with doctors."[7] The Hebrew version of this treatise, in contrast to the earlier Greek and Latin versions, added the first quality necessary for a midwife: "God-fearing" was a Jewish essential, found in the Hebrew text only. A Jewish midwife had to be pious, like Jochebed and Miriam. The treatise went on to describe in detail everything a midwife should know about conception, pregnancy, birth, and the postnatal period. It advised that a midwife should have three intelligent helpers during birthing and instructed on the management of difficult births, embryotomy, removing the afterbirth, and cleaning the woman after the birth. In addition, the text provided recipes for medicinal lotions, potions, and suppositories made from ingredients known since talmudic times and named tools required for embryotomy. We do not know whether medieval Jewish community midwives were generally as knowledgeable as the author of this text, but they may have been, for they enjoyed a good reputation.

A nineteenth-century midwifery handbook and ethnographic accounts of the practice of midwifery in early twentieth-century Jewish communities allow us to build up a picture of the midwife's functions in the days before modern medicine. As soon as a woman believed that she had conceived, she summoned a midwife. An experienced midwife could foretell the expected date of birth merely by placing her hand on the woman's belly. At first, the midwife visited once a week, and eventually she came every day, to reassure the pregnant woman.

When labor began, the midwife arrived with a little bag of equipment. Such a bag contained a clean apron, some clean gauze and cotton wool, vials of medicine, and a few tools in individual linen bags for cleanliness. The composition of medications that a midwife carried with her varied from region to region, as did the sophistication of her tools. Women of the house helped the midwife however they could. The midwife cared for the newborn, too; she was an expert at bathing and swaddling the infant. Her duties extended to care and treatment of postnatal ailments for a week or more after the birth. She knew how to staunch postnatal bleeding and offered remedies if the new mother became feverish. She advised on foods that ensured a healthy supply of milk and knew what compresses to apply when a woman did not breast-feed or developed cracked nipples.[8]

In addition to their many practical skills, midwives were often specialists in folk remedies and incantations. The old midwife, the *bubbeh* (Yiddish for "granny") who served the Jews in the shtetl a century ago, kept her incantations a closely guarded secret, for fear of destroying their potency. When a baby girl was born, the Yiddish-speaking midwife had one more task to perform on the first day: she pierced the baby's ears with a plain needle and some red thread, or she tied a red thread around the baby's wrist to ward off evil. This practice was customary, even though since talmudic times rabbis had condemned the tying of a red thread on mother or baby as a heathen super-stition.[9] In North Africa and the Middle East in the early twentieth century, midwives treated the baby's eyes, painting the lids with carbon black, using a little silver stick. Like the salting and swaddling that a midwife performed (described in Chapter 11), this cus-tom was not specifically Jewish; it was done medicinally to prevent sore eyes, but Jews believed that the black gave brilliance to the child's eyes and enhanced their beauty.[10]

In most Jewish communities since antiquity, a midwife called on the assis-tance of a doctor only when a birth proved particularly difficult and she knew that both mother and baby were in mortal danger. The situation changed in the West only in the late nineteenth century, when the middle class often called a doctor to deliver the baby, although poor families continued to rely only on a midwife. The change came later in Middle Eastern and North African countries.

Spiritual Care

A book of ethical sermons, *Shevet mussar*, first published in Constantinople in 1712, includes advice to Jewish midwives in the form of a prayer for a midwife to recite on her way to a woman in labor. In this prayer, she supplicates God that she shall cause no harm and pleads for mercy for the birthing woman. On her arrival at her client's house, she helps the laboring woman to stand up and put her faith in God before sitting on the birthing stool and explains that safe delivery depends not on the midwife, but on divine mercy. She instructs the pregnant woman to perform some charitable act by way of atonement, such as a donation to the synagogue, because if she committed any sin, God will remember this during birth. The text further advises that, after the delivery, the midwife wash and clean herself and the new mother before both offer prayers of thanksgiving. This book, popular among the Sephardic Jews of the Ottoman Empire, was translated into Yiddish for the use of the Ashkenazi Jews as well.[11] An Italian woman's prayer book, written in the late eighteenth century, includes advice to a midwife in Italian that follows the recommendation of this ethical sermon closely. It also includes a prayer in Hebrew for the midwife to recite, again in the spirit of *Shevet mussar*.[12]

A Jewish midwife in Morocco in the early twentieth century offered a prayer of thanks after a safe delivery. She stood by the doorpost and held the swaddled infant in both hands stretched out toward the mezuzzah. The words she uttered were not written down; they were straight from her heart. This was the custom among Moroccan Jewish midwives, and each midwife expressed her thanks in her own way, in Judeo-Arabic. She did not sit back in satisfaction over a job well done; while grateful that all went well, she thought of another woman still in need of help and yearned for better times with the coming of the Messiah. For example:

> My Gracious Lord! Just as you saved this lonely woman from her great anguish [of labor] and brought her happiness, so may you redeem all the people of Israel from this exile and bring us the Messiah to redeem us and bring us to Jerusalem.
>
> Just as You have seen this miserable poverty, notice the miserable barren women. Do not withhold your blessing for a miserable woman, x daughter of y; open her "belt" and the inside of her womb. Notice her distress and do not cull the blood of her life.
>
> May Your Great Name be blessed for saving this [baby's] soul from another [fate] and may the boy who was just born be a Torah scholar, dear to his parents and to the whole of the Jewish nation. Amen.[13]

Such a midwife hoped that her own small actions would contribute to the well-being of the whole Jewish people.

COMMUNITY MIDWIVES

The Bible tells that "the king of Egypt spoke with the Hebrew midwives" (Exodus 1:15), implying the existence of midwives who served the Hebrew community in ancient times. As discussed earlier, rabbinic tradition favors that Jochebed and Miriam were the community midwives, and the names Shiphrah and Puah merely referred to the jobs performed by midwives in ancient times.

In talmudic times, Jewish society highly respected the "wise woman." Her authority was such that women in childbirth did not argue with her: an old Jewish proverb warned that "while the midwife and laboring woman are quarreling, the child is lost." While fulfilling her duty to save human life at all cost, Jewish midwives of talmudic times labored on the Sabbath: they traveled any distance to deliver a baby; they kindled a light and cut the umbilical cord. On delivering twins, midwives asserted which twin was first-born, an important fact in some matters of inheritance and Jewish ritual observance. Rabbis accepted the testimony of midwives in court at times when women were rarely given a hearing. In addition, midwives could charge for their services.[14]

In medieval times, families who could afford to remunerate midwives for their services did so, but the community sometimes gave these women emoluments to attend the poor and not only the rich. The oldest record of such emoluments, found among the fragments of the Cairo *Geniza*, dates from the tenth century.[15]

From the seventeenth century onward, Jewish communities sometimes contracted midwives on the basis of salary or social benefits. For example, some Jewish community registers from Germany and Eastern Europe documented the wages paid by a community to Jewish midwives. Sometimes midwives were offered free lodging or tax incentives; sometimes a high salary was paid, with the proviso that anything earned privately be given to the community; sometimes a specific amount was given for each baby delivered in the hospice for the poor; and sometimes midwives set their own terms, especially if they had been recruited in one community to work in another.[16] The records of the German town of Fürth for the end of the eighteenth century tell of a midwife who opted for a low wage because she assumed that she would make a tidy sum from her wealthy clientele. However, the following year she fell ill and could not work; she became so poor that, after selling off all their furniture, her husband applied to the Jewish community for a donation.[17]

In Jewish communities, especially in North Africa and the Middle East, where there were no formal contracts with midwives in the early twentieth century, each birthing woman paid according to her means. The midwife received food, presents, and even board and lodging for some days after the birth. Visitors during the lying-in period also left a few coins for her. The midwife received a much larger reward when a son was born. When the birthing woman was very poor, the midwife sometimes went from door to door asking for charity for her client or obtained a donation from community funds.[18]

Jewish midwives generally maintained the high ethical standards expected in Judaism and enjoyed good reputations. For example, in the Middle Ages before the expulsion of Jews from Spain in 1492, Jewish midwives in Castile and Aragon gained positions in the royal courts.[19] In the eighteenth century, Jewish midwives were actually sought by Gentiles in southern Holland in preference to their own midwives because Jews gave priority to the mother's life in a difficult delivery, whereas local Catholic doctors gave priority to the baby's life.[20] The considerable status of the Jewish midwife did not dwindle until the twentieth century.

MOTHER-IN-LAW AS MIDWIFE: A FOLKTALE

Often the senior woman in the household was well versed in childbirth management by virtue of her own experiences as well as the wisdom passed on from her own mother or mother-in-law, and she, rather than an outsider, helped in the deliveries of her daughters or daughters-in-law. In the Sephardic and Middle Eastern communities especially, it was common for a woman to live with her husband's family a century ago. A folktale popular in Sephardic communities tells of the tensions between a woman and her mother-in-law when the time comes to give birth. The husband is in a difficult position, negotiating between the two powerful women in his life; will he sympathize with his wife or his mother?

In this story, a queen, seated at the entrance to her palace, writhed with birth pangs that she could scarcely endure. If only she could give birth at her parents' house, she moaned. Oh, if only she could have her mother at her side, who would pray for her safe delivery.

Her mother-in-law overheard her from her rooms high above. She has-tened down the stairs to the travailing woman and told her to go and give birth at her mother's home, as she wished. "When your husband comes home," she added, "I'll give him chicken for his supper and capons for his breakfast. I'll feed his horse and his hawk. And now I'll throw bones to his dog, so he'll not follow you."

So the queen left to give birth at her mother's home. Her pains grew worse with every step she took, and as she arrived, she delivered a fair son.

When the king returned home he looked for his wife. His mother informed him that she had left to give birth at her parents' home, adding: "She called me 'whore' and you a 'son of an evil father.'"

"I shall go and kill her, or may I die on my own sword!" he fumed. Just as he uttered these furious words, however, messengers arrived with good tidings.

"Your wife gave birth to a son with a golden arrow in his hand and a dia-mond star: may it bring you good fortune."[21]

In the Castilian (early Spanish) and later Moroccan versions of this tale, the husband brutally kills his wife. In versions from the Eastern Mediterranean, the angry husband swears to take revenge on his mother. In this nineteenth-century version from Salonika, however, the wife's fate remains ambiguous; the good omens accompanying the birth of the son diffuse the tension and render the women's fate unimportant. Like the Iraqi tales of false pregnancies, this story is a healing tale, for those who suffer mother-in-law problems.

THE DANGERS OF MIDWIFERY

Witchcraft and Anti-Semitism

In the face of the dangers of childbirth, a skilled midwife, Jewish or not, was preferable to an unskilled woman helper. For this reason, when the community had no professional midwife, Jews sometimes employed Gentile midwives, suitably supervised by the women of the household. Reflecting the atmosphere of mistrust, both the Talmud of the land of Israel and the Babylonian Talmud warn that, when this happens, the non-Jewish woman must never remain alone with the birthing woman, lest she harm the baby.[22]

Throughout history, until the advent of modern medicine, people told stories of women who cast spells to open or close the womb. Because some midwives used incantations, amulets, and special recipes for their practice, it was not surprising that one who muttered incomprehensibly and used suspicious materials risked accu-sation of black magic if the delivery ended tragically.

When a pregnancy or delivery ended in tragedy, some families blamed the midwife for incompetence or, worse, for invoking evil powers. As long as a midwife worked in her own community, where her employers knew and trusted her, such accusations were unlikely. When a Jewish midwife worked for unknown Gentiles, or a Gentile midwife worked in a Jewish home, however, she was vulnerable to nasty accusations that sometimes had serious consequences.

During periods of overt anti-Semitism, Jews and Gentiles avoided hiring each other's midwives, and local legislation sometimes expressly forbade them to do so. For instance, in 1366, the Synod of Avignon prohibited Gentiles from employing Jewish midwives, and an order issued in Regensburg, Bavaria, in 1452 forbade Gentile midwives from helping Jewish women.[23]

In the late fifteenth century, the Pope approved the publication by two inquisitors of a grim book about witches, detailing directions for their detection, conviction, and punishment, including a chapter entitled "How Witch-Midwives Commit Most Horrid Crimes when they either Kill Children or offer them to Devils in Most Accursed Wise [sic]." This text provides examples of the terrible deeds of witchcraft practiced by midwives in the Diocese of Strasbourg and of Basle.[24] The book enjoyed immense popularity, went through thirteen editions in less than forty years, and was reissued repeatedly in Germany and France in the following two hundred years. The witch craze spread through Europe, where midwives accused of being witches were burnt at the stake. Christians suspected witches, and Jews, of using the blood of newborn babies in their rituals and accused some Jews of being witches.[25] Jewish midwives working in Europe between the fifteenth century and the late seventeenth century must have feared accusation of being a witch-midwife. Among the ample documentation about witch-midwives, however, this study revealed no evidence of a single accusation that a Jewish midwife was a witch, perhaps because Jewish midwives took care not to work for Gentiles.

True Stories

In 1584, the tense atmosphere between Jews and their non-Jewish neighbors led to a midwife's appearance in front of the magistrates in Worms. One day in June, a German woman found a dead infant girl, half-buried under the city wall in the Jewish cemetery, with drops of blood on her forehead. The woman concluded that the baby did not die a natural death and summoned a physician. He found seventeen pinpricks on the baby's knees and feet. Witnesses reported having seen a Jew bury the infant and immediately suspected a ritual murder. These events culminated in a court of inquiry on the same day, and the leaders of the Jewish community were summoned. The Jews revealed that twin girls had been born ten days previously in the Jewish hospital and that one had died and had been buried the day before the inquiry by the Jew in charge of the hospital. Predictably, the court called on the midwife to testify before the magistrates. She confirmed that she had delivered the twins and reported that one had been very weak at birth but had become stronger. The midwife mentioned that she knew the parents quarreled and suggested that such a quarrel may have led to child abuse and infanticide. The court then called in the infant's father, who denied any knowledge of the injuries. Nevertheless, the court held the father in custody. The next day, the magistrates entered the ghetto to question the infant's mother. She was bedridden and weak, yet she identified the dead baby as hers. She too denied any knowledge of the injuries and suggested that the baby received these during burial. The town records concluded the case with the apparently unfounded statement that the mother was guilty of the baby's death, without revealing what became of the parents. What began as an investigation of suspected ritual murder by a Jew was no longer of interest to the town archivist once ritual murder was ruled out and it became clear that the affair was a domestic problem within the Jewish community.[26]

Despite their mistrust, some Jews did employ a professional Gentile woman in the hope of safe delivery when no Jewish midwife was available. When the outcome was tragic, however, the experience only served to reinforce the mistrust. For example, in his memoirs, a German Jew described the death of his first wife in 1720, after their son was stillborn: ". . . it was known that the Gentile midwife harmed her with sorcery [may her name be obliterated] until she died of her great affliction . . . after a hundred days of sorrow."[27]

Demonic Danger

When babies were delivered at home, a husband or neighbor went to call the midwife when labor began. To be summoned in the dark of night by an unfamiliar man may well have been frightening to a midwife. Moreover, every birth held an unknown potential danger. The following Kurdistani folktale verbalizes these fears:

> My grandmother, bless her soul, was a midwife who worked for love, seeking no reward. She was sure that her payment would come when she died and went straight to heaven. There were no doctors in her town of Zakho in Kurdistan, and my grandmother never lacked for work.
>
> One day, as she sat outside her house, relaxing over some embroidery, she saw a beautiful cat stealing into the house, sniffing as she went, as though looking for food. My grandmother was taken with the cat and fetched her something to eat. She noticed the cat was pregnant and wished that she could deliver her babies.
>
> Some days passed, and one stormy night a knock at the door awakened my grandmother. She dressed hurriedly and opened the door to a tired and perspiring man. "Grandma," he said breathlessly, "come with me, my wife is in labor. There is nobody to help her, and if you come you will be rich."
>
> Grandmother rejoiced, for such a great task, at such an hour and on such a night would be like fulfilling all six hundred and thirteen commandments at once. She followed the man along the main street, but wondered why she could not hear his footsteps. Then she noticed that they had walked out of town and were now in uninhabited land, in a field. She trembled as she realized that the man leading her must be a demon.
>
> "Lord have mercy on me," she said to herself, not daring to make a sound. Soon they reached a stone bridge, and then the man told her to enter a huge cave, where the birth was about to take place. Grandmother's heart pounded in fear when she saw in the cavern many horned demons, mewing like cats.
>
> The demon with the longest horns addressed her with a warning that if the newborn were male, he would reward her with everything she

desired, but God forbid if it were a daughter! My grandmother remained speechless in her fear. The demon showed her to the confinement room, and there she recognized the beautiful cat that had visited her a few days before. She quickly set to work, and soon a male cat was born.

The demons' cries of happiness reached heaven, and their leader called my grandmother to offer her whatever she desired, up to half his kingdom. She refused, however, and said that she did not charge for a good deed. The incredulous demon warned her to take something, according to their custom, and my grandmother realized that she could not leave empty-handed. She asked for some garlic that she saw hanging in the corner of the room. The demons stuffed her pockets with it and accompanied her home.

Exhausted by her night, she emptied her pockets of garlic by her door and sank into bed. Her grandchild visited in the morning and awoke her with his questioning; "Where did you get so much gold, Grandma?" As she opened her eyes, she saw that the garlic had turned to gold. She gave it all away, to her children, her grandchildren, and all the family. To this day, each of us keeps a bit of the golden garlic that she received as a reward.[28]

A Kurdistani storyteller may even show the audience a little golden garlic, as proof that it was his own grandmother's story. The Judeo-Spanish rendering of this popular folktale has a sinister switch, referring to the midwife as a witch named Brusha or Lilith who delivered the desired son and was paid in gold coins that then turned into garlic.[29] An Ashkenazi version of this story makes the hero a circumciser rather than a midwife.[30]

Another Danger

Midwives have needed to be wary of unknown men who summon them in the dark, even if delivering a baby is a mitzvah. In Jerusalem, at the turn of the twentieth century, a young and pretty lady arrived from Prussia with a diploma in midwifery. One night, two men called her out for a delivery. Rather than lead her to a laboring woman, they led her elsewhere and raped her. She reported the crime, and the police found the criminals, who were duly punished.[31]

HOSPITAL MIDWIVES

In the Middle Ages, some Ashkenazi Jewish communities supported a *hekdesh*, a Jewish society for the very poor, for the sick and for birthing women. The *hekdesh* usually consisted of one or two rooms with a maximum of six beds, where charitable women nursed the patients and a doctor occasionally visited. Itinerant pregnant women who stopped there to give birth and to lie-in shared a room with the poor and sick. The community midwife attended these women. When no midwife was available, the *hekdesh* saw to their needs. Conditions were often squalid.

The transition from disease-infested *hekdesh* to a place where medical services were routinely available began in the eighteenth century in large Jewish communities in certain European cities, although some *hekdeshim* were still functioning in Eastern Europe in the nineteenth century.[32] As with the *hekdeshim*, one of the main functions of the early Jewish hospitals was to provide maternity care for poor Jewish women, for the itinerant, and for inhabitants of outlying villages.[33] Jewish communities continued to maintain charitable societies to provide free midwifery services, lying-in facilities, and food for these people, as well as provision for circumcision. Thus, the early maternity wards were for women who did not have, or could not afford, the option of giving birth at home. Hospital regulations regarding qualifications for admission show that these facilities were in popular demand. An unusual incident occurred in the Jewish hospital in Frankfurt-am-Main, in 1783, when a Jewish woman, who had conceived extramaritally, begged for admission. The hospital refused, claiming that it lacked space. Apparently this was not the only reason for refusal, however; the hospital administration feared that patients would suffer from contact with such an immoral character.[34]

The Training of Midwives

By the eighteenth century, reason and enlightenment had eradicated the witch scare, and local authorities initiated standards for the practice of midwifery. European hospitals established formal training for midwives. National and local directives to enforce the standards of the profession demanded that Jewish communities send women to pass qualifying examinations in midwifery. Because only Jewish midwives would understand the religious needs and language of their own people, local authorities deemed it preferable for Jews to continue their custom of maintaining community midwives, but insisted that these midwives be properly trained.[35] State registration of midwives began only in the late nineteenth century in Europe and not until the twentieth century elsewhere.

Jewish midwives trained in midwifery schools in Moscow in the late nineteenth century were among the privileged few exempted from the residence restrictions imposed on Jews. Anti-Semitism quickly escalated as the century drew to its close, however, so Jewish midwives lost these privileges and could no longer qualify in their profession. In the early twentieth century, many Jewish women traveled to Vienna from as far away as the United States and Palestine, to qualify for a diploma in midwifery. Most Jewish women living in Arab lands did not have access to such training centers until well into the twentieth century, however. In Arab countries, a woman became a midwife by apprenticeship to an experienced midwife or simply by virtue of her repeated attendance at births, her intelligence, and her accumulated knowledge.[36]

From Home Birthing to Hospital

Until the late nineteenth century, mainly underprivileged women gave birth in hospitals, but in the first decades of the twentieth century, this pattern began to change.[37] For example, in 1896, a Jewish charity set up a nursing home in London that was modeled on one set up by Jews in Frankfurt-am-Main. Infant mortality was high in the appallingly overcrowded tenements of the immigrant Jews in London's East End, and the new nursing home was an attractive proposition for birthing mothers. By 1920, the Jewish maternity home had expanded to offer prenatal care, and soon new wards and a postnatal clinic were added as well. Delivery in a maternity ward guaranteed better hygiene than at home, it offered some privacy, and it enabled a mother to rest a little after the birth.[38]

In 1927, the percentage of all women in England giving birth in a maternity ward was still low; ten years later, about one of every three women gave birth in a maternity ward, whereas by midcentury, half of all women did so. By this time, the British government had provided many more maternity beds with accompanying subsidized midwifery services. In the hospital maternity ward, however, the midwife no longer enjoyed the special status of community midwife; she was now subordinate to the doctors in charge.[39]

Further east, in Palestine, the change from home birthing to hospital birthing was slower. Sephardic and Ashkenazi midwives, as well as Christian and Muslim midwives, served the local population of Jerusalem, each in her own ethnic community.[40] In the early twentieth century, academically trained Jewish midwives arrived from Europe, but by the 1920s, women were able to qualify locally. Mrs. Havah Karlan, over ninety years old when interviewed in 1988, graduated in midwifery at Hadassah Hospital, Jerusalem, in 1926 and subsequently spent many years struggling to introduce "modern" ideas of childbirth management into Jewish homes in Palestine, where old women monopolized her profession. In those days, a midwife sent only her most complicated cases to the hospital, and by the time a laboring woman arrived there, it was often too late to save either mother or baby. A woman in the throes of a prolonged and difficult birth knew that her end had come if the midwife or local doctor sent her to a hospital. During her training at Hadassah, Mrs. Karlan had seen horrific cases of women who arrived too late.

Mrs. Karlan began her career in the community by bribing pregnant women to call her in good time to deliver their babies; she gave the women presents of American diapers that she obtained from Hadassah Medical Organization. Supported by a good salary from Hadassah and dressed in her nicely starched uniform, Mrs. Karlan soon won herself respect and status in the Jewish villages. She ensured cleanliness, persuaded women to give birth on a bed and not on the floor in the corner of a shed or outhouse, and called a doctor for help in good time, if the case looked complicated. From 1928 until her retirement in old age, she remained a community nurse-midwife, providing prenatal and postnatal care in a mother-baby clinic, in addition to delivering babies at home.[41] As in London, by the 1950s, the Jewish state had maternity homes and maternity wards in the general hospitals, enabling the majority of women to give birth safely with medical supervision.

In Europe and the United States, the change from home delivery to the hospital labor ward occurred in the cities in the first half of the twentieth century; in outlying villages, and in the Jewish communities in Arab lands, the transition was slower and occurred later. The gradual change, from the norm of home delivery for the general Jewish public to the norm of hospital delivery, occurred the world over

as hospitals made better use of medical discoveries and technology to reduce maternal and infant mortality and to relieve the pain of childbirth. A midwife delivering a
woman of a baby at home today does not have the expertise of an anesthetist, nor
does she have the equipment available in a modern hospital.

   This change has had its price, however. When a woman labored at home,
the midwife usually relied on many helpers who busied themselves not only with the
physical preparations for the baby's arrival, but also with spiritual concerns and emotional care. Childbearing was not a private event: female family members and neighbors
participated. Similarly, the men of the community joined the worried husband in
prayer, in another room or in the synagogue, so he was not alone with his anxieties, and
he knew what was expected of him. When childbirth was transferred to the maternity
ward, hospital midwives neglected the emotional needs of both the parturient woman
and her husband. The status of the midwife dropped from a dignified professional
employed in the community to a special form of nurse, on a low rung of the hierar-
chical ladder of the medical establishment. As people noticed these shortcomings,
changes again began to take place: today, there is a return to home deliveries with a
familiar midwife of the parents' choosing; hospitals allow the husband, mother, or other
relative or friend to stay with the birthing woman, for emotional support; fathers are
learning how to help during childbirth; and in some places, nurse-midwives once again
have their own practice.

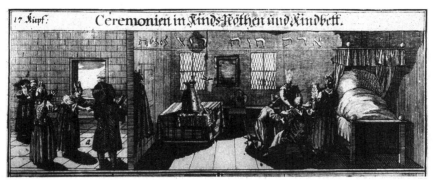

Plate 12. Childbirth scene. Husband and others praying outside the door; Torah in the birthing room. Kirchner, J.C., *Jüdische Ceremoniel,* (Nüurnberg: 1726) 148.
Jewish National University Library, Jerusalem.

Chapter Eight

Giving Birth

PAIN OF CHILDBIRTH

"In pain shall you bear children" (Genesis 3:16) is God's punishment to Eve for her sin in the Garden of Eden. Jews have interpreted this verse, like other biblical verses, to extract lessons for human behavior; in this case, the verse has been used to rationalize the pain of childbirth.

God punished Eve with the pain (*etzev*) of childbearing, but also punished Adam for having eaten of the forbidden fruit: "By toil (*be-itzavon*) shall you eat of it all the days of your life" (Genesis 3:17). Both these Hebrew words refer to suffering: Eve would suffer when she labored to give birth, whereas Adam would suffer when he labored to provide food. The translator interpreted that the two would suffer in different ways, through the experience of pain in one case and toil in the other. Neither type of labor need necessarily involve pain, however. One can work hard, exert oneself physically, and perspire without experiencing pain. Although it is probably true that in the past most women suffered in childbearing, some women have given birth easily, without pain.[1]

The Book of Genesis actually makes no mention of Eve's suffering when she was delivered of her three children.[2] Nor does it mention pain associated with other births, except in the case of Rachel, who died giving birth to her second son, but she was destined to die for having stolen her father's idols.[3]

Metaphors of distress in the Books of the Prophets refer to the discomfort of a laboring woman and reveal the way people understood childbirth in antiquity. For example, "They shall be seized with pangs and throes, writhe like a woman in travail" (Isaiah 13:8); and "Like a woman with child approaching childbirth, writhing and screaming in her pangs" (Isaiah 26:17). Thus, *tzirim* (*tzir* is a hinge) are a woman's twists and turns ("throes" in the first quotation) during labor, like a door on its hinges. *Ḥavalim*, meaning "bindings," are contractions ("pangs" in the foregoing verses); the abdomen indeed tightens as though bound from the inside. The travailing woman, *ḥolah*, "writhes" (in pain), and other words are used to describe her straits (*tzarah*, "distress"), as well as her groaning and crying.[4]

This vocabulary led, in the fifth century, to the view that a pregnant woman is like a house, with locked doors that prevent the embryo from leaving. God unlocks these doors, which open on hinges when a woman kneels to give birth.[5] Talmudic sages imagined that the cry of a woman in childbirth could be heard from one end of the world to the other, and that the pain was worse when a woman bore a girl than when she had a boy.[6] The sages also assumed that when birth was unbearably painful, a woman vowed never again to have sexual relations with her husband.[7]

The talmudic rabbis rationalized that the righteous were excluded from God's decree to Eve. They imagined that Jochebed, mother of Moses and most exemplary of righteous women, experienced no pain when giving birth.[8] Conversely, they taught that women died in childbirth on account of their own sins, in particular their failure to observe their religious duties.[9] This teaching influenced rabbinic advice for easing delivery. Their exegesis of "in pain shall you bear children" concluded that this verse referred to the whole process of conception, pregnancy, birth, and child rearing; a woman suffered in bringing up her children.[10]

One sage of the early talmudic period elaborated on the nature of God's decree to Eve and imagined it to have ten dimensions, including the affliction of menstruation, the pain of giving birth (after seven or nine months), the necessity to nurse for two years, and the affliction of menopause. (The remaining afflictions related to a woman's subservience to her husband and to her eventual mortality.) In an eighth-century rendering of the nature of this decree, nursing and menopause were replaced in the list with the more general pain of rearing children.[11]

Through the ages, Jews have continued to study, teach, and develop the biblical and talmudic ideas about birth. Medieval Jewish mystics in Spain also took an interest in this biblical verse and interpreted it in terms of their view that all that happens on earth has a divine context. They examined the supernal mystery of the scene in the Garden of Eden to discover what happens at birth. Thus, the Zohar envisaged a female dimension of the godhead (the Shekhinah) as a pregnant hind that gives birth only when the supernal snake, which is the "Other Side," responsible for evil, bites her to open her birth canal. The snake's bite causes her pain, without which birth cannot take place. This supernal source of evil opens the path for the soul's descent to the human baby in the earthly world. Thus, the Other Side, in the form of the snake, causes bodily pain yet enables a woman to give birth both in the world above and in the world below. When a soul is destined for a pure and holy body, the snake does not tamper with the birth, and therefore righteous women have painless deliveries.[12] The birth scene unfurls simultaneously on earth and in the divine realm.

The zoharic mystical interpretation developed from earlier Jewish myths of the evil snake and the God-fearing hind. Of course, the evil snake in the Book of Genesis tempted Eve to bite the apple and thereby commit the sin for which God issued the decree. The Talmud depicts the snake lusting after Eve after her fall and even impregnating her. More important, in another context, it tells that God prepares a snake to bite open the womb of a hind crouching to give birth, to permit the delivery of her offspring.[13] In Jewish tradition, the hind symbolizes the prayer of the righteous; "Like a hind crying for water, my soul cries for You, O God" (Psalm 42:2). This zoharic mysticism influenced kabbalistic remedies for easing childbirth, as discussed later.

Although medieval physicians believed that there were physical reasons for labor pains, such as fetal presentation and a narrow pelvis or closed birth canal, or astrological reasons (the configuration of the planets and stars were thought to influence these pains), medieval rabbis used the threat of death in childbirth to encourage piety in day-to-day life.[14] They forbade gossip about sins the laboring woman may have committed in the past, and at times the sins of the father were also suspected of causing pain during childbirth.[15]

In the centuries that followed, physicians made little progress in elucidating the pain of childbirth. In contrast, rabbis continued to face the problem. In the early seventeenth century, a Yiddish ethical text, a book of biblical homilies, *Tze'enah u-re'enah*, popularized the connection between the suffering of a woman in childbirth and Eve's sin in the Garden of Eden.[16] The author, Jacob ben Isaac Ashkenazi of Yanov (1550–1625), stated that all women must suffer in childbirth for Eve's sin, even though they themselves were more righteous than Eve and, in her place, would not have tasted the forbidden fruit. This book, first printed in 1616 and reprinted at least twenty-five times before the end of the seventeenth century, and some two hundred times since, influenced millions of Yiddish-speaking women (in Central and Eastern Europe, and eventually in the United States and the Holy Land) for four and a half centuries. Another very popular Yiddish ethical text, the *Brantspiegel*, by Moses ben Hanokh Yerushalmi (c. 1546–1633) associated the blood of childbirth and menstruation with the impure venom that the serpent injected into Eve.[17]

In the eighteenth century, a pious Ashkenazi Jew acknowledged that his wife's great suffering in childbirth was due to Eve's sin, but nevertheless he reasoned that perhaps there were additional influences for such suffering, such as the stars. Perhaps, he wondered, the star under which a woman was herself born dictated the extent to which she would eventually suffer in childbirth.[18]

Even in the twentieth century, a rabbi, who appeared more interested in female morality than in physiology, stressed the idea that a woman's sufferings in childbirth reflected her piety.[19] Agonizing shouts in the labor ward of "Mother, what have I done?" were common not long ago among women who were not offered pain relief and show that the idea of suffering as punishment for sinful behavior survived the ages.[20] In 1984, a young Jewish woman who felt guilty about having conceived before her wedding considered the unexpected extreme pain of childbirth as retribution and was convinced that she would not survive the ordeal.

Although, in the past, women pregnant for the first time knew about the pain of childbirth from observing their mothers or sisters, women today are less likely to have observed travail or delivery. Nonetheless, in modern times, "in pain shall you bear children" is one of the best-known biblical phrases among Jewish women, and many fear childbirth. Although childbirth is now relatively safe, their fear is based on helplessness, on the feeling that the events of birthing are beyond their own control.

EASING DELIVERY

Methods for easing delivery, like remedies for barrenness and preventing miscarriage, depend on the perceived causes of the problem. Believing that the pain of childbirth has divine causes, Jews have prayed, repented, and made donations to charity in the hope of obtaining God's favor toward a laboring woman. At the same time, they have tried medical remedies to relieve pain and hasten delivery. When neither spiritual nor physical methods have produced results, Jews have sometimes resorted to magic.

Prayer and Atonement

Prayer and atonement are two duties in the daily life of a Jew. Those who are accustomed to pray, repent, and give to charity in their daily lives also do so during childbirth.

In the talmudic period, the sages encouraged women to pray for God's mercy to ease the decree that God issued to Eve. In later centuries, rabbis continued to stress the need to pray for a woman giving birth. Some supplicatory prayers, recited before and during labor, beg that her sins may be considered atoned for.[21]

A Wife's Prayers

Jews have recited psalms, especially Psalm 20 (a psalm of supplication), to ease delivery, since the gaonic period.[22] Psalm 20 begins with the words "A psalm of David. May the Lord answer you in time of trouble . . ." (Psalm 20:1–2). In one custom beginning in the fourteenth century, a helper recited Psalm 20 while the woman in labor focused her thoughts on a certain magical name of God. This procedure was repeated nine times, or more often twelve times. The psalm's nine verses corresponded to the nine months of pregnancy, and the seventy words that make up the psalm symbolized the seventy pangs of labor.[23] Remedy books and prayer books, from the early seventeenth century onward, directed the reader to vary systematically the vowels in the tetragrammaton each time it appeared in the psalm. This medieval method of meditation, practiced by kabbalists, required the meditator's prior purification and peace of mind (not specified in our texts and both unlikely in a delivery room). Because women would not have known how to meditate in this way, it was surely originally the husband's job to meditate on this psalm while his wife was in labor. In Italy in the late eighteenth century, the birthing woman herself recited this psalm, three times only, while she was in labor. When no progress was made, the woman assisting her pleaded with the angel governing the womb for divine help with delivery.[24]

Prayers dating from the seventeenth century sometimes invoked Psalm 118:5 ("In distress I called on the Lord; the Lord answered me and brought me relief") in the hope of easing delivery.[25] Moreover, Rabbi Nahman of Bratslav (1772–1811) reputedly advised reciting Psalm 100 (a psalm praising God), whose words and letters were calculated, using *gematria*, to be particularly relevant for easing childbirth.[26]

Since the fifteenth century, if not earlier, Jews have composed special prayers specifically for a woman to recite for easy delivery. Some of these prayers stressed the connection between the woman's suffering and Eve's sin, and a few related to Hannah and a woman's religious duties, whereas others recalled God's mercy to the biblical matriarchs during childbearing.[27] All these formulas established continuity between the woman's experience of childbirth and her Jewish ancestry.

The *Tze'enah u-re'enah* stressed the importance of piety and charity as well as the punishments awaiting the sinful. The author of this treatise assumed that the Tree of Knowledge in the Garden of Eden was an *etrog* (citron) tree and taught a woman to pray for easy delivery while biting off the end of the *etrog*.[28] This prayer connected the suffering of birth to Eve, yet protested that biting the fruit was no pleasure. The prayer over the *etrog* was a precaution, recited on the seventh day of Sukkot (Hoshanah Rabbah), when God seals the verdict of each person, judged on high on the Day of Atonement. The popularity of this book must have enhanced the spread of this custom. In the late eighteenth century, non-Jews also made use of this "Jewish object with magical powers," known to ease delivery. In Berlin, in 1795, the birth of Frederick William IV of Prussia was eased with a "paradise apple." Perhaps a Jewish midwife made the suggestion, or this remedy may have been common knowledge among non-Jewish birth helpers. Jews in nineteenth-century Holland and Bavaria used an *etrog* to ease delivery, sometimes preparing a potion from this fruit after the festival, and the potion was kept as a remedy to help a woman give birth easily and without pain. Jewish women in Poland bit off the end of this fruit for the same reason, on the last day of Sukkot, but without reciting the prayer.[29]

Although many Jews probably accepted without question that women suffered in childbirth for Eve's sin, not all did. For example, an eighteenth-century book includes a woman's prayer admitting that no one (certainly not the humble woman reciting the prayer) would question God's distribution of mercy, yet suggesting the unfairness of extending Eve's punishment to all women.[30] A later prayer asks God to protect a woman from the decree against Eve, because the supplicant had observed her religious duties scrupulously.[31] (The talmudic sages had taught, after all, that the righteous do not have painful births.)

Women's childbirth prayers sometimes mention Hannah, because the initial Hebrew letters of a Jewish woman's three duties—separating the dough offering (in memory of the priestly tithes), *hallah*; maintaining sexual separation during menstruation, *niddah*; and kindling the Sabbath lights, *hadlakat nerot*—spell her name. For example, Sore bas Toyvim, who is thought to have lived in seventeenth-century Ukraine, allegedly wrote many supplications, including one to recite during ritual immersion, before conception occurred. The supplications stressed that women needed to keep the commandments properly, to benefit as Hannah had benefited; they had to take special care to observe the laws regarding menstruation, because then they would have an easy delivery. Otherwise, they could be judged during childbirth, God forbid.[32]

One prayer, composed in German by Fanny Neuda (1819–1894), was popular in Central Europe. The following English translation was published in Vienna (c. 1900):

> God, with trembling do I go near my confinement; the pains take over and my delivery is near. I shudder at the pains that are before me, at the danger that threatens me! Lord and God, let me not succumb under my pains! Give me strength to endure the pains. Remember not my sins in the hour of danger, and save me for thy mercy's sake. God be near to me in the hour when all human abilities and human art are as nothing, and only Thou can help. Let my confinement be easy and without danger, save me from severe and heavy pains, God be near to me in the hour of pain and danger, and let thy thought rest upon thy aid and protection, to strengthen me, that my soul may not stumble, and that I may not be the prey of the danger that I have

before me. God and Lord! I trust in thee. Thou shalt wake upon my
life, Thou shalt not let me be the prey of my pains. Amen.[33]

This prayer was written by a woman who had experienced childbirth.
She alluded to the ancient idea that her sins could affect her birthing experience and
asked God's mercy and help. Her tone differs from that of earlier prayers for easing
delivery that were written by men, however. Instead of a plea such as "Bring blessing
upon her, for her eyes depend on You, as a maidservant's eyes depend upon her mistress," Neuda's prayer asserts the strength of her faith; she speaks the last line in con-
fidence rather than in servitude. With these words, she gives herself, and surely many
other women, too, the strength to cope.[34]

A Husband's Prayers

When a woman was in labor, it was usually her husband's role to pray for
relief of her suffering and for her safe deliverance and that of their baby. An early legend (some two thousand years old) about the birth of Cain shows that the husband's
prayer was considered more effective than the wife's. The legend tells that Eve was
heavy with child when one morning she felt pain in her belly. She felt all her mus-
cles stiffening and her back ache. The pains increased, and she lay helpless on the hot
earth, praying to God to help her, but her supplications were ignored. She cried out
for Adam to plead on her behalf, but to no avail, because he was reaping a meadow
to the east. Eve never imagined such agony. She was sure that if it lasted much longer
she would die; she closed her eyes and, in one last effort, let out a piercing scream.
Adam heard the scream and rushed to Eve's side, fearing that she had been bitten by
the evil snake. With all his soul, Adam prayed to God for help. God immediately dispatched a dozen angels who encircled her while the archangel, Michael, passed his
hand over her body, from her face to her breast, and told her that, in response to
Adam's prayers, he had been sent to help her. Then her son was born.[35]

A husband's supplications can be particularly poignant, reflecting the torment of the moment: his wife is crying out in pain, and two lives are in danger. He
calls on God to ensure their safety. Jews have believed that if a husband prays in the
company of a quorum of righteous men, his prayer is likely to be all the more powerful, but such prayers are not part of the synagogue liturgy.

Since medieval times, the husband of a birthing woman has recited the
Shema (the prayer Jews recite twice daily, composed of three verses from the
Pentateuch declaring the unity of God), psalms, verses from the Prophets, and other
biblical verses when seeking spiritual help. The choice of verses recited has varied
from place to place.[36] The husband may pray aloud outside the door of the birthing
room, near the mezuzzah, accompanied by household members, or in the synagogue,
with friends and relatives.[37]

Intercessors' Prayers

When it is apparent that such prayers have had no effect, a husband may
request help from a holier person, known to be gifted for having his prayers answered.

As discussed in Chapter 2, Jews have called on such people for help in other situations as well. By requesting a man more pious than himself to intercede, a husband hopes to relieve his wife's distress; at the same time he does something positive to relieve his anxiety and shows others that he is trying to help.

Moshe Leib of Sasov (d. 1807) was an Eastern European hasidic rabbi who helped to ease the delivery of birthing women. One story about the rabbi took place in a small village near Lvov, where a woman had been in travail for days, to no avail. Her distraught husband sent a messenger to the rabbi of Sasov, to beg him to pray for God's mercy. The messenger set out immediately and arrived in Sasov in the middle of the night. The town was asleep, yet a light still burned in one house only, and he approached it. Neglecting the late hour because his task was urgent, the messenger knocked on the door. An old man answered, listened to the messenger's speech, and invited him inside. The old man insisted that it was too late at night to disturb the rabbi. The message would have to wait until morning. The exhausted man did not need much persuading and accepted something to eat, a glass of brandy, and a bed and was soon sound asleep.

When the messenger awoke in the morning, he was immediately remorseful that he had not completed his errand the previous evening. He did not have time to fret, however, because the old man greeted him with the happy news that the village woman had given birth to a healthy boy. The messenger hurried off to spread the news among her relatives and soon discovered that his host, the old man, was none other than the venerable rabbi of Sasov.[38]

The rabbi of Sasov was a *tzaddik*, a man extraordinarily gifted with holiness. One assumes that, as soon as the messenger fell asleep, the rabbi prayed for the woman and she immediately was delivered of her child.

Issachar Dov Roke'ah (1854–1927) of Belz was another Eastern European Hasid with a reputation for helping to ease childbirth. In *The Family Poem*, Yiddish poet Melech Ravitch (1893–1976) told of the sleepless nights when his wife was in agonizing labor and her cries echoed through the well-lit house. Half the town, three doctors, and her ninety-year-old grandmother waited up fearfully. Eventually, a cable was sent to Issachar Dov Roke'ah, "Hindeh, child of Blumeh, labors: beg for mercy!" A son was delivered eventually, after the intervention of the Belzer rabbi (one assumes, as the poem does not specify).[39]

Many Jews have believed that the spirits of the dead have access to the divine realm and have asked the dead to act as intercessors. Thus, in some communities, when a birth was particularly difficult, the woman's relatives visited the cemetery to plead for her delivery from danger. The practice, known in Yiddish as *k'vorim reissen*, was common among the Jews of Eastern Europe, who composed prayers for this purpose. *K'vorim* means "graves," and *reissen* means literally "to tear." Jews visited the grave of a holy person with a piece of string that could later be used as a wick and measured the grave with this string; then they tore up the string to make wicks for candles, which they burned in the synagogue.[40] Sephardic Jews have also made pilgrimages to the grave of a holy person to plead for an easy delivery, often in the ninth month of pregnancy, before the onset of labor; some rabbis have done this for the woman's sake.[41]

Atonement and Charity

Because "charity saves from death" (Proverbs 6:2), pregnant Jewish women have given to charity. Although giving charity is a biblical commandment, talmudic sages added that almsgiving atoned for sins and ensured the giver wise, wealthy, and learned sons.[42] Almsgiving has always been important in Jewish life, throughout a person's life, not only during childbirth. Rabbis sometimes thought it necessary to issue a reminder, however, and printed this directive in some prayers for late pregnancy.[43]

The existence of a rabbinic ruling concerning alms for this purpose, dated 1687, from a Jewish community in Lithuania, suggests that the sum collected from birthing women may not always have reached the correct destination. The ruling warned the collectors of dues to ensure that no charity box was passed around, other than the boxes of the official collectors of the community. The midwife was obliged to deliver to these officials all contributions made by women who vowed money during childbirth. Moreover, the collectors of dues had to give this money to the fund for poor birthing women.[44]

In the early twentieth century, Sephardic Jews sent a dish of oil with the laboring woman's vow to give alms to charity to the synagogue for use in the eternal lamp: they hoped that the oil for this lighted lamp, which symbolizes life, would facilitate the emergence of new life, and the act of charity would save the mother from death.[45]

Also in the early twentieth century, Kurdistani Jews expiated a laboring woman's sins, in the hope of easing delivery: they swung a hen in circles over the head of a woman in labor, like the expiatory custom performed on the eve of the Day of Atonement.[46]

Physical Remedies

Since ancient times, midwives have used oil for massaging the lower abdomen of women in labor, to try to relieve pain, and to lubricate the lower end of the birth channel to ease delivery.[47] Midwives also ensured that the birthing room was kept warmed, and they helped the travailing woman to take a hot bath to ease her suffering and hasten delivery. A hot stone wrapped in cloth served as a warm compress to relieve pain, much as we use a hot-water bottle today.[48]

Birth attendants concocted many different potions for easing childbirth.[49] These were herbal, animal, or mineral, often a combination, sometimes not kosher, prepared for swallowing, for insertion into the birth canal, or for producing vapors to induce sneezing (in the hope that the force of the sneeze would expel the baby). One remedy, from a medieval medical encyclopedia by the Spanish rabbi, Meir Aldabi (c. 1310–c. 1360), has no Jewish content but offers advice that remains of interest today:

> If the pregnant woman has difficulties in labor, she should bathe in water in which fenugreek or sprouts, and flax and barley seeds have been cooked, and let her press her hands against her two sides and loins, and rub on her hips soft, wet oils, such as sesame oil or wild

beechnut oil and the like. Make her sneeze with incense, and help her walk slowly up and down a slope. Let her drink saffron pulverized and mixed in water, the milk of a bitch, peanut oil in warm water, warm water alone, or [take] the juice of leek and its leaven, and dip into it unwashed wool and insert it into her womb.[50]

A warm bath with strengthening ingredients, massage with soothing oils, help with walking up and down, and a harmless potion to induce labor could suit birthing women today. Aldabi's advice was actually followed for many centuries: a fifteenth-century Yiddish remedy book recommended bitch's milk mixed with wine or honey for inducing labor. Other popular remedy books in Eastern Europe published later advised the use of this potion as well as burning incense.[51] Burning incense and taking snuff were both intended to induce sneezing and thereby expel the baby. Sometimes the laboring woman was helped to walk around her bed, inside a protective magical circle, or to step to and from over burning incense, in the hope of opening the birth canal and hastening delivery.[52]

Magical Remedies

Attempts to secure God's help in easing delivery sometimes involved harmless magic.

Ritual Objects

Jews used objects pertaining to Jewish ritual, in the hope that magical beneficial effects would ease childbirth. For example, in Europe, at least since the sixteenth century, the Torah was sometimes brought to the birthing room for added spiritual strength, "for perchance the merit of the Torah will protect her, and not as a charm."[53] If this was impractical, the Torah cover, phylacteries, or even the key to the synagogue served in its stead. In the nineteenth and early twentieth centuries, Yemenite Jews and Sephardim in Georgia and Turkistan covered the birthing woman's head with the *parokhet*, the covering of the Ark in which the Torah is housed, to create proximity between the Torah and the suffering woman, in the hope of easing labor. Sometimes a travailing woman drank water in the cup-shaped Torah finials (*rimonim*) that crown the staves of the scroll. With the same principle in mind, Jews in Galicia brought the community minute book (*pinkas*) to the birthing room. In some communities, the shofar was sounded as the ultimate appeal to God if the woman's life remained in serious danger and prayers had proved to no avail.[54] In Ouezzan, Morocco, a laboring woman borrowed the belt of Rabbi Amram ben Diwwan, a holy man who lived in the eighteenth century. This sacred belt, preserved for many years, had a reputation for facilitating delivery. Elsewhere in North Africa, Jewish women used the staff or coat of other esteemed rabbis who died long ago, for this same purpose.[55] The use of the *etrog* as a charm for easing delivery is a variation on the same idea.

To hasten delivery, some Ashkenazi Jewish women in Eastern Europe and some Sephardic women in the Holy Land in the early twentieth century held on to a string, which was tied at its other end to the Ark that housed the Torah scroll. At each uterine contraction, the travailing woman pulled on the string, opening the Ark in the hope of opening her womb. The opening of the Ark was a Jewish form of sympathetic magic, a version of another custom common among Gentiles, too, in which everything that could be opened was opened (such as buttons, knots, cupboards) so the womb would do likewise. In Lithuania, a person who entered a house and found open chests and drawers would ask jokingly whether someone were in labor.[56] Opening the Ark and blowing the shofar were not only means of asking for God's attention, but many Jews believed that these acts also frightened away demons capable of killing the woman in her frail condition.

Incantations

Many Jews have assumed that incantations, as a form of magic or sorcery, are strictly forbidden by biblical law. In talmudic times, the sages warned that people who recited magical incantations, such as the reciting of biblical verses for a child's well-being, would lose their share in the World to Come. Nevertheless, the reciting of biblical verses became a popular method of coping with a difficult situation, and Jews, mainly women, but some rabbis also, used incantations remedially in the talmudic period, especially when life was at risk.[57] Many centuries later, Maimonides accepted the reciting of biblical verses as incantations only to heal the soul, for soothing and reassuring (nevertheless important during childbirth), and he firmly objected to the recitation of biblical verses for curing bodily ills.[58]

In ancient and medieval times, Jews sometimes inscribed a magical text in Hebrew or in Hebrew lettering on the inside of a bowl to give magical strength to water poured into it, which the travailing woman drank as a remedy to ease delivery.

Two biblical verses were often used in birth incantations: ". . . 'Depart, you and all the people who follow you!' After that I will depart . . ." (Exodus 11:8) and "Like a hind crying for water, my soul cries for You, O God" (Psalm 42:2). Exodus 11:8 was invoked in a popular medieval incantation for easing delivery, which was "tried and proved" according to a Judeo-Arabic remedy book.[59] Since the fifteenth century, Ashkenazi and Sephardic remedy books recommended the recitation of this verse, which was soon incorporated into the texts of prayers for birth attendants to recite when a woman was in labor.[60] The recitation of Exodus 11:8 could have been a simple request to God for a quick departure of the baby from the womb, just as the Jews made their exodus from Egypt. It could also have been an address to the evil spirits: once all these left the area, the baby could be delivered safely.

Yiddish, Sephardic, and Judeo-Arabic remedy books enlarged the incantation, blending this verse with the early legend about Eve's pain in childbirth and the zoharic metaphor of the birthing hind. The enlarged incantation tells of the arrival of Michael, the archangel, in response to the cries of a hind in labor and ends with Exodus 11:8 in full (italicized below):

> Michael, the archangel, was walking on Mt. Sinai when he heard cries and screams and asked God, "What are these cries and screams that I hear?"

God answered that a hind was giving birth and crying.

"Go," said God to Michael, "Go and tell her 'go out, go out, go out' for the earth wants you. *Then all these courtiers of yours shall come down to me and bow low to me, saying 'Depart, you and all the people who follow you!' After that I will depart . . .*"[61]

The enlarged incantation revealed that the archangel Michael would be sent to enable the delivery if God approved of the birth: the thinking was that when God judged that a woman giving birth was not particularly righteous, the evil [snake] of the Other Side caused painful delivery. Moreover, when explaining the supernal mystery of birth, the Zohar quotes from Psalm 42:2 ("Like a hind crying for water") and evokes the supernal hind to represent God's female element (the Shekhinah).

Italian Jewish birth prayers in the late eighteenth and early nineteenth centuries quoted Psalm 42:2 and then enlarged on this theme within the prayer: a hind was kneeling to give birth when contractions came upon her. The animal reached out for God with her antlers and cried out with bitter cries, groaning and pleading for mercy before the Throne of Glory. God in heaven heard her cries and opened her womb.[62]

As mentioned previously, the hind represents the Shekhinah. Thus, a woman reciting this prayer may hope that the supernal birth will facilitate the birth of her own earthly child. In the eighteenth-century text, but not in the nineteenth-century version, an added Aramaic incantation adjured the angels, and not the Other Side, to influence the decree on the new soul and its birth.

Amulets

Through the ages, most Jewish books of charms and magical remedies have offered ancient formulas for inscribing on amulets "for a woman having difficulty in birthing." Jews have tied such amulets on the foot, thigh, belly, or forehead of the travailing woman, in the hope of easing delivery. Amulet makers have copied Hebrew letters bearing magical significance, often in Assyrian script, onto a kosher parchment or a new pottery shard. They have chosen magical names of God, have used a magic square, and have invoked specific angels. Sometimes the user has been warned to remove the amulet immediately after childbirth, for fear that the mother's entrails could also be expelled by the amulet's phenomenal power.[63]

Eleazar of Worms (c. 1165–c. 1230), one of the Hasidei Ashkenaz, was apparently well-versed in amuletic formulas. A mystical book, *The Book of Raziel* (*Sefer Razi'el*, first published in Amsterdam in 1701), that includes formulas for amulets to ease childbirth, was derived partly from the writings of Eleazar of Worms and partly from another, much earlier mystical text, *The Book of Mysteries* (*Sefer ha-razim*) with magical formulas. One "tried and proved" formula in *The Book of Raziel* involves writing on deer parchment permutations of an Aramaic word, *pok*, meaning "get out" or "come out," and tying this parchment to the birthing woman's navel while whispering the verse of Exodus 11:8.[64]

The Book of Raziel was not the only text to draw on medieval sources: *Toldot Adam* attributes one formula for easing childbirth to Nahmanides, whereas other formulas in this eighteenth-century collection had been kept for generations as closely guarded secrets by practicing kabbalists.[65] These formulas for easing birth were not only handed down from generation to generation, but also they traveled from one community to another, appearing in Jewish remedy books in use in distant places, such as Amsterdam, Cracow, Damascus, Yemen, and Baghdad.[66]

As discussed in earlier chapters, Jews attributed remedial powers to red stones, by virtue of their association with the biblical Reuben, and Jewish women used these stones to ease delivery, as they did to cure barrenness and to protect against miscarriage. The eighteenth-century rabbi, physician, and encyclopedist, Isaac Lampronti (1679–1756), reported that the wife of a well-respected and wise man almost died in difficult labor in the early winter of 1685, but was saved by the advice of a blind rabbi of Reggio, in southern Italy. The blind rabbi had recommended that the woman drink some red wine containing the powder of a stone called *rubino* (ruby), of the size of about two lentils.[67] Lampronti may have heard this story from his own mother, or it may have been advice offered to his wife when she was in difficult labor. This type of recommendation for a remedy known to have been tried and proved by the wife of a respected and wise man was just what Jews valued. A treatment known to have helped someone trustworthy was tried optimistically by others over and over again.

Another Italian Jewish physician recommended jasper for easing delivery; the Bible tells that, in the breastplate of the high priest, jasper is the stone of Benjamin, whose mother died when he was born.[68]

In the early twentieth century, a Polish rabbi recalled how his late father had given those wanting to ease delivery a "tried and proved" amulet that he had received from his forefathers:

> There was just one square inscribed on this amulet, with the words *Ha-Shem* (The [Holy] Name) and *eled* (I will give birth), and this was tied on the forehead of the laboring woman. When giving this amulet, my father would stand praying, with great devotion, a secret prayer that he would never divulge to me, even though several times I implored him to do so.[69]

In fact, a Hebrew remedy book published in Poland in the early twentieth century included a formula for a similar amulet, for tying on the forehead of a laboring woman. It showed a special combination of the letters of the tetragrammaton and warned that, because the kabbalist learned this formula by divine revelation, it had to be used with utmost care and prepared only by someone who understood kabbalistic combinations.[70]

Like Gentiles, Jews have fashioned amulets out of herbs, animal parts, and other minerals with no Jewish significance, so they are not discussed further here.

JEWISH PRENATAL CLASSES

Nowadays, Jewish prenatal classes, where they exist, combine an exploration of the Jewish values of parenting with breathing and relaxation exercises, and only sometimes the spirituality of birthing.

Women who have faith in God find comfort in the traditional religious methods of coping with the pain and fear of giving birth, especially if they pray, repent, and give to charity at other times in life. For other women, prayer gives the experience of labor some spirituality, a feeling of closeness with God or a feeling of sharing pain and concern. In addition, a gift to charity may be a satisfying way of expressing gratitude for the successful outcome of childbirth.

Women in labor can choose from many different prayers, or they may write their own, as done by women in the past. The prenatal class can study existing prayers and can examine the phrases that the participants find meaningful with a view to composing a new personal or group prayer, to reinstate Jewish content into an experience that, for some, has become a purely medical procedure. Prayer may put a person in touch with God. Prayer may also put a person in touch with others who have been or are in pain and may thereby reduce the loneliness of suffering. In addition, a prayer may give a person strength to cope.

Today, an ultra-Orthodox woman may pray for her childless friends over and over again when she is in labor. When the woman no longer has the strength to verbalize her supplication, her mother, who is near her, continues the recitation for her in her ear.[71] In such a community, a woman in pain, even in danger, who pleads for another who suffers, rather than pleading for herself, is considered truly righteous; the hope is that God will grant mercy to both women.

Nowadays, other psychological methods of coping with pain exist that are not religious, and the prenatal class can explore ways to infuse Jewish spirituality into these methods. A woman can recite together with her companion a psalm, a prayer, or, if preferred, some nonreligious Jewish verse, poem, or song. She can meditate on a word or a phrase (for example, with vowels or letters systematically changed over and over again) and even control her breathing with this verbal exercise.[72]

The prenatal class can devote some time to considering the rabbinic interpretations of Genesis 3:16, although the traditional assumptions about the pain of birth that were handed down from generation to generation are outdated. Anesthesia effectively reduces the suffering of labor and delivery, and women who opt for natural childbirth can try to overcome their pain with relaxation and breathing exercises. Clearly, in the secular world today, giving birth is no longer a day of judgment, Eve's original sin is almost forgotten, and a woman's three duties appear irrelevant. Nevertheless, the triangle of suffering, sin, and atonement still lurks: in the absence of scientific explanation of why a birth should be particularly difficult, some people still comfort themselves by rationalizing it as an atonement for some sin, real, imagined, or unknown.

The prenatal class may look at how men share the suffering of childbearing. This could be done, for example, by studying the prayers that address the whole process of childbearing and thereby examining the many stages at which a mother or a father could experience pain and suffering. An examination of the expectations of suffering would necessitate also a study of creative methods of coping with this suffering, as already suggested, and, in counterbalance, an examination of the joys of becoming a parent![73]

Jewish tradition has proffered a pattern for living. Through the ages, rabbis have taught that if one followed the commandments scrupulously, one would not suffer in childbearing, and the children of the righteous would also be blessed. This teaching leads us to question to what extent we ourselves can control our experiences of childbirth and to consider which behaviors promote our own well-being and that of our children. Prenatal classes do address these questions, from a religious or a secular angle. When the approach is secular, it is still worthwhile to study Jewish sources and to glean inspiration from them.

In 1996, one woman, who was expecting her third child and actively seeking a spiritual dimension in childbirth, expressed the following opinion:

> One can "prepare" for childbirth in many ways: by gaining information (re: psychological processes, medical measures, etc.), by speaking about one's fears and expectations, by examining one's relationship within the family, with one's spouse, and with God. For me, the "spiritual" aspect of childbirth has a lot to do with my own aspirations and potentials in perspective and redefining who I am as a partner, mother, Jew. I believe that all the energy and attention one has devoted to honest introspection comes to one's aid in moments of trial. To ignore such matters makes one much more vulnerable to feelings of helplessness, guilt, undirectedness.

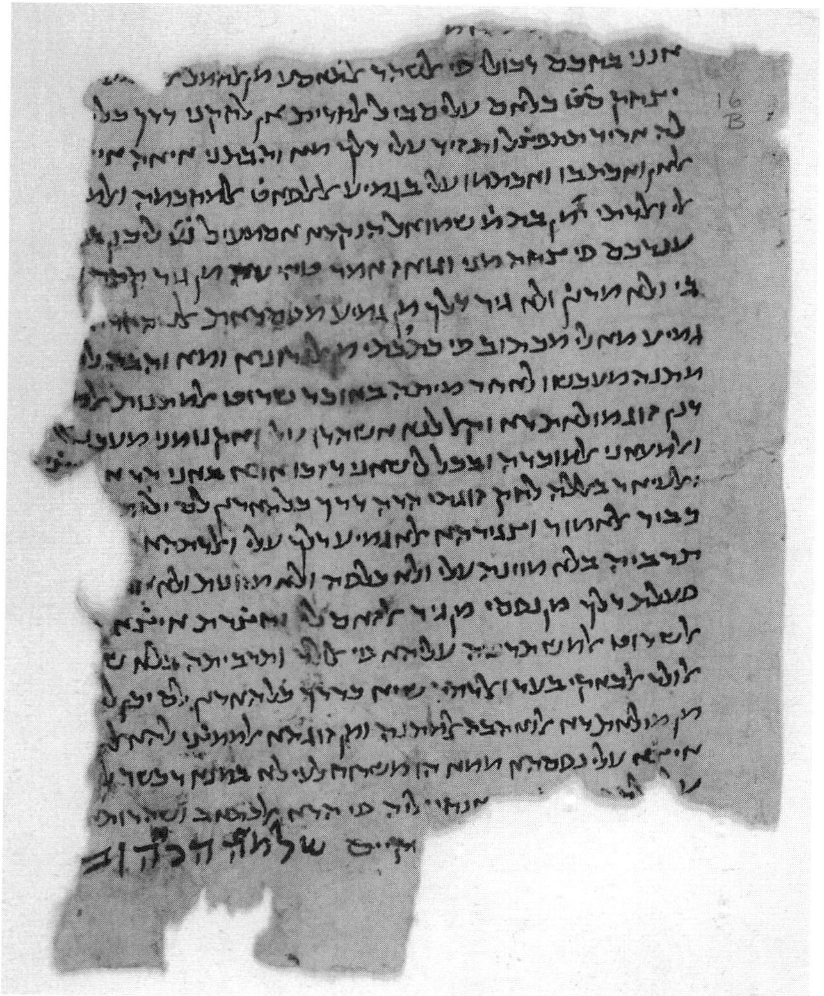

Plate 13. Will of a pregnant woman in case she died in chidbirth.
c. 1090. Preserved in the *Geniza* in Cairo, 1090.
Jewish Theological Seminary, New York; ENA 4101 f.16b.

Chapter Nine

Death in Childbirth

Until the twentieth century, when modern medical discoveries were able to reduce the rates of maternal and infant mortality, childbirth was often fatal. Sometimes there was nothing a midwife could do to prevent a double tragedy.

MATERNAL DEATH

Of all the biblical women, Rachel suffered most for the sake of bearing children and died when giving birth to her second son.[1] Rabbinic tradition attributed her death to an unintentional curse that her husband uttered against her.[2]

Rachel may have died because of her husband's angry words, but (as discussed in the previous chapter) the Mishnah teaches that a woman's death in childbirth may be her own downfall, if she has neglected to observe meticulously her three religious duties: to observe the laws regarding menstruation, to prepare the Sabbath loaf, and to light the Sabbath candles.[3] Through the ages, Jewish women have been familiar with this teaching. On occasion, however, even the most righteous women died in childbirth, and Jews looked for other explanations. Sometimes a physical explanation, such as an illness or unusual physique, was obvious, but sometimes Jews suspected witchcraft or demonic involvement.

The Talmud teaches that when a mother dies before the baby is born and there remains a chance that her baby is still alive, "one may bring a knife and cut her womb open to take out the child" (*B. Arakhin* 7a), even on a Sabbath. One wonders whether a midwife would have been willing to do such a thing many centuries ago, however. It was more likely a surgeon's job.

The talmudic sages reasoned that when the "drop of poison from the Angel of Death" entered the mother's body, the baby inside her died first, because the baby's life was more fragile than the mother's. The sages pointed to a case in which, after the mother's death, the baby was observed to move three times in her womb. They wondered whether this was a sign that the baby had outlived the mother or whether the baby had died and its movements were like those of an amputated lizard's tail.[4] If the latter proposition were correct, it would not have been necessary to use a knife on the dead woman.

The talmudic ruling was in line with the Indian medical treatise, *Susruta* (this text probably originated in the last centuries B.C.E. but was fixed in its present form by the seventh century C.E.), which recommended that the baby be cut out of the mother's womb if she died and there was a sign of life within. This recommendation was also in line with early Roman law, which decreed that a baby had to be removed from the mother before she could be buried, to prevent a living baby from being buried alive (even in the womb). (The use of the term "caesarean" to describe this particular method of delivery was coined only in the late sixteenth century; it arose from many centuries of guessing the etymological origins of the word "Caesar" and eventually led to the hypothesis concerning the manner of birth of Julius Caesar.[5])

Hebrew funerary inscriptions and ossuaries dating back to the first or second century C.E., studied by archeologists in Israel, reveal several women who died in childbirth, including one, Salome, daughter of Saul, who was buried with her infant still inside her.[6]

In medieval times, the Church forbade the burial of an unbaptized baby, even if it were unborn. In those days, some European Jews also believed it ominous to bury a woman with a baby inside her. Rather than use a knife on the dead woman and desecrate her body, however, medieval midwives attempted various physical manipulations to ease out the baby, resorted to magical methods in the hope of expelling it, or extracted the fetus limb by limb (embryotomy) if necessary. In 1902, a pregnant Jewish woman died in a shtetl near Smolensk. It took the midwife two days of great effort to extract the baby, but she succeeded and enabled the corpse to be buried before the Sabbath. Remedy books offered ample advice of this sort. If the midwife failed to remove the fetus, a surgeon was sometimes consulted.[7]

Jews living in Moslem lands may not have had a problem burying a pregnant woman, as long as they were sure that the baby was dead before the burial. In the sixteenth century, the head of the Jewish community in Egypt was shocked to discover a means for making sure that a fetus was dead before a pregnant mother was buried: when, after a woman died in labor, her distended belly revealed signs of life in the womb, the midwife hit it with a broomstick until the movements stopped. We do not know whether this was an extraordinary case or whether it was a local custom. It may have been a non-Jewish custom, because some Gentiles performed this brutal act a few centuries later.[8]

Usually, Jews cleanse their dead and wrap them in a shroud for burial, without a coffin. Eighteenth-century Ashkenazi Jews, however, buried a woman who died in childbirth, unwashed, in her soiled clothes, with a shroud placed over her, in a coffin that was well sealed. When her newborn also died, the baby was washed and clothed and buried in the same grave, but not in the mother's coffin. When a woman died in childbirth with her baby still unborn, a diaper was buried with her so she could care for her baby in the grave.[9]

The peculiar attitude of eighteenth-century Jews to women who died in childbirth is evident in another custom. In Endingen and Lengnau, Switzerland, near the German border, and in some Dutch communities, too, Jews kept a section of the cemetery for the burial of women who died in childbirth. Clearly, the dead women's ritual impurity influenced this attitude, because the Bible dictates that the blood of childbirth is impure. The mishnaic idea that a woman dies in childbirth for her sins may also have encouraged this special treatment, however; by this reckoning, her death indicated that she was neither pious nor righteous.[10]

In the late nineteenth century, when remedies to remove the fetus did not help, some Sephardic Jews apparently buried the pregnant woman with her fetus inside, but only after performing a small ritual. Three holy men, well-versed in Torah and halakhah, visited the dead woman and decreed that she release the child; when this did not happen, they promised her to name the child, to enable it to participate with her in the redemption in the World to Come.[11] One wonders how they decided which name and sex to choose and whether the bereaved father was informed of their decision.

A Woman's Will in Case She Died in Childbirth

In the Middle Ages, a wealthy Jewish woman who was realistic about the chances of dying in childbirth may have written a will in favor of her unborn child, in the hope that her baby would survive her. She dictated her desires regarding the distribution of her personal fortunes just in case her worst fears were realized. She wanted to make sure that her surviving baby—and not her husband or any child of his by a future marriage—would inherit her personal fortune.

Two wills, dictated by women in their ninth month of pregnancy, were found in the Cairo *Geniza*. One, c. 1090, is torn at the side, but the other, dated 1137, is fully legible. Both were legal documents in the formulaic Judeo-Arabic used by the Jews of the Mediterranean in the Middle Ages, and both involved the transfer of money and property among the pregnant woman, her husband, and her own mother, in the interest of the expected child. The author of the later will was the daughter of the well-established and important head of a Jewish community in Egypt, whereas her mother's family were refugees from the Holy Land. The pregnant woman had apparently received a house and money from her father when she married. In the event of her death in childbirth, she spelled out exactly the arrangements that she wanted made between her husband and her mother so the expected child would receive the house and some money. She also made provision in her will for money to be transferred after her death to the poor and needy of Cairo and Fustat, some to her sister's daughters, and some to her brother, a *cohen* (priest) in the religious high court.[12]

PRIORITIES: MOTHER OR CHILD?

Jewish Law

The question of priorities regarding human lives at risk is not a recent problem of medical ethics, but one the sages discussed in talmudic times. In the special case of birth, when labor was unduly difficult and human life was at risk, there was no doubt in their minds about whether the mother's or the baby's life had priority, because the Mishnah stated the law on this matter:

> If a woman is in hard travail [and her life cannot otherwise be saved], one cuts up the child in her womb and brings it forth, member by member, because her life comes before that of [the child]. But if the

greater part has proceeded forth, one may not touch it, for one may not set aside one person's life for that of another. (*Oholot* 7:6).

In difficult labor, when the baby shows no sign of emerging and the mother's life is clearly at great risk, it is left to the midwife's or the physician's discretion to remove the baby to save the mother's life. In the past, when the mother was also killed during this procedure and witnesses claimed the practitioner's negligence, the practitioner could be exiled.[13] Therefore, embryotomy was regarded seriously; the great care taken by Jews to preserve a mother's life enhanced the good reputation of Jewish midwifery.

As discussed in Chapter 3, Jews have likened the fetus' endangering its mother's life to a criminal attempt to kill another person: if an onlooker (in this case the midwife or surgeon) observes that a person (the mother) is likely to be murdered by an attacker (the baby in the womb), then the onlooker may save the victim (the mother) by killing the aggressor (the baby).[14] The talmudic rabbis insisted, however, that once the baby is born, or half-born, there is no way of telling who is pursuing whom, so neither may be killed to save the other.[15] Despite the objection that the fetus cannot be held responsible (not yet being a person), Jewish physicians and scholars have favored the pursuer-aggressor justification for embryotomy (as well as for abortion earlier in pregnancy, as mentioned in Chapter 3).[16]

Caesarean Section

Historical Perspective

Surprisingly, the Mishnah, written almost two thousand years ago, considers caesarean section, not only on dead women, but also on live women. It seems unlikely that ancient physicians had the technical knowledge to deliver a baby successfully by cutting open the womb of a live woman and enabling both mother and baby to survive. The Mishnah implies that this may indeed have been the case, however. In a discussion of primogeniture, the Mishnah rules that a first child brought into the world not by normal birth, but *yotze dophen* (by way of the [abdominal] wall), does not enjoy the inheritance rights of a first-born child: only the baby born normally, subsequently, enjoys these rights. The Mishnah refers to "*yotze dophen* and he who is born after him" (*Bekhorot* 2:9), implying that a mother could survive a caesarean section and later have another child by normal birth. Another implication that Jewish physicians may have known how to perform this operation in the second century C.E. lies in the mishnaic discussion of the purification laws: a woman delivered by *yotze dophen* who survived need not observe the special purification laws that apply to normal birth.[17]

Later, the Talmud uses the phrase *yotze dophen* more than half a dozen times, but without defining it. Furthermore, no description of this method of delivery has survived from late antiquity. These facts indicate that the phrase was commonly understood at that time. Because no report states that the operation was actually performed on women in talmudic times, however, it is quite possible that the procedure was performed successfully on live animals and was merely hypothetical in the case of human patients.

In the talmudic era, Greco-Roman physicians performed caesarean sections only when they thought the mother had died, and (so far as we know) never on a live woman. We can assume, for example, that Soranus, a leading Greco-Roman obstetrician in the second century, did not consider the possibility of caesarean section on a live woman; he only discussed embryotomy.[18] It therefore appears that the knowledge of the technique of such a delivery, if it existed at all, did not come from the Greeks or the Romans, but may have come from an Eastern civilization. Jews in Babylonia after the destruction of the First Temple and during the talmudic period undoubtedly learned some Eastern medicine.

The earliest account of a mother's being anesthetized (with wine) and of the survival of caesarean section by both mother and baby comes from eleventh-century Persia, in rhyming couplets describing the wondrous birth of the Persian hero, Rustam.[19] Unfortunately, one cannot deduce from this source that such an operation was actually possible, although the description is plausible. Only five centuries later, a French physician was the first to offer a reliable account of a successful caesarean section.[20]

How did medieval rabbis and physicians explain the mishnaic *yotze dophen*? The rabbis who addressed this problem were puzzled, because they did not know how a baby could be delivered through the abdominal wall of a live mother such that she could survive. In the eleventh century, Rashi (Rabbi Solomon ben Itzhak; 1040–1105) suggested that surgeons may have opened the woman's abdomen by means of a caustic drug and then used a knife to extract the fetus, but he admitted that he did not know whether this had ever been done. Even the great physician Maimonides was at a loss to understand how a woman could survive a caesarean section; to his knowledge, the woman inevitably died.[21] The Tosafot commentary (dating from the twelfth to the fourteenth centuries) regarded this operation as purely hypothetical.[22] Rabbis in the fifteenth and sixteenth centuries wrote that surgeons did not perform this operation, because no one could really be sure that a woman was dead and that her baby was still alive. These rabbis pointed out that if the woman were merely unconscious, the operation would kill her.[23]

Medieval Hebrew medical texts, sometimes adaptations of Latin, Greek, or Arabic treatises, ignored the possibility of concluding a difficult birth in this way. These texts addressed the topic of "difficult births" (a separate category from "natural" births and "unnatural" presentations), characterized by a fetus "that cannot emerge and tortures the mother and oppresses her," leading to the mother's protracted "anguish and . . . anxiety." By way of solution they offered various manipulations by the midwife, popular medicinal remedies, and eventually embryotomy.[24]

In 1581, the publication in Paris of some successful reports of caesarean section performed on live women, together with bold advocacy for the procedure, caused an uproar among physicians. The author, François Rousset, entitled his book *New Treatise of Hysterotomotokie [sic], or Caesarean Birth*, with the verbose and optimistic subtitle of "Extraction of the child through a lateral incision of the belly and womb of a pregnant woman not able to give birth otherwise. And this without detriment to the life of one or the other, and without hindering subsequent maternal fecundity." The idea horrified most contemporary physicians, who doubted the authenticity of the cases cited and considered Rousset's claim both absurd and incredible. Jews studying medicine at that time were aware of the controversy. For example, Rodrigo de Castro and Isaac Cardoso each published a Latin text on gynecology and obstetrics and discussed the possibility of a caesarean operation on a live woman, as described by Rousset. De Castro believed that this procedure should be done only in extremis. Whereas de Castro's analysis was devoid of Jewish sources, Cardoso did refer to these sources, quoting the Mishnah and Talmud on the subject.[25] In the early eighteenth century, another Jewish physician, Tobias Cohn (1652–1729), considered this fashionable, new medical issue in light of the talmudic references. In contrast to the *Marrano* de Castro (who had converted to Judaism), Cohn had received a traditional Jewish education in Poland. He wrote a Hebrew encyclopedia, *Ma'aseh Tuvya* (Venice, 1707), in which he described delivery by *yotze dophen*:

> Sometimes it is not possible to remove the fetus by the efforts of the midwife, nor by any medicine, and the only way is by skillful removal through the walls of the womb. This is [done] for one of three reasons. . . . First, if the woman is already dead. Second, if the woman is alive and the baby is dead. Third, even if the woman and the baby are alive but there is a great delay preventing the exit of the baby through the vagina. Then one calls the specialist who cuts one of the abdominal walls. (. . . This seems strange to the learned reader of this chapter as this practice is not done on Jewish women, may God protect them. Yet our learned fathers mentioned this in the *Gemara* [commentary on the Mishnah] and now I am explaining their words.) And now I will give you to understand correctly that when a woman dies she does not need [magic] tricks, as the midwife can extract the baby by a tear with her hands. And when the fetus has died in the womb and the mother is still alive, it is not with ease that one performs the tear; it is the custom of the doctors to extract it with a drug that expels it, or to remove it limb by limb using in their hands an iron tool with a chain [shown in an accompanying illustration]. However if despite all these [methods] the birth is prevented and the baby delays there [in the womb] for many days, then it is necessary to perform the cut. This is apparently the deed done by Mathieu C . . . on the woman whose baby died and remained in her womb for four years and in the end was removed through the wall without any damage. Many books [mentioned] such actions but for the love of brevity left out [the details].[26]

Tobias Cohn went on to describe the necessary equipment and precautions for performing a caesarean delivery and gave step-by-step instructions for the procedure. He ended his chapter with quotations from the Talmud regarding the purification laws that pertained to a woman delivered in this way.

Modern Times

Only in the twentieth century, with improvements in hygiene, anesthesia, obstetrical knowledge, and surgical techniques, has the procedure become reliably successful, and the frequency of caesarean deliveries has risen steadily. One reason for this increase was the medical theory that if a woman gave birth once by caesarean section, any subsequent babies she bore had to be delivered in the same way. Physicians today, however, appreciate that the Talmud was correct in assuming that some women can indeed give birth normally after a caesarean section, although it remains difficult to imagine that this would have been possible two thousand years ago.

In 1879, an anthropologist named Felkin observed a successful caesarean operation in an isolated community in Kahura, Uganda. The woman was anesthetized with wine, like the mother of Rustam.[27] This observation suggests that a caesarean section performed in this way could also have been possible among other peoples long ago. Thus, Jews may have performed this operation successfully in the talmudic period.

Jewish law regarding mother-baby priorities became relevant in a recent case. In early 1992, the district court in Jerusalem (a secular and not a religious court) ruled that a doctor should deliver a certain baby by caesarean section if the mother died, in the hope of saving the infant's life. The mother was in her seventh month of pregnancy and comatose, and her doctor expected her to die shortly: her opinion could not be obtained. The court ruling went against the father's and grandparents' objections, which were based on their belief that they could not take on the responsibility of caring for a premature baby who was likely to suffer severe developmental difficulties. The legal question was whether the unborn baby's rights to life had priority over the family's desires. The district court referred to Jewish law in reaching its decision to save the baby's life, but before the ruling could be carried out, the baby was born naturally, and the mother's condition improved noticeably.[28]

DEATH OF THE FETUS OR INFANT

Explanations

It is human nature to seek explanations for events in our environment, especially for traumatic events. In the past, infant mortality was more common than today, often the result of poor maternal health and diet, lack of hygiene, protracted labor, and lack of medical expertise. Jews have looked for medical explanations and therefore have studied the natural causes and physical conditions that could inhibit a safe delivery. At times, they also blamed midwives for carelessness and, if these midwives were non-Jews, for inflicting malicious harm. Jews have also turned to God and wondered why innocent newborns should die, if God is merciful and just.

The theological problem of why the innocent suffer, while those who are wicked seem to live long and happy lives, has worried many Jewish philosophers. Could it be that the tragedy of stillbirth is a test by God of the faith of the bereaved parents? The Psalmist taught that a person is humbled to learn God's law, and Job's faith was tested by the death of his children.[29] Or is the reason for an infant's death that the parents are not wholly righteous? The Bible attributes the death of the newborn son of King David and Bathsheba to David's adultery. The Mishnah attributed maternal death to a woman's failure to observe her religious duties, as discussed previously. Sa'adia Gaon (882–942) rationalized that the death of the innocent baby could bring a reward in the World to Come.[30]

In medieval Spain, the Zohar taught that a baby's soul was blemished by the sins of its parents. God foresaw the blemish and allowed the infant to die. God enabled such a baby to die at the hands of Lilith, a female demon, before it lost its sweetness.[31]

The Hasidei Ashkenaz, in medieval Germany, believed that an infant died on account of the father's sins, its mother's failure to observe the purification laws, the name chosen for it, or evil spirits in the family's place of residence. *Sefer Hasidim* tells of a man who went to his rabbi and begged him to pray for his wife to conceive, if the infant would survive. If the rabbi could see that the infant was fated to die, however, the man wanted the rabbi to pray that his wife not conceive. He clearly knew the pain caused by an infant's death and feared it. The rabbi replied that an infant, whether alive or dead, redeems his parents from death. He consoled the man by telling him that some parents are fated to suffer, but such suffering is redeeming.[32]

In 1597, the wife of Hayyim Vital imagined that the souls of her sons who had died in infancy became sparkles of light in a pool in a great courtyard that was due to be their father's share (when his time came) in the Garden of Eden.[33]

Mourning

In Jewish tradition, parents are not obliged to observe the mourning ritual (described in Chapter 6) after stillbirth or the death of an infant within thirty days of birth, and therefore, in the past, it was not customary to mourn this loss formally.[34] A baby who survived for thirty-one days and then died has always been ritually mourned, however, because by this time he or she deserves the "dignity of the departed." The time factor stems from a biblical ritual whereby a first-born son is redeemed only one month after his birth, and the talmudic sages therefore concluded that he acquired viable status only at this time.[35] In modern times, Jews have questioned this tradition because a baby born at full term can be viable and yet die for some unforeseen reason within one month, whereas another baby sustained in an incubator for several months before dying does not become independently viable even after thirty days. The Jewish mourning ritual disrupts everyday life—work stops for a full week—and Jews clearly had to draw a line somewhere concerning the mourning of a lost baby, when this was a common occurrence. How does one not mourn a stillborn baby or an infant who survived birth and died soon after, however? One wonders again, as with pregnancy loss, whether through the ages the sages and rabbis did not mourn a stillbirth or an infant who died within a few days or weeks of delivery. Did they simply decide not to express their grief? The answer appears to be that Jewish fathers felt little emotion at the loss of a newborn, unless perhaps they still had no heir. Rabbis have explained that the lenient approach to the mourning laws in this case was so as not to add sorrow to the occasion, to allow a parent to forget the episode quickly. Maimonides generalized that parents' love for a newborn is not so great as it is for a one-year-old child, and especially a father's love for a newborn is weak, unlike his feelings when the child reaches the age of two or three years. Maimonides' choice of words, first mentioning parents, and then focusing only on the father, leaves one wondering whether he had perhaps observed a mother's distress at losing her newborn and knew that women suffered more than men in his day.[36] A father had had no time to create a bond with his infant, whereas a mother had already nurtured the child for months.

Like ritual mourning, circumcision, naming, and burial of a lost infant preceded rabbinic rulings on these behaviors, and customs have varied from one community to another. The Bible and Talmud tell that a stillbirth was not accorded a formal burial; it was cast into a pit or hidden in the ground without a grave. The Talmud, but not the Bible, explains what to do when an infant younger than thirty days old dies: with only two men for company, a woman carries it out in her arms and buries it. If a baby dies when it has lived a full month or more, but less than a year, it is buried ceremoniously, but in a small coffin, and formally mourned. (If the infant is more than a year old, it is wrapped in a shroud, taken to the cemetery on a bier, and buried without a coffin.) The Jews in Babylonia in the gaonic period introduced the custom that a baby boy who was stillborn or who died within the first week of life be circumcised and named before burial, without blessings, for fear that, without circumcision, the infant's soul would go to Gehenna. (The Midrash tells that Abraham sits at the gates of Gehenna to save the circumcised from entering.) Rabbis in medieval France advocated this custom to avoid the shame of leaving the foreskin in place. Although the custom of circumcising a dead fetus was controversial in medieval Europe, this practice was eventually incorporated into the Shulḥan Arukh. One of the medieval antagonists, a thirteenth-century circumciser in Germany, wrote that a premature baby who died was not to be circumcised because God would send an angel to remove the infant's foreskin and give it to a dead Jew who had sinned, to prevent him from entering Gehenna. Some later Ashkenazi and Sephardic rabbis also objected to circumcising an infant "who never saw the light," on the grounds that these infant foreskins benefited sinners by enabling them to escape perdition (in Gehenna). In the eighteenth and nineteenth centuries, circumcision was not always done on an aborted fetus; it was a matter of local custom.[37]

At the turn of the twentieth century, the Sephardic chief rabbi in Hebron ruled that a daughter who was miscarried or stillborn be named before burial. Nevertheless, not all Jews have followed this custom, either.[38]

Traditionally, Jewish parents have not attended the burial of their newborn infant; the burial society makes all necessary arrangements, and still today many advise parents against attendance. Some Jewish burial societies bury the infant with an older person, whereas others bury the infant in an unmarked grave. Some burial societies do not inform parents where the infant is buried; others do.[39]

The death of an infant is a distressing and traumatic experience for all members of the family, not only for the mother and father. In 1978, Judith Lasker's first-born daughter was stillborn, and she wrote a book, together with Susan Borg, whose first-born son had died two weeks after his birth, to discuss openly the feelings and methods of coping with the tragedy of losing a baby, as well as the social implications of these experiences. These women described how some people found comfort in religion, mourned in their own way, and said the *Kaddish* prayer every year on the day that their baby died, whereas others found themselves questioning or rejecting God as a result of their loss. In 1985, Shelly and Jeffrey Allon's first-born child was stillborn; they discovered that a support group in which they could share their emotions with other couples was an important factor in coping with the tragedy in their lives. Because there was no such group where they lived, they started one, which continues to offer support to others who meet with such bereavement today.[40]

Although traditionally the Jewish community has had a social conscience and has helped those in need, no positive attention was paid in the past to the needs of a couple who lost an infant at or soon after birth, even though children have always been so important to the community. Now some Jewish communities are offering support groups, in which members can mourn as Jews as well as share their emotions and learn skills to help them cope with family, with society, and even with attempting a new pregnancy.[41] Some recent personalized alternatives to the Jewish mourning ritual are offered in Chapter 6.

Stillbirth

Stillbirth can be traumatic. The story of a woman who "lost her youth" from the experience was told in a jewelry shop over a necklace of pearls, perhaps a century ago, in Vitebsk:

> "My mother used to have a string of pearls . . . Hers were old and yellow. They'd belonged to my grandmother, and must have got dull against the old woman's wrinkled neck. My mother was left an orphan very young. But someone put the string of pearls around her neck at her wedding. It was the only thing that had come down to her from her own mother . . . My mother brought nine children into the world," Mrs. B. went on, "and for each birth she wore the pearls. She believed it would bring her mother to her bedside to bless her and the newborn infant. 'The pearls shine brightly,' said my mother, 'and they'll make my children bright and beautiful too. Aren't you as lovely as a pearl?' she used to say to me."
>
> A bashful smile passed over Mrs. B.'s face, then vanished. She sighed, and her voice grew sadder too.
>
> "Once my mother had a child that was stillborn. She didn't know it was dead, but she asked the people looking after her to see what was the matter, because she felt as if ants were swarming all over her. They found the pearls scattered in the bed. The string had broken. She couldn't take her eyes off them. She was bathed in sweat, and they looked to her like tears.
>
> 'The baby's dead, isn't it?' she said.
>
> She lost her youth at the same time as the necklace. She didn't have any more children. . . . You see the power pearls have?"
>
> Mrs. B. looked up.
>
> "And now I shall have my own string of pearls. I'll wear them always. Perhaps I'll bring something beautiful into the world too. I'm still young."[42]

Elegy to a Dead Infant

On January 18, 1943, in the icy Vilna ghetto, the Yiddish poet Abraham Sutzkever (b. 1913) mourned the loss of his infant son in the following elegy, entitled *To My Child:*

Because of hunger
or because of great love—
your mother will bear witness—
I wanted to swallow you, child,
when I felt your tiny body
cool in my hands,
like a glass
of warm tea.

Neither stranger were you, nor guest.
On our earth, one births
only oneself, one links
oneself into rings and the rings into chains.

Child, the word for you would be love
but without words you are love,
the seed of dream,
unbidden third,
who from the limits of the world
swept two of us
into consummate pleasure.

How can you shut your eyes,
leaving me here
in the dark world of snow
you've shrugged off?

You never even had your own cradle
to learn the dances
of the stars.
The shameful sun, who never shone
on you, should shatter like glass.
Your faith burned away
in the drop of poison
you drank down as simply
as milk.

I wanted to swallow you, child,
to taste
the future waiting for me.

Maybe you will blossom again
in my veins.

I'm not worthy of you, though.
I can't be your grave.
I leave you
to the summoning snow,
this first respite.
You'll descend now
like a splinter of dusk
into the stillness,
bringing greetings from me
to the slim shoots
under the cold.[43]

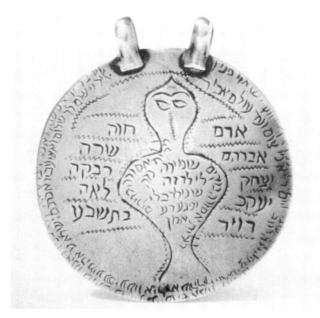

A

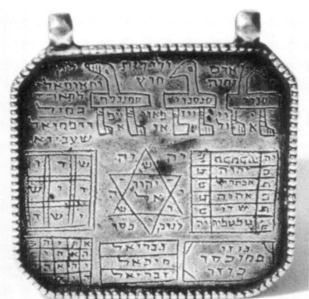

B

Plate 14A and B. Protective childbirth amulets. Silver, Persia, nineteenth and twentieth centuries. Collection of Itzhak Einhorn, Tel Aviv. A, Lilith, with adjuration "Lilith is bound" inscribed inside the demon's figure, and statement that this amulet protects the newborn from harm. B, Protective inscriptions against Lilith, according to *The Book of Raziel.*

Photos: Yacov Brill, Beth Hatefutsoth Photo Archive.

Chapter Ten

Lilith, The Demon Who Threatens Women in Childbirth

The myth of Lilith in all its various forms—in rabbinic commentary and biblical exegesis, in Hebrew literature and mystical prayer books, on pottery bowls and silver lamellae, in an ethical will, in remedy books, and in old wives' tales—was no mere local superstition, legend, or fairy tale, nor was it magic. It was a reflection of reality; it offered an explanation for the common phenomenon of death in childbirth.

The myth of a bloodthirsty demon who preyed on women in childbirth and who sought to strangle newborns was common in non-Jewish cultures in the past, but as the myth developed among Jews, it acquired Jewish characteristics. Lilith, who was given this role, eventually featured in Jewish cosmology as a demon that God created at the same time as Adam. She became queen of evil, whose lust was awakened by Eve's sin in the Garden of Eden and who was out to avenge herself on Eve and all Eve's female descendants.

The earliest expressions of fear that this demon would harm a woman in childbirth appeared in written incantations. Throughout the ages, Jews fashioned protective amulets to ward off this danger.

ANCIENT ORIGINS

Lilith originated in the spirits of ancient Mesopotamia. The single mention of Lilith in the Bible (Isaiah 34:14) depicts her resting in the wilderness, amid wildcats and jackals. This scene came from local myths: around 2000 B.C.E., the ancient Sumerians of Mesopotamia feared a female demon named Lillake, who had fled to the desert. Soon after, cuneiform incantations in ancient Babylonia told of demons named Lilu, Lilitu, and Ardat Lili ("maid of the night"). One of the Lili, Lamashtu, was a wicked female who slew children, drank the blood of men, and caused nightmares. Also in biblical times, the Assyrians fashioned amulets for protection against such dangers, in the form of winged figures or representations of the head of the demon; a cord threaded through holes in the demon's ears enabled these amulets to be worn. Sometimes, these amulets bore incantations against the demon, or a version of the myth about the evil spirit. In addition, a winged demon was featured on a Phoenician-Canaanite incantation text for safe childbirth, dating from the seventh or eighth century B.C.E., found in northern Syria.[1] Thus, in biblical times, local non-Jews feared that a demon caused the death of a woman or her infant in childbirth.

In the sixth century B.C.E., when the Jews were exiled to Babylonia after the destruction of the First Temple, they must have heard these local myths explaining death in childbirth. A few centuries later, Alexander the Great conquered Babylonia for the Greeks, and soon a Greek version of the myth emerged: Lamia ("The Devourer") was said to have enjoyed a short affair with Zeus, whose jealous wife, Hera, robbed Lamia of her children. In her fury, Lamia killed and devoured every child she could find. Like Lamashtu, Lamia was known also to seduce sleeping men, to suck their blood, and to eat their flesh. Like the ancient Babylonian demons, Lamiae were sometimes referred to in the plural, as harmful spirits.[2]

TALMUDIC PERIOD

A Greek manuscript, *The Testament of Solomon*, which is an amalgam of Jewish, Christian, Hellenic, and Eastern material, written some time in the first centuries of the Christian era, relates that King Solomon met a female demon who roamed the night visiting women in childbirth and who sought to strangle newborns:

> And I adored the Lord God of Israel and . . . there came before me a spirit in woman's form, that had a head without any limbs, and her hair was disheveled. . . . She said, "I am called among men Obizuth, and by night I sleep not, but go my rounds over all the world and visit women in childbirth . . . and if I am lucky, I strangle the child . . . for I am a fierce spirit of myriad names and many shapes. . . . But, as now, though you have sealed me round with the ring of God, you have done nothing. . . . You will not be able to command me. For I have no work other than the destruction of children. . . ."[3]

Solomon's ring, with the Ineffable Name inscribed on it, was the king's primary source of power over the demons. In the foregoing passage, however, the demon declares herself to be immune to the power of this ring, so the king must discover what other power will prevent her from inflicting harm.

The text continues, revealing how Solomon cunningly learned from the evil spirit the name of the angel that frustrated her action. This was an angel of God called Afarof, which (by *gematria* on the Greek letters of this name) was Raphael (one of the archangels, whose name means "God is healing"). The evil spirit revealed that when this name was written on a woman in childbirth, she could not fulfill her bloodthirsty purpose.

Solomon proved his supremacy in his cunning; he had the evil spirit tied, bound, and displayed near the Temple to all the children of Israel so, as they passed by, they could see her and glorify the Lord God of Israel.

The talmudic sages wanted to discourage the practice of magic, so the Talmud refers only briefly to Solomon's familiarity with magic. Because the sages explained death in childbirth as a punishment for sins, it is no wonder that the Talmud makes no mention of a female demon who strangles children. It warns, however, of a demon named Lilith, a winged female with long hair, who for sexual pleasure seizes men sleeping alone, and it mentions spirits and demons named Lilin, allegedly begotten by Adam during his long separation from Eve after the murder of Abel.[4]

Although the Talmud excludes the myth of a demon who preyed on women in childbirth, the myth did not disappear. Another magical handbook dating from the early talmudic period, *The Book of Mysteries* (*Sefer ha-razim*), written in midrashic Hebrew, includes some Greek magic and warns how to guard against an evil spirit so that it would not visit a woman in childbirth and kill her baby. This text advises writing the names of angels on four silver lamellae and hanging these on the four walls of the room during childbirth.[5] Archaeologists have excavated such amuletic silver lamellae in Israel.

GAONIC PERIOD

During the gaonic period, Jews in Babylon used magic bowls to protect against a child-killing demon. Such bowls, excavated at Nippur, Mesopotamia, and dating approximately from the sixth to the eighth centuries, were buried under the threshold of houses for protective purposes. Some of these bowls were specifically used for protecting women during childbirth and lying-in. Such bowls had an Aramaic incantation against the demon, telling the fearful legend and naming the women requiring protection, written concentrically around the inside of the bowl, sometimes surrounding a drawing of a female figure. One bowl describes the physical appearance of Lilith; others tell of a wicked demon named Sideros, who had killed all twelve sons of a certain woman. The woman fled to a mountain, where she fashioned copper and iron for her protection, but Sideros nevertheless found her and killed her last newborn son. The woman then invoked four angels, Swny, Sswny, Sngru, and Artiku, who chased the demon and found it in a great sea, Pelagos. The demon swore in the name of God (quoting Isaiah 40:12) that she would have no power wherever the names of the angels appeared. The text restrains all demons, including one named Lilith, by pronouncing them bound and ends with a quotation from Song of Songs (3:7–8): "Encircled by sixty warriors of the warriors of Israel, all of them trained in warfare, skilled in battle, each with sword on thigh, because of terror by night."[6]

Israeli archaeologists discovered almost the identical legend inscribed, also in Aramaic, on a thin sheet of silver excavated in Israel. This amulet was not Babylonian, but local to Israel, and the names cited showed a Greek influence.[7]

Medieval Christian versions, in Ethiopic, Coptic, Syriac, and Greek, of a demon who kills newborns suggest the existence of an earlier Greek form of the story.[8] Instead of the name Sideros (meaning "iron" in Greek), the demon in the Ethiopic version is Verzelya, from the Hebrew and Aramaic words for iron (*barzel, parzela*). A Coptic story, in Arabic, relates an episode in which Saint Susniyus killed his sister, a demon who preyed on newborns. The Syriac version of this story depicts a witch who tried to kill newborns, was chased into the sea, and promised to desist if the names of the three angels were written on an amulet. Several late medieval Greek manuscripts relate a legend similar to the earlier Aramaic versions, with helpers named Sines, Sisinnios, and Saint Senodoros.[9]

The Jewish myth of Lilith was developed in a midrash, *The Alpha Beta of Ben Sira*, of Eastern, possibly Persian, origin some time in the latter half of the gaonic period. This midrash portrays Lilith as Adam's first wife, who quarreled with him over their manner of sexual intercourse and refused to lie beneath him because they were both equal; God had formed them both from the earth. Uttering the Holy Name of God, Lilith flew away in anger. At Adam's request, God dispatched three angels to bring her back, if necessary by force. As in the legend on the bowl and the story on the silver amulet, the angels found her in the sea. She swore in the name of God that the names of the three angels—Snwy, Snsnwy, and Smnglf—would frustrate her harming newborns.[10] The aim of the tale was apparently to instruct readers on how to make an amulet to protect a woman in childbirth; that the angels failed to return Lilith to Adam was of no consequence to the story.

Ben Sira inserted several new elements into our tale. By portraying Lilith as Adam's first wife, he gave a reason for the demon's vile purpose. He did this knowing that the first chapter of Genesis indicates that God created a female at the same time as Adam, and therefore Eve was not Adam's first partner.[11] Some Jewish sages in Palestine in the fifth century agreed that the first female that God created may not have appealed to Adam,[12] but the quarrel over the couple's style of sexual intercourse was Ben Sira's addition, in keeping with his penchant for lascivious stories.[13] Similarly, his idea that Adam's first sexual partner was the infamous demon Lilith—not Eve— was an elaboration of the already well-known rumor that Adam had coupled with female spirits, including some called Lilin, after the death of Abel. Moreover, although the talmudic Lilith was winged, Ben Sira enabled her to fly only when she uttered the magic name of God. Thus, he cleverly added threads of his own as he wove together Jewish legends about Adam with existing myths about Lilith, to create a plausible and interesting reason for the use of amulets to protect women in childbirth.

Ben Sira's was the first Hebrew rendering of the story known today. A later version of *The Alpha Beta*, known in Europe since the eleventh century, repeats the full story, yet addresses the problem of why the angels did not return Lilith to Adam as he had requested. When the angels demanded that Lilith return, the later version adds, she told them that she had been defiled when sleeping with the Great Demon and therefore, according to Torah, could not return to her husband.[14] This invention set the scene for the zoharic embellishments of Lilith. More than a hundred versions of Ben Sira's story have been preserved, in Hebrew, Arabic, Persian, Latin, and Yiddish.

MEDIEVAL KABBALAH

Lilith gained popularity in Jewish circles also through the Book of Zohar, in which earlier elements of female demonology appear in the many depictions of Lilith. Child killer and seductress, Lilith is also portrayed as the immortal queen of the forces of evil (the Other Side), partner of Samael, the Great Demon with whom she coupled in the later version of Ben Sira's tale.[15] An evil spirit since the beginning of Creation, she waited in the depths of the sea until Adam and Eve had sinned, then roamed the world seeking to snatch the souls of babies.[16] In a moralistic tone, the

Zohar teaches that Lilith cannot harm an infant conceived in holiness, because in such circumstances God assigns angels to supervise its divine studies during pregnancy (as described in Chapter 5). If a man is not holy when uniting with his wife, however, he draws a spirit from the Other Side, and Lilith comes and plays with that child. If she kills him, she takes away his soul.[17] Following the rabbinic line, the Zohar explains that tragedy in childbirth occurs as a result of some impiety on the part of the parents, but adds that Lilith carries out the job. This text does not mention Snwy and his partners or any protective amulets.

Another passage in the Zohar relates that Lilith collaborates with God to destroy newborns destined to be evil or blemished. While such a newborn is still small and sweet, Lilith torments the infant and removes it from the world while it is sucking innocently at its mother's breast.[18] She feasts off the body, freeing the soul, if it is pure, to soar "to the topmost heaven," where God redeems it. If the soul is not pure but blemished, Lilith takes it to the Other Side, where only the coming of the Messiah can redeem it. The Zohar suggests that parental impiety, the sins parents accumulated in previous transmigrations, and the overall number of sins in the world are all reasons for the claiming of a newborn's soul by the Other Side.[19] Thus, the Zohar views Lilith as having a positive role in God's great plan for the world, because she helps to bring about death when this is an infant's destiny.

LATER KABBALISTIC VERSIONS

A fourteenth-century manuscript of practical Kabbalah includes the Lilith legend in the medieval Greek version, with Greek names. A century later, a Greek Christian version, in which a witch on her way to harm newborns meets Saint George, was adapted by the Jewish community of Crete. In this Jewish rendition of the story, the evildoer is renamed Lilith, and, instead of the saint, she meets the archangel Michael. Later Jewish versions replace the archangel with the prophet Elijah, who cancels the demon's evil powers with an adjuration. Sometimes alternative names, influenced by local versions of the legend, were given to the evil spirit, and display of these names (instead of those of the angels) provided the protection from harm.[20]

In a manuscript, *Paths of Life*, an ethical will from Venice in 1544, Rabbi Eleazar the Great warned his son about Lilith:

> Do not leave an infant in his cradle alone in the house by day or
> night, nor pass thou the night alone in thy abode. For under such cir-
> cumstances, Lilith seizes man or child in her fatal embrace.[21]

Scholars have tried to guess which Eleazar this might have been, suggesting namesakes in the ninth and eleventh century, but the rendering of Lilith at the same time as a child killer and succubus suggests familiarity with the zoharic portrayal, and therefore it is unlikely that the foregoing warning antedates the thirteenth century.

In the sixteenth and seventeenth centuries, Lurianic kabbalists elaborated further the legend of Lilith. Naphtali ben Elhanan Bacharach (early seventeenth century) repeated the zoharic warning that Lilith tampered with sperm from improper sexual relations.[22] Hayyim Vital cautioned that Lilith could appear in the form of a black cat, a goose, or another animal, and therefore advised that animals be kept well away from the birthing and lying-in room. He also warned that the danger of Lilith's harm extended for forty to sixty days after birth (in contrast to eight days after the birth of a boy and twelve in the case of a girl, in Ben Sira's version).[23] He taught that an infant who laughed in its sleep should be tapped on the nose, because Lilith could be playing with it and the tap would avert such a danger.[24] These ideas soon became established as Jewish folklore.[25]

Two other kabbalists (David Lida, a rabbi in Amsterdam around 1700, and Hayyim Yosef David Azulai [1724–1806], a rabbi in Hebron who traveled widely) retold the story of Lilith, with gory details, in their instructions for writing childbirth amulets.[26] In these instructions, the display of esoteric names of the female demon, and not the names of the angels, provided protection against harm, as in the medieval Greek versions.

The version on many eighteenth-century paper amulets extant today is as follows:

> In the Name of the Lord, God of Israel, whose Name is great and awesome; Elijah the Prophet, remembered for good deeds, was on his way when he was confronted by Lilith and her cohorts. He said to her "You wicked, impure spirit, and all your impure entourage, where are you going?"
>
> "My lord Elijah, I am going to the house of (x daughter of y) who has just given birth, to give her the sleep of death and to take the newborn son to drink its blood and suck the marrow of his bones and eat of his flesh."
>
> Elijah the Prophet, of blessed memory, replied: "You shall be excommunicated and stopped, by the blessed Name; you will become like a silent stone."
>
> "For the sake of God's Name, remove this curse from me and I shall cease [this activity] and swear to you by the Name of God, Lord of Israel, to leave the lying-in woman and her newborn; as long as I hear my names, I am restrained [from this activity] and now I shall inform you of my names and for as long as they are mentioned I and my cohorts shall have no evil power to enter the house of a lying-in woman and do harm. These are my names: Lilith, Abitu, Abizu, Amzarfo, Hakash, Odem, Ikpodu, Iylu, Tatrota, Avinukta, Satruna, Kalicatiya, Tulatuy, Piratsha."

Scholars have tried unsuccessfully to trace the origins of these names. Some of them are similar to names mentioned in earlier Greek versions.[27]

A folktale from Kurdistan provides yet another version of the myth of Lilith in Jewish folklore. The story tells of a time, more than a hundred years ago, during the Ottoman Empire, when Jews lived peaceful and fulfilling lives, carrying out their duties as written in the Torah:

A Jewish woman felt that she was about to give birth. She called for the elderly midwife, who had learned her skills from generations of mothers and grandmothers before her.

The midwife immediately set to work and prepared an infusion to ease delivery. She gave it to the laboring woman, who took one look at it and fainted, collapsing on the earthen floor. To her horror, the midwife saw a long hair in the drink that she had just prepared. She fished out the hair, put it in a leather bottle of milk, and tied the neck of the bottle tightly. With all her strength, the midwife hit the leather bottle with a stick. Suddenly a shout was heard from the bottle. It was a woman's voice screaming, "Help, help, I ask for pity!" Carefully, the midwife opened the mouth of the bottle and the head of a female demon popped out.

"Evil one, what are you doing in this house?" asked the midwife.

"It is our custom to visit the house of a woman about to give birth. We smell the scent of the newborn. We steal the woman's womb and give it to our children to eat. Then she dies." It was Lilith in the bottle.

The midwife grabbed Lilith by her hair and told her, "We shan't let you go until you tell us how we can save this woman from your powers."

Lilith told her to take some saliva from the unconscious woman and put it in a pail of water. The demon blew on it, and the woman awoke from her faint. The midwife recited incantations from an amulet on her necklace and delivered the woman of the baby safely. Later, the men of the house checked the mezuzzot on their doorposts and found some that needed replacing. The new kosher mezuzzot kept Lilith away.[28]

In this story, the demon revealed to her captors how to curb her powers as she had done in *The Testament of Solomon* hundreds of years earlier, in Ben Sira's story, and in amulet versions through the ages. Here, too, she was kept away by a protective amulet, by the mezuzzah on the doorpost of the house.

PROTECTIVE AMULETS

Since antiquity, many Jews believed, like other peoples, that they could avert harmful powers with amulets inscribed with magical formulas. The large numbers of childbirth amulets that have survived the ages reveal that this custom was part of Jewish life until the advent of modern medicine. Jews fashioned amuletic pottery, jewelry with engraved incantations, and parchment, paper, or cards with amuletic inscriptions for multiple protection against the dangers of Lilith, the Evil Eye (a demonic force that could strike at any time, at the height of one's good fortunes—a force attributed to witches, magicians, demons, or even another's envy, especially after the birth of a boy), and any other demonic forces.

In the nineteenth and early twentieth centuries, some Persian Jews engraved or painted protective inscriptions on stone, and Jews in the Ottoman Empire embroidered a name of God (Shaddai) and the names of the protective angels (Snwy and partners) on cloth, for example on the headdress that a woman wore when lying-in.[29] Some Jews buried amulets below the floor of the room where a mother gave birth; others tied their amulets on themselves and on their newborn infants, and yet others hung them on doorposts, walls, or curtains of the room or on the bed and cradle.

Since talmudic times, amulets for protection against Lilith, like those used for other purposes, often bore adjurations, magical names, biblical quotations, even an illustration, and a personal dedication. A person needing the amulet was usually identified by the mother's name and not the father's, the custom also when Jews prayed for a sick person.[30] (In contrast, a person is usually identified paternally in Jewish ritual.) When an amulet was passed on to another who needed it, a new dedication was sometimes superimposed over the first owner's name, or the amulet was merely copied out for reuse.[31] Although kabbalists warned that only persons properly initiated in practical Kabbalah should issue such amulets, any literate craftsman or scribe could follow instructions in a book of charms, without necessarily understanding the magical secrets of the words and symbols. In the early twentieth century, printing houses in Jerusalem mass-produced amulets for protection in childbirth and in the home. A circumciser who recommended the use of certain amulets kept exemplars in his register.[32]

Adjurations

An Aramaic fragment discovered among the Dead Sea Scrolls, probably dating from the first century C.E., consisted of an adjuration against a male poisoning demon and a female poisoning demon, for protection in childbirth (and prevention of disturbing dreams in sleep). The inscription repelled the demons "by the Name of He who forgives sins and transgression."[33] We do not know whether it was used by Jews or by the earliest Christians in the Judean desert.

As discussed earlier, *The Book of Mysteries* (Palestinian, talmudic period) gave instructions for making a childbirth amulet that followed a similar form of adjuration against an evil source. Moreover, the magic bowls from Babylonia featured a more detailed form of adjuration, spelling out the nature of the danger and pronouncing the demonic force to be bound and restrained.

A Jewish woman about to give birth in Egypt in the Middle Ages also made use of a protective amulet with adjurations to ward off all sorts of demons and demonesses, male and female evil spirits, Lilin and Lilitin (the latter being the plural of Lilith). The adjuration was pronounced "in the name of El Shaddai [Almighty], from whom you tremble, and of whom you are afraid, and in the name of Michael [the archangel], your master, and in the name of Ashmedai [Asmodeus, king of the demons]."[34]

The Book of Raziel, which combined cosmological material from *The Book of Mysteries* with medieval practical magic, offered an esoteric formula in the name of God, followed by an adjuration:

I adjure you, First Eve, in the name of God who created you, in the name of the three angels whom your creator sent after you, and the angel in the isles of the sea, to whom you swore that wherever you will find the names of you and your cohorts and your servants, no harm will happen. Whoever will carry their names and the seals of their names written here, I adjure you and your cohorts and your servants that you cause no harm to the woman in childbirth, x daughter of y, nor to the child who was born to her. . . .[35]

This adjuration was attributed to Eleazar of Worms (1176–1238) and was probably used by the Hasidei Ashkenaz, but it may be a version of an earlier text. It was preserved, perhaps edited, and eventually published in the foregoing form, in 1701. Since then, it has been reprinted frequently.

Divine Names

Jews commonly inscribed on amulets various names for God, such as El Shaddai, previously mentioned, others made from combinations of the four letters of God's name (the tetragrammaton), and yet other magical names made of twelve, forty-two, and seventy-two letters.[36] Some of the names for God, as well as the names of the angels, date from two thousand years ago. Over the centuries, the Jewish mystical tradition devised more and more magical names. The esoteric derivations of some of these are now unknown.

Kabbalists believed that the magical names of God carried the effective power, but because of the angelic liaison between God and mankind, the names of angels were essential features of protective childbirth amulets. Thus, the charm recommended in *The Testament of Solomon* invoked Raphael, and the medieval amulet preserved in Egypt called on Michael (both these sources mentioned other angels, too). The silver lamella and the bowls invoked the triad associated with Lilith (Swny and partners).

The Book of Raziel offered an amuletic formula, attributed to Eleazar of Worms, which invokes seventy named angels, reminiscent of the seventy ministering angels mentioned in the Apocrypha.[37] It also depicted the figures of the three protective angels, three birdlike creatures, "as Adam saw them and drew them . . .", with their names (Snwy, Snsnwy, and Smnglf) inscribed on their bellies, and three other esoteric images with the same angels' names above. Both sets of drawings had "Adam and Eve" and "Out Lilith" written in Hebrew above them. These were frequently copied onto paper or metal and used for protection in childbirth and lying-in.[38]

Biblical Quotations

As discussed earlier, the Babylonian bowls included biblical quotations in their incantation texts. The medieval Egyptian amulet included a long magical name made up of the first letters of each word of Psalm 91. Since talmudic times, Jews have considered this psalm, also called *Shir shel pega'im* ("song against evil spirits") or *Vi-hi no'am* (the last two words of Psalm 90), antidemonic. By quoting only a few of its sixteen verses, the reason for this attribution is clear:

> That He will save you from the fowler's trap, from the destructive plague. . . . You need not fear the terror by night, or the arrow that flies by day, the plague that stalks in the darkness, or the scourge that ravages at noon. . . . No harm will befall you, no disease touch your tent . . . (Psalm 91:3–10).

Through the ages Jews recited this as an incantation to ward off evil spirits, so it was a natural choice for protective amulets.[39] A verse of this psalm appears in a "tried and proved" formula in *The Book of Raziel*, for an amulet to protect mother and newborn from sorcery, the Evil Eye, and wicked demons. The verse was inscribed between two circles, together with the names of protective angels, "Adam and Eve," "Out Lilith," and "First Eve."[40]

A popular handbook of Jewish magic, *The Use of Psalms* (*Shimmush tehillim*), dating from the gaonic period, recommends Psalm 126, *Shir ha-ma'alot* ("a song of ascents"), for protection in childbirth.[41] In Yiddish-speaking communities, however, Psalm 121, also a song of degrees, was so commonly inscribed for protection during and after childbirth that Jews referred to such an amulet as *Shir ha-malot-tsetl*, "the charm of the song of ascents." Again, by quoting a few verses, the reason for choosing this verse for protection becomes apparent:

> The Lord is your guardian, the Lord is your protection at your right hand. By day the sun will not strike you, nor the moon by night. The Lord will guard you from all harm; He will guard your life (Psalm 121:5–7).

Jews sometimes also included the Priestly Blessing on childbirth amulets, for protection against the general harm of the Evil Eye:

> The Lord bless you and protect you! The Lord deal kindly and graciously with you! The Lord bestow His favor upon you and grant you peace (Numbers 6:24–6).

Similarly, Jews often chose extracts from Jacob's blessing to provide immunity from the Evil Eye: "I wait for Your deliverance, O Lord!" and "Joseph is a fruitful bough . . ." (Genesis 49:18, 22).

The verses of Deuteronomy 6:4–9 ("Hear, O Israel! The Lord is our God, the Lord alone . . .") and 11:13–21, professionally inscribed on kosher parchment, have featured in a special form of amulet, the mezuzzah. Since biblical times, Jews everywhere in the world have followed the injunction of Deuteronomy 6:9 to fix these verses to the doorpost of rooms in which they live. Many Jews believe that the mezuzzah is generally protective. By the end of the gaonic period, Jews added the divine name Shaddai to the reverse of the parchment. A letter of congratulation on the birth of a son, written by a professional scribe during the Middle Ages, told that he had written an amulet ("a protection, but the Protector is God") for the safety of mother and newborn and also sent a mezuzzah, certainly destined for the lying-in room.[42] Shaddai amulets have been used for general protection in all Jewish communities, but in Italy, especially, ornate ones were fashioned specially for protection of newborns and were kept by the child as a protective charm throughout his or her life. When a woman gave birth, she hung her amulet on her bed. The previously described folktale from Kurdistan revealed the popular belief concerning the protective powers of the mezuzzah, even against Lilith.

Iron Motif

Belief in the power of iron to protect women in childbirth was common among non-Jews in Palestine during the early talmudic period, because the sages of the era found it necessary to warn against this practice.[43] This belief was referred to in the inscriptions on the Babylonian bowls, too. The medieval amulet from Egypt included an interesting reference to iron, however. It warned: "If you should abrogate this, my adjuration, I will beat you with the iron rods of those four holy matriarchs, Bilhah, Rachel, Zilpah, Leah."[44] In this case, the iron was associated neither with pagan superstition nor with the demon of the bowls whose name (Sideros, "iron") had no relevance in Jewish tradition, but with the four biblical women (who bore Jacob's sons), whose initial Hebrew letters spell the Hebrew word for iron, *barzel*. The association of these four women with the magical power of iron was not limited to the medieval Jews in Mediterranean lands; it was accepted in the practical magic of the Hasidei Ashkenaz, among German Jews in the late Middle Ages.[45] The four biblical women gave Jewish character to a particular form of pagan magic. In later centuries, Jews in Germany and Alsace, North Africa, Bulgaria, Palestine and Syria, and Afghanistan continued to use iron, fashioned into the blade of a sword, knife, or sickle, for protection after childbirth.[46]

In Morocco, until recently, the iron blade featured prominently in a ritual to exorcise Lilith called *tahdid* (*hdid* being the Arabic word for iron). Moroccan Jews performed this ritual nightly during the first week after the birth of a son, until the circumcision. Family and neighbors gathered in the lying-in room after dark and recited a verse from the story of Noah, stating that "male and female of all flesh [were in the ark with Noah] and the Lord shut him in" (Genesis 7:16). At this point, the door of the lying-in room was closed, and the baby's father brandished the bare sword about the walls of the room. Recitations of the Priestly Blessing, the usual excerpts from Jacob's benediction, and Psalms 91 and 121, as well as Proverbs 3:24, followed. Women prolonged the ritual into the night, telling stories and thereby maintaining vigilance over the lying-in woman and baby. *Tahdith* is the Arabic word for telling stories.[47]

Fowl Motif

In some communities in the early twentieth century, Jews displayed a symbolic form of a fowl among charms for protection during or after childbirth.

Some Moroccan Jews slaughtered a cock after the birth of a boy and hung the head near the mezuzzah until after the circumcision, in the belief that the cock's head averted demons and evil spirits. Iraqi Jews hung the legs of the cock above the woman's bed.[48]

The figure of a fowl with a cock's head, limbs, and feathers bearing Hebrew letters with magical significance was featured on some childbirth amulets printed in Jerusalem. Jews throughout the Ottoman Empire as well as in Eastern Europe used these amulets in the early twentieth century.[49] These are different from the birdlike figures representing Lilith on Persian Jewish amulets and those representing the three angels in *The Book of Raziel*.

A colorful parrot on a childbed amulet from Alsace and two ornamental birds on protective cut paper amulets from southern Germany and from the Carpathian mountains, all made in the nineteenth century, probably reflect local folk motifs and have no magical connotations.[50]

"Tried and Proved" Amulets

An amulet that had been "tried and proved" by one person was often handed to another person with the same need. Writers and editors of remedy books knew the importance of this weighty recommendation, and by noting it for specific amuletic formulas, they contributed to the survival of these formulas through the ages. "Tried and proved" formulas, such as those in *The Book of Raziel*, were reproduced on childbirth amulets in almost every Jewish community worldwide since the book's first printing.

Pinhas Katzenellenbogen, a Jew who lived in the early eighteenth century in what is now southeastern Germany, wrote about such a "tried and proved" childbirth amulet. Soon after his wife, Sarah Rachel, died in childbirth, Pinhas met a kabbalist, Binyamin Binesh, whose book of charms and remedies, *Amtahat Binyamin,* was already popular in Germany and Eastern Europe. Fearing that his daughters would also have difficulties bearing children, the widower asked the wonderworker for a charm to prevent death in childbirth, because the advice in the book had not helped Sarah Rachel. Binesh wrote two words in Assyrian letters on a piece of white linen five fingers wide and seven fingers long—*p'nim* ("in"), on the side of the cloth that would face the woman's navel, and *hutz* ("out"), on the other side of the cloth—and explained in detail the proper position of the charm and when to remove it.

Pinhas remarried, and in due course his second wife learned of this charm. She lent it to all her friends, to safeguard their deliveries. One day, however, one of Pinhas' colleagues asked for the charm for his daughter who was in labor and never returned it, claiming that it was torn. Pinhas eventually found a scribe who made a copy according to Pinhas' descriptions. When his daughter eventually gave birth to a son, she had an easy delivery and did not need the magic charm, but perhaps Lilith was present after all because the daughter died after the baby's circumcision.[51]

The inscription of the two Hebrew words in Assyrian lettering follows an old kabbalistic custom and attests to the lingering belief in the power of ancient Near Eastern magic. These words probably had magical significance: the use of *p'nim* and *ḥutz* may refer to the custom of including Adam and Eve and excluding Lilith on amulets. Pinhas' friend, Binesh, was a *baal shem*, "Master of the Divine Name," someone who practiced a form of magic using holy names.

Amulets of Rabbi Eybeschutz

In the early 1750s, it was said that few women died in childbirth in Hamburg. The eminent talmudist and kabbalist, Jonathan Eybeschutz (1690/5–1764), was the rabbi of the community, and women believed that the amulets he made were particularly effective. However, he was accused of invoking on these amulets the name of the false Messiah, Shabbetai Zvi, whose apostasy had severely shaken Jewish communities less than a century earlier. Great arguments ensued between Eybeschutz (and his followers) and famous rabbis in many parts of Europe. The controversy eventually reached the civil court of the King of Denmark, and the king ruled in Eybeschutz's favor, but the repercussions of this scandal permanently damaged faith in amulets in the West, and their use waned.[52]

MODERN TIMES

As objective reasons for death relating to childbirth were identified, and as medical procedures were implemented to avoid such death, the need for mythic explanation and amuletic precautions dwindled. Nevertheless, amulets are still in use, pinned on a baby's clothing or hung on its cradle, among Jews born in North Africa, Syria, Ethiopia, and Yemen. Such amulets are used in Israel, as well, in hasidic communities, probably now more out of a lingering unease toward the Evil Eye and a feeling for tradition than from any real fear of Lilith.

Whereas in the past this myth provided an imaginative explanation where one was needed, today our knowledge overwhelms our imagination, and we are tempted to dispose of the myth. This myth still offers some insight into what to expect from life, however. Like other myths, it reveals the nature of what C.G. Jung called the collective unconscious, or the psyche. It admits some deep archetypal fears: our ever-present concern for our babies' survival; our own existential anxieties; and our fears of a partner's unfaithfulness. It expresses the shadow side of human nature— our animal instincts, our seductive and destructive appetites, which are dangerous if uncurbed. Lilith also provides a scapegoat for the destruction inherent in nature and for human evil.[53]

The myth of Lilith has gained new popularity among Jewish feminists. These women have highlighted certain elements of the myth to portray Lilith as a model of a powerful woman. They admire her struggle for independence, her courage in taking risks, and her claim of equality with Adam, in the version of *The Alpha Beta of Ben Sira*. They stress her power over men (achieved by playing with their potency, robbing them of their wives, and killing their babies) and point out that men have chosen to demonize powerful, threatening women.[54]

Part IV

Welcoming the Newborn

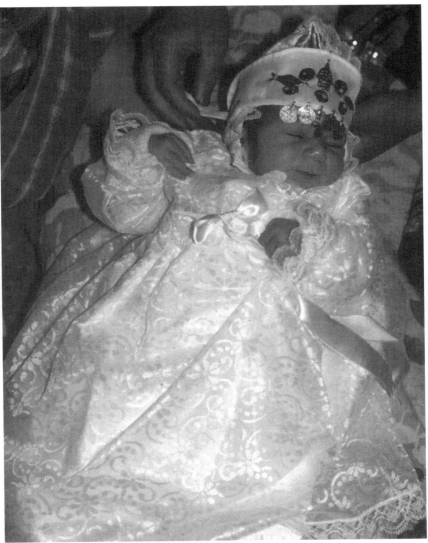

Plate 15. Baby with protective amulets, dressed for circumcision. Djerba, 1983.
Copyright: Keren T. Friedman Photography.

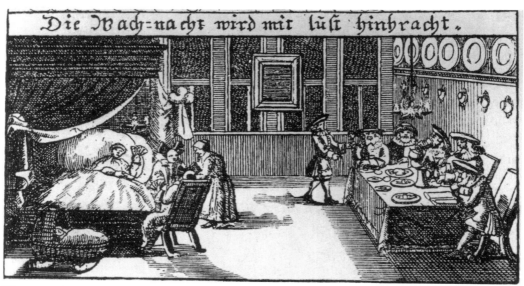

Plate 16. Lying-in scene. Peter Fehr (1981–1740).
Etching and engraving on paper. Schudt, J.J., *Jüdische Merkwürdigkeiten* (Frankfurt and Leipzig: 1714–1717). Jewish National University Library, Jerusalem.

Chapter Eleven

The First Week

CARE OF THE NEWBORN

Jewish legend tells that the baby's first cry is the cry of its soul forced by God to enter the vile matter of the impure world after its blissful existence in the womb.[1]

Receiving the Newborn

The obstetrician or midwife cuts the umbilical cord with a sharp tool, cleans the baby, and disposes of the placenta; in the past, the midwife also salted and swaddled the infant.

From biblical times until the early twentieth century, salting and swaddling were common practices in many Jewish communities.[2] Women thought that the salting of newborns was vital for the baby's skin, to thicken and harden it and thereby protect the inner organs, and to prevent rashes. Salt may help the navel to heal, but since biblical times it has been a well-known protection against the Evil Eye. Yemenite women in the early twentieth century added salt to the infant's bath in the hope that it would give taste to his future words and actions. Moroccan Jewish women today recall dropping a raw egg and a few gold bangles into the water, for strength and good fortune; they only wiped and cleaned the newborn in the first week and bathed it on the eighth day.[3] Eastern European Jews in the early twentieth century always washed a newborn in an old tub used previously for other babies who had grown up healthy. After the baby had been washed, the father and visiting relatives threw coins, *bodgelt*, into the bath, which the midwife kept for herself.[4]

Midwives swaddled babies, binding their bodies in a long cloth or strips of soft linen, to restrict their movements and straighten their limbs. In talmudic times, in Babylon, when a baby was at least a month old, midwives swaddled also the baby's head, to shape it. Later, in most communities, women swaddled a baby only from the shoulders down, covering the head with a little cap.[5] The age-old practice of swaddling continued into the twentieth century; today, hospital nurses often wrap a newborn tightly to restrict its movements. This swaddling effectively reduces the amount of time a newborn cries.[6]

Special customs surrounded the disposal of the afterbirth. Through the ages, people believed the placenta to be an extension of the baby and feared that if a stranger somehow acquired it, this person would gain control over the baby. Thus, the Talmud recommends that it should be hidden, a practice that remained prevalent among some Jews at the beginning of the twentieth century, when birth usually took place at home. The Talmud reports that rich people preserved the placenta in oil while the poor wrapped it in soft rags or straw, then buried it in the earth, just as the child who was once attached to it would also be buried eventually.[7] Until around 1900, the Jews of Palestine buried the placenta of a baby girl near the hearth, in the hope that she would remain housebound when she grew up: a wayward daughter was "one whose afterbirth was lost."[8] Sometimes the midwife exploited the placenta for its curative powers before burying it, for example, by allowing a barren woman to sit on it in the hope that she would absorb its nurturing force and conceive or for stimulating the newborn's breathing by rubbing the placenta on the infant's chest.[9]

Nursing by the Mother

Jews, like other peoples, have believed that a mother has a natural desire to nurse her baby and that any woman who is well enough should do so. In the past, however, women who were wealthy or who had twins often hired a wet nurse.[10]

Two talmudic homilies reveal that God enables the milk to come forth. One tells that, when Abraham arranged a banquet for the weaning of Isaac, he invited many people, but no wet nurse, and a miracle happened; Sarah's breasts filled with milk, and she suckled all the babies at the celebration (proving her motherhood, to counter rumors that Isaac had been adopted). The other story describes the straits of a man whose wife had died in childbirth and who was too poor to pay for a wet nurse; God filled his breasts with milk to feed the infant.[11]

Through the ages, Jews have insisted that a nursing woman maintain a good, healthy diet. For centuries, until the early modern period, they accepted the Greco-Roman idea that milk derived from retained menstrual blood. Therefore, to encourage and increase milk supply, a woman drank warming infusions (in wine or honeyed water) believed to thicken the blood and avoided cooling foods, such as cucumbers, melons, onions, garlic, and salty foods. Medieval obstetric treatises and later remedy books offered advice for both increasing and reducing a mother's breast milk. Until recently, Yemenite Jewish lying-in women drank hot milk with honey and clarified butter, Indian Jews preferred sweetened coconut milk mixed with dill seed, and Tunisian and Persian Jews favored black beer for increasing breast milk in the first week after birth. Ashkenazi Jews encouraged eating sweet and fatty foods, as well as meat.[12]

The Talmud also preaches discretion to nursing women; a husband could divorce his wife if she shamed him by suckling her infant in the street. An early eighteenth-century Ashkenazi remedy book quoted anonymous "moralist sages" who advised women not to bare their breasts to nurse in front of strangers lest the milk be harmed for "several reasons"—the expected harm was from the Evil Eye cast by the glance of others. In contrast, a rabbi in Baghdad in the early twentieth century said that when a woman is suckling, her breast is like her hand or face (that is, a functional part of the body): it is indecent to expose it only when she is not feeding an infant. Although one cannot generalize from these examples, other reports from the nineteenth and early twentieth centuries imply that perhaps Ashkenazi Jews were more prudish about suckling a hungry infant in public, whereas Sephardic and Middle Eastern Jews were relaxed about this practice.[13]

The medieval rabbis advised that a mother begin nursing with her left breast rather than her right, because the left breast is nearer the heart, the seat of wisdom. A few rabbis in the sixteenth and seventeenth centuries said that this advice applied only to sons, who have to become wise to understand the Torah, and not to daughters, who would not need this wisdom.[14]

Throughout the ages, the usual duration of breast-feeding was eighteen months to two years, but often longer, sometimes even five years; Jewish women traditionally nursed a sickly child for longer and weaned boys earlier than girls. In the nineteenth century, however, many Jewish mothers weaned their sons after one year, for fear that extended nursing would reduce their intelligence.[15]

For almost two thousand years, most Jews maintained that a mother who was breast-feeding a child should stop if she conceived, because her milk would be affected by pregnancy and could harm the nursling. As discussed in Chapter 3, the talmudic sages permitted a woman who was nursing to use a contraceptive tampon, because they feared that a new pregnancy would harm the milk and cause the death of the suckling infant.[16]

The same fear lies behind the mishnaic law that a nursing woman who has been widowed or divorced may remarry only after the infant she is nursing is eighteen or twenty-four months old (the usual duration for breast-feeding). One talmudic sage said a woman could remarry three months before she stopped nursing, because it would take three months for her milk to be affected if she conceived again after her wedding. Another sage said that a woman who is not nursing her newborn should wait three months before remarrying.[17]

Early in the eighteenth century, rabbis turned to these Jewish sources when a Jewish widow in Hamburg applied to remarry while her infant was being wet-nursed. She had lost her first three children in infancy and, when pregnant with the fourth, had been advised to hire a wet nurse for her next baby, for fear that her milk had poisoned the infants. She did this, and her next four children had been wet-nursed and survived. Her husband had died soon after the birth of the last child, and not long afterward, she chose to remarry. The rabbis disagreed among themselves about how long she should wait before remarrying, even though the mother was not nursing, and they argued long enough to delay the marriage.

Years later, in Prague, Rabbi Eybeschutz met the lady who had been the topic of this controversy. Impressed by her good health, he doubted the wisdom of the alleged medical reason for the wet nurse and consulted the medical faculty of Prague University for an expert opinion on whether a mother's milk could poison her baby. The reply was that the baby could be disturbed if a mother were upset, or if her diet were too rich or too thin, but a mother's milk could not harm her baby.[18] Nevertheless, in the nineteenth century, many Jews still believed that a mother's breast milk could harm her baby and even cause its death, and in such cases her husband had to hire a wet nurse.[19]

In the early eighteenth century, a Sephardic rabbi formulated a prayer for Jewish women to recite when nursing an infant, on the assumption that a good Jewish mother nursed on demand. This prayer was copied out into a woman's personal prayer book. In this prayer, the nursing mother asked God to grant her as much milk as her infant needed and the time and patience to nurse until the baby was satisfied. She asked God to lighten her sleep and sharpen her hearing so she would wake instantly when the infant cried. (She also prayed that she not smother her infant in her sleep, God forbid.)[20]

An ethical treatise written in the early nineteenth century, by Eliezer Papo (d. 1824) of Sarajevo, summarizes advice about nursing that men needed to know, because it concerned marital relations, breast-feeding on demand, a nursing woman's nutrition, and the baby's intellectual stimulation:

> If a woman lies with her husband, she should not breast-feed her son until half an hour has passed.
>
> If the child should cry for a quarter of an hour from some complaint connected with nursing, usually the reason is not known, but try to understand. . . . Certainly those women who leave their nursing children to cry for a long time, until they have finished doing everything they need to do, will be judged when the time comes.
>
> Books have warned not to nurse boys a long time as this causes them to become stupid. . . . these are things that have no meaning, because if the baby is weak, one should not hurry to wean the child or he will remain weak forever. It is said of a great man [that his soul] transmigrated a few years after he died; he had to suffer this punishment for having weaned his son before time, for fear the son would be stupid, but the boy was weak all his life.
>
> The nursing woman must take care with her own nutrition, so that she eats foods that encourage good milk. She must not eat foods that are bad for her milk and for the child's nutrition. And while she is nursing the baby her and her husband's minds should be on Torah . . . and he should study next to the boy so that his ears will become accustomed to the words of Torah. . . .

Whoever did not heed this advice, Papo warned, could suffer in the World to Come. Papo's advice to wait at least half an hour after sexual relations was classic; the Zohar had made the same recommendation more than five centuries earlier. In these ways, he encouraged fathers to take an interest in their babies. Furthermore, Papo's advice was particularly relevant for fathers who held the pursestrings, who needed to be aware that a nursing wife or wet nurse had to eat well. In the case of a wet nurse, Papo stipulated that the father not dismiss her until the infant was strong enough for weaning.[21]

Through the ages, Jewish women were encouraged to feed their infants on demand, as much as the babies desired. In the nineteenth century in some parts of Europe, and in the twentieth century elsewhere, however, medical advice changed, and infants became accustomed to fixed feeding times. A Hebrew handbook, published in Lemberg in 1821, taught how to raise a child according to "medical wisdom"—to nurse at fixed intervals. A century later, *Falksgesundt*, a Yiddish paper about health published in Vilna, instructed mothers to wake their sleeping infants to nurse them at the correct times. Jewish mothers living in Moslem lands and in Asian communities nursed on demand until they met with modern Western medicine, sometimes only recently.[22]

A woman born in Jerusalem in 1905, of Yemenite parentage, talked in 1969 about the changes she noticed in the younger generation regarding nursing:

> The strongest sign for me that women today are not really mothers is that they do not have milk even for their first child. How can that possibly be? Is there a single organ in the body that God made for no reason? Can it be that God brings a baby into the world and stops up its mother's breast? No, heaven forbid, this is not God's doing! It is the fault of the women: today they do not nurse with their heart and soul and therefore their milk goes away. The milk in our body is not a standing store, not a package that you open and use whenever you need it. . . . it is a living source, like a spring, which begins in a woman's heart. If a woman does not want to breast-feed, the source dries up.[23]

The woman repeated the ideas maintained in Jewish sources, that God fashioned the female breast for the purpose of nursing and that milk comes from the blood. Yet by involving her heart and soul, she also revealed the spirituality that she found in suckling her infants.

Nowadays, we know that some toxic substances, such as drugs and alcohol, pass through breast milk and affect the baby; we know, too, that a woman's milk flow can be reduced if she is tense, but it should return to normal if she relaxes, rests, and eats well. Moreover, medical fashion has returned to breast-feeding on demand. This natural female function, vital for an infant's survival until recent times, has become an art that some women do not want to learn or for which they cannot find the time. Of course, today many women use infant formula, to enable others to feed the baby and thereby free themselves for work.

Because breast-feeding usually delays the resumption of ovulation after childbirth, it often provides a natural form of contraception for a few months. Ultra-Orthodox Jewish women who choose not to nurse conceive again quickly and have large families, fulfilling the duty of being fruitful.

Wet Nurses

The Bible states that Rebekah and Joash were wet-nursed, and the Talmud reports the hiring of a wet nurse when twins are born and when a mother dies leaving a surviving infant. The Talmud also reveals that a wet nurse should be paid a fee and should eat nourishing foods, but nothing that could harm the baby.[24]

A medieval Hebrew handbook about childbearing repeats classical advice about choosing a wet nurse:

> A good wet nurse to wean a child is a woman who has given birth twice, whose skin coloration is pleasant and good, whose chest is

wide, and whose breasts are not dried and wrinkled, also not bigger or flatter than is seemly, and whose breasts do not have ruptures. Her body should not be short and small and she must be wise and diligent, patient and compassionate, clean and charming.[25]

In addition, the author of this handbook advised that a wet nurse needed to eat healthily, wash regularly, and desist from sleeping with a man.

In the sixteenth century, a medical case study involved a wet nurse. The case study actually concerned the treatment of syphilis. Amatus Lusitanus (1511–1568), a *Marrano* physician, wrote of a man infected with syphilis, whose wife bore him two healthy boys. During her third pregnancy, she developed ulcerations and lumps in her breasts and gave birth to an infant with a syphilitic rash. The mother was unable to nurse her newborn, and a wet nurse was employed. Within one month, the infant had infected the nurse, who infected her husband and two other infants she was suckling, who in turn infected their mothers. Amatus Lusitanus treated all the patients with mercury. The baby who had been born with the illness and his father died, but all the others were cured. This story provides a good reason for choosing a wet nurse known to be healthy and for checking out the health of any other babies she was nursing. These conclusions were not drawn by the physician, however, whose interest lay only in the treatment of syphilis.[26]

Since antiquity, when a Jewish wet nurse was unobtainable, a Gentile one was found and came to live with the baby's family. Alternatively, the baby was sent to live in the Gentile's home, a fate no Jewish mother wanted for her child, but sometimes the only solution. The wet nurse could become a good family friend, but she wielded power because she could leave, or claim that her milk would be affected, if she did not have her own way.[27] Parents therefore needed to take care when choosing a wet nurse, although in small communities they may have had little choice.

Relations between Jews and their non-Jewish neighbors sometimes led to legal problems when the baby and wet nurse were of different faiths. For example, according to a thirteenth-century document, a Moslem family in Egypt employed a Jewish wet nurse and sought permission to buy meat for the household from a Jewish butcher so the wet nurse could eat with her employers. In another record from the same period, a Jewish woman agreed to nurse a Moslem boy while nursing her own son. She died, and it was impossible to establish which infant was Jewish and which was Moslem.[28]

In medieval Europe, anti-Semitic Church rulings sometimes extended to the employment of wet nurses. In 1366, for example, the Synod of Avignon renewed an already existing interdiction against Gentile wet nurses taking employment from Jews and forbade Gentiles to employ Jewish wet nurses.[29]

Some Jewish communities eventually issued legislation and favored contracts stating the conditions for employment of wet nurses. These contracts were sometimes documented in community records. Contracts stipulated the fee, and sometimes also the sleeping arrangements of the wet nurse or of the baby. For example, in Lithuania, in 1637, the local Jewish council stipulated that a wet nurse's hiring depended on her marital obligations. She was expected to live with the baby's family and therefore could be employed only if her husband were away or if she were widowed. The ruling further stipulated that a woman could work as a wet nurse against her husband's will only if a doctor decreed that this would be a lifesaving act.[30] In Cracow, a wet nurse was hired in 1650 with a written agreement between the father of the newborn and the husband of the nurse, stating the fee to be paid and the condition that the baby would be nursed until weaned.[31]

The sterile teats and infant formula that became available in the twentieth century finally enabled women to dispense with wet nurses and all their associated problems when, for whatever reason, a mother did not nurse her child.

CARE OF THE MOTHER

Delivery

As discussed in earlier chapters, until recently, childbirth was a time when a woman, and indeed all her family, feared she would die. The danger did not pass with delivery. "Childbed fever," which developed in the days after giving birth, was frequently fatal. Talmudic rabbis thought that the sickness was due to catching cold on the birthstool and offered a warming remedial potion of herbs cooked in beer. The fever was more likely a sign of a septic infection, however. Severe uterine bleeding was also common, and the Talmud offers a potion for this, too. In later centuries, many remedy books provided recipes for curative potions for childbed fever and bleeding. Midwives bound parturient women's abdomens tightly in the hope of stopping such bleeding, but often these remedies were to no avail, and women died "even while conversing."[32]

The Talmud acknowledges that a woman who has just given birth is in mortal danger and therefore advocates treating her as an invalid for the first thirty days.[33] In talmudic times, she was attended by other women, who believed that her limbs were disjointed from the immense physical strain of labor and delivery.[34] They kept her room warm, prepared chicken soup and warm infusions for her to drink, and helped take care of her baby. These women prepared food for her that was intended to reduce uterine bleeding, heal and strengthen her, and increase her supply of breast milk.

Bitter experience strengthened the association between birth and death, however. Jews acknowledged their proximity in various ways—in song, in prayer, in ways of addressing a woman after birth, and in clothing.

A welcoming song of the Jews of Sana'a, Yemen, verbalized the presentiment of death after a birth:

If only you could know, oh sisters,
What I perceived at the moment of birth.
I felt relaxation in my bones
I sensed the taste of death.[35]

Soon after the birth, when strong enough to attend services, a Jewish mother sometimes offers prayers in synagogue, including a benediction thanking God for showing kindness in her deliverance from mortal danger, *birkat ha-gomel.* This talmudic prayer is also recited on other occasions when a Jew has narrowly avoided death. Sometimes a new mother also recites verses of Psalm 116, some praising God for showing compassion and some affirming the close scrape with death, for example:

> The Lord is gracious and beneficent; our God is compassionate. . . .
> You have delivered me from death, my eyes from tears, my feet from
> stumbling. I shall walk before the Lord in the lands of the living
> (Psalm 116:5, 8–9).

In addition, the mother has often added a prayer that the child grow strong and wise, live according to Jewish law, become a worthy member of society, and comfort and support her and her husband in old age.[36]

In the early twentieth century, many Jews referred to a new mother by a special name in local dialect, reflecting her precarious state of health, even her closeness to death. Thus, Yemenite Jews referred to such a woman as one who had been reborn, North African Jews spoke of one who had undergone deliverance, and Eastern European Jews named her as one who needed to be indulged in everything.[37]

In Yemen until recently, a woman who had given birth wore a ceremonial gown when first receiving her guests on a Sabbath after the delivery. The gown was richly embroidered with traditional symbolic patterns and was borrowed from an older woman who wore it again on the eve of the Day of Atonement and finally on her deathbed.[38]

Today, an element of fear surrounds birth, but the experience of tragedy is rare enough that women do not usually believe that they will die at this time. Thus, specific prayers for childbirth are often omitted from modern prayer books, we are no longer congratulated for our deliverance, only for the baby's safe arrival, and few women own a ceremonial gown. Ashkenazi Jews serve lentils and chickpeas on the first Sabbath after a birth, however, the custom also after a funeral, to console the new mother for the baby's loss of the knowledge learned from the angels while in the womb.[39]

Postnatal Depression

The arrival of a newborn is a moment that parents long anticipate, and for many parents it is a happy time, but not for all. It is important to differentiate between life-threatening psychotic breakdown and the depression of a woman who has little or no help, who is exhausted, lonely, overwhelmed, and despairing that she cannot cope with the demands of motherhood, or the depression of a woman who feels rejected by her husband for bearing him a daughter or a child with a serious health problem. A woman who had expected joy on first seeing her newborn may be too exhausted from the trauma of birth to feel anything but a desire to sleep. She may not feel a bond with her baby until she begins to nurture the child, a natural process that may be delayed, destroyed, or rejected, when the infant is cared for by someone else—in the past, when it was wet-nursed, but nowadays, when the infant is removed for special care. Miriam Shomer Zunser described a mother's feelings about her newborn's arrival in a crowded household in Russia in the late nineteenth century. Dinneh had just delivered her fifth child, and the turbaned midwife told her gently that the infant was a boy. Dinneh did not cheer at this news, however. Four times she had brought a child into the world, but each one had departed to an early grave. Dinneh's body was sore and sick, and her soul was low and lost in the dark world about her. She had not seen her husband for months, and she had no money with which to call a doctor or to buy the medicine she sorely needed. Her father, too, was away on business. Her mother was overwrought and begrudged her the extra work she caused; Dinneh dared not ask her for anything.

Dinneh begged the old servant Sosche to bring her secretly a little extra soup from the family pot and to buy her a bottle of ergot (to reduce her bleeding), although she had no coins with which to reimburse her. Old Sosche soon came back with the medicine and soup and tried to cheer up poor Dinneh, who lay in bed despairing over how she would keep her newborn alive, after her four others had died. Dinneh had no idea how she would find money to buy swaddling clothes and to pay the wet nurse. (She never thought of nursing her own baby.)

The next day, Sosche brought her a letter from Vilna. Dinneh was not interested: she no longer expected anything from her husband. As she opened the envelope, however, two Polish rubles dropped out. From her husband, two new Polish rubles! Dinneh sat up and smiled. Two rubles seemed a vast fortune to her. Perhaps her husband could and would provide for her and her newborn after all. For the first time in ages, Dinneh dared to hope for a better future. She cradled her infant in her arms, and her tears fell on his tiny face.[40]

Emma Goldman (1869–1940), who worked as a midwife among Jewish immigrants in an overpopulated neighborhood of New York before she became a famous anarchist, noticed the terrible depression of lying-in women whom she visited. At a loss to help alleviate their predicament, she decided to teach and lobby for birth control.[41]

Acute postnatal depression occurred sometimes after the birth of a daughter when a son was anticipated, and a stigma often accompanied the birth of a girl, especially in Middle Eastern and Asian Jewish communities. In these societies, some husbands snubbed their wives when a girl was born instead of an expected son and heir.[42] This problem was first documented in the early nineteenth century, although it must have existed earlier. Eliezer Papo was moved by the misery and neglect of a woman who had borne a daughter. He wrote how foolish it was for a husband to refrain from greeting and visiting his wife at such a time, because "it was not as if she had gone to market to choose him a girl and not a boy."[43] Yosef Hayyim (1834–1909), a rabbi of Baghdad, also noticed the suffering of such women:

> A woman who bears only girls will be neglected and in her great distress can harm herself [immediately after] the hour of birth. She is in a critical condition, and the damage will not be effaced. Her family and friends, husband and in-laws deride and scorn her as if she had committed a terrible crime.[44]

In Israel, some thirty years ago, some immigrant fathers from Morocco and Kurdistan refused to visit their wives in the hospital when they had given birth to daughters.

Since medieval times, many Jewish communities have organized benevolent societies to help lying-in women, by offering food, clothes for the baby, and provision for circumcision in the case of a newborn boy. Some Jewish communities still offer postnatal help today, especially in ultra-Orthodox neighborhoods where the birth rate is high. Such a community may provide a special rest home where a woman can recover quietly, away from her family, granting her perhaps the only real chance she has to rest. The community may also have a fund offering financial aid with the expenses of birth and circumcision.[45]

Of course, some countries now distribute postnatal aid through municipal social services. Money may not be enough, however, because when a woman has the added stress of poor relationships with members of her household, like Dinneh, she may be less able to cope with her newborn than if she were in an emotionally supportive environment.

In the nineteenth and early twentieth centuries, doctors and midwives sometimes labeled a woman's feelings of unreality, delusions, hallucinations, and even infanticidal impulses after giving birth as psychosis of exhaustion, the result of extreme physical exertion. The family dismissed signs of psychological problems during pregnancy as "caprices of pregnancy" and did not find these signs unduly worrying; perhaps they pampered the woman more as a result. When her mental condition collapsed after childbirth, however, more often than not, the woman's family as well as society declared her insane.[46] A talmudic sage reported that a nursing woman once killed her baby to remarry sooner than the accepted time for her wedding, and the Talmud declares that no sane person would do such a thing. We do not know the woman's story. In the twentieth century, however, rabbis as well as psychiatrists have come to recognize the threat to mother or infant posed by postnatal psychotic breakdown and the need to find a cure for this malady.[47]

CELEBRATING THE FIRST WEEK

Greeting the Newborn

Since antiquity, the mother learned of the safe arrival of a boy or a girl from the exclamations of the women attending the delivery: "When a child is born, everyone rejoices, and more so when it is male" (*Leviticus Rabbah* 27.7).

A father recited a traditional blessing on hearing the good news of his baby's safe delivery. For a son, he recites: "Blessed are You, Lord our God, King of the Universe, who are good and beneficent." For a daughter, he recites: "Blessed are You, Lord our God, King of the Universe, who has granted us life and sustained us and enabled us to reach this day" (*B. Berakhot* 59b).

These blessings are said also at other happy occasions in Jewish life.

For as long as births took place at home in many North African and Middle Eastern Jewish communities, the birth of a boy was announced with great fanfare by the ululating of women. Every member of the community made the effort to congratulate and bless the proud father personally. When a girl was born, however, the women attending the birth reported that mother and baby were well, wished a blessing of good fortune on the daughter, and often added the hope that, with God's help, the next child would be a boy.[48]

Welcoming verses sung in some Jewish communities reveal the mixed emotions that often accompany a baby's arrival. For example, a welcoming song popular among Sephardic Jews in the Balkans until the early twentieth century combined blessings to mother and baby, praise to God, and some words about relationships:

"Woman-giving-birth, may God guard you from all harm and cherish you, according to the desire of your mother's heart! You have given birth to a baby boy; angels, protect him from all harm!

Not for nothing were your pangs of labor, you gave birth to a handsome son. We are thankful to Him that He has awarded us this happiness.

The newborn will be a good omen! Look at the door, new mother, and see. Pretty maidens entering, each saying to each other: who will give us such a one!

We thank the Lord who privileged you with this celebration."

The new mother answered:

"Summon to me my husband and I shall complain to him of the many pains he caused me. Summon to me the midwife so that she won't alarm my mother. Summon to me my brother to give me a gift—a fowl to make soup."[49]

The last verse shows the woman's resentment toward her husband, her care for her mother, and her expectations of help from her brother.

Yemenite Jews sang a similar type of welcoming song until the middle of the twentieth century in the form of a dialogue between the lying-in woman and her visitors. Here the new mother mentions her close scrape with death and her relief at her deliverance; the song lists her immediate needs and the itemized blessings of all her extended family.[50]

Some twenty years ago, in Chicago, Daniel and Myra Leifer could not find an appropriate Jewish expression for their feelings after the birth of their child, which had been a profound religious experience for them both. They wanted to share their blessings and their joy, immediately and privately. Two hours after the birth, when they were alone with their newborn, the couple said together the seven wedding blessings in Hebrew and English with a cup of wine. This was not traditional, but it was meaningful for them.[51] The Leifers looked only to the rabbinic sources for religiously celebrating birth and were apparently unaware of the welcoming songs sung in some Jewish communities, whose words and melodies are also part of Jewish tradition, part of the oral heritage handed down from mother to daughter.

Unfortunately, for most of us it is too late to ask our mothers or grand-mothers to teach us these welcoming songs, because they themselves do not know them. However, musicologists are taking an interest in this special type of folk music and are trying to preserve it.[52]

Specific Celebrations

If mother and baby are well, the first week after delivery is a time for cel-ebration, and family and friends visit the new parents. The "week of the son," cele-brated since talmudic times, culminates with the circumcision, although Jews have also celebrated the first week after the birth of a daughter.[53] Traditionally during this week, the father hosted festive meals for the visitors, who brought gifts or money for the midwife or nurse and sometimes for the baby, too. It was customary for candles and lamps to burn all week: the light was an expression of rejoicing, as well as a pre-caution against harmful demons, who worked in the dark.[54]

Most celebrations in the first week have focused on the Shabbat. Shabbat is a day of rest and of happiness, and the birth of a baby adds to the atmosphere of happiness and rejoicing. Many Jews have marked the birth of a son by a celebration on the first Friday evening. This celebration is known as *shalom zakhar*, from the tal-mudic saying "as soon as a male (*zakhar*) comes into the world, peace (*shalom*) comes into the world" (*B. Niddah 31b*). Friends and relatives fill the home or synagogue and join the family in prayer and a festive meal, or after the meal, for fruits and grains. The feast has been called *yeshu'a ha-ben*, the salvation of the son, to rejoice in the baby's salvation from the mother's womb.[55]

Asian and North African Jews have celebrated *Shabbat avi ha-ben* ("the son's father's Shabbat"), in which the father is the center of the festivities in the synagogue; well-wishers join him in prayer and singing on the Friday evening and on the Shabbat morning. The songs include blessings for father, mother, and baby, expressions of hope that the boy will grow up wise, and *piyyutim*—liturgical poems. The father feasts the guests at his home after the synagogue and gives the children sweets. If he is wealthy, he gives money to charity on this occasion; if not, others give money to provide for the circumcision expenses. Until the middle of the twentieth century, Jews in Eastern com-munities also celebrated at the end of the first week. Thus, Jews in Kurdistan, Iraq, and India gave a party for children on Friday night, although more commonly on the sixth night after the birth, the "Night of *Shashah*," a noisy occasion with much singing and feasting, when children were given popcorn. Jews in Yemen celebrated the first or sec-ond Shabbat after a delivery, depending on the mother's condition. Men visited with the father while the women sat with the new mother for a short while.[56]

Celebration of the first Friday night has not been customary among all Jews. Since the late middle ages and until the early twentieth century, some Sephardic Jews visited a lying-in woman during the first week and gathered in her home on the night preceding the circumcision (see later in this chapter and the discussion in Chapter 12), but not on the first Friday night.[57]

Many Jews have also celebrated the first Shabbat after a daughter's birth.[58] They honor the parents in the morning service, and then the parents make a festive *kiddush*—a prayer recited over wine before the meal to consecrate the Sabbath and the happy occasion. Family and friends share in this festivity. If the mother cannot attend services on the first Sabbath after giving birth, this celebration is sometimes postponed to a later Sabbath when she can attend.

Although all Jewish communities have celebrated the first week after a child's birth, local differences have been reported. The visits during the first week have primarily been social expressions of joy: in the early fourteenth century, Jews in southern France sang and danced in the home of a lying-in woman, while sitting vigil with mother and baby (boy or girl) every night of the first week.[59] This noisy celebration was not customary in every medieval Jewish community, however, and certainly not among the Ashkenazi pietists, or among Jews in North Africa, who would have celebrated the "week of the son" but not of a daughter.

Ashkenazi Jews in the Rhine valley and in the region of Fürth in Germany, but apparently not elsewhere, practiced a custom in the early fifteenth century that was derived from the need for candlelight before and during the circumcision ceremony.[60] The candle made for burning during the circumcision was known as *Yidschkerz*, or *Yidish-kerts*, derived from the German word for candle, *Kerze*. On the fifth day after the boy's birth, the synagogue beadle announced in the streets of the town "*Zu der Yidish kerts!*" because it was time to prepare the circumcision candles. Female relatives and friends visited the lying-in mother and then sat in her house to make the candles that would be necessary for the circumcision. First, they prepared a large wax candle that was to remain lit until the third day after the ritual, and then they made twelve plaited candles representing the twelve tribes of Israel. They said a little blessing or a prayer as they picked up the wick and rubbed the wax over it, just as they did when making candles for Yom Kippur. The women told legends about the sons of Jacob who fathered the tribes of Israel. They knew which characteristics were desired in the newborn boy, and they hoped that as he grew up he would be a pride to his family and community.[61] This custom died out in the nineteenth century.

Sometimes Jews have added religious and protective nuances to their social gatherings. For example, the recitation in the lying-in room of the *Shema* prayer, "Hear, Oh Israel; The Lord is our God, the Lord alone . . ." (Deuteronomy 6:4–9), has provided religious content to the occasion. Traditionally, a woman who had just given birth did not recite this prayer, and therefore, family and visitors gathered in her room every evening to do so. Its protective value against demons, recognized in talmudic times, gave added relevance to this custom.[62] In the last three hundred years, in Eastern European communities and in the countries to which Eastern European Jews emigrated, yeshivah boys have briefly visited lying-in women and their newborn sons to recite the *Shema* every evening of the first week. This custom has replaced the nightly celebrations in Orthodox families. The boys are rewarded with honey, cakes, and sweets. (Girls sneak to the door to try and obtain some goodies too, because they are excluded from the gathering.) The custom has spread outside Eastern Europe, because Jews in Debdo, Morocco, also recite the *Shema* and invite yeshivah boys to recite psalms in the lying-in room on the days preceding the circumcision.[63]

As described in Chapter 10, Moroccan Jewish women gathered on the third or fifth day of the first week, to bless the newborn infant in local fashion, in addition to the nightly *taḥdid* gathering of men. Although the *taḥdid* was originally a ritual to keep away evil spirits, in the twentieth century it became a religious occasion, with participants studying the Zohar and reading Psalms.

In the first half of the twentieth century, Jews in India celebrated the fifth or sixth night after a birth, visiting the new mother and bringing gifts for the baby. Foods symbolic of fertility were laid out, and the women feasted and sang.[64]

These home celebrations in the first week became less appropriate when women started spending this week in hospital maternity wards. Orthodox Jews limited the visit of yeshivah boys for reciting the *Shema* to the night before the circumcision. A new father still often celebrates the birth of his child on the first Shabbat, and friends and family visit during the first week, but many Jews now limit celebrations to the circumcision and, in the case of a daughter, to a *kiddush* in the synagogue, or to some other form of party, described in the next chapter.

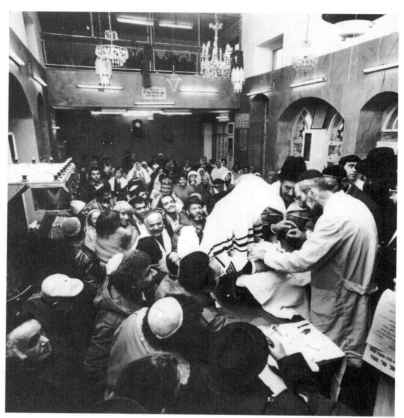

Plate 17. Circumcision ritual. Old Persian Synagogue, Bukharan quarter, Jerusalem, 1984.
Photo: Werner Braun.

Chapter Twelve

Ceremonies of Welcome: Rituals

The Bible prescribes certain postnatal rituals. Therefore, Jews traditionally circumcise their newborn sons, and, when the child is the mother's first-born, some perform a redemption ritual. Some Jews hold a joyous welcoming ceremony to name and bless a newborn girl, but this custom does not stem from the Bible. Biblical law dictates that a woman ritually purify herself after giving birth. In addition, the Bible mentions a weaning celebration, which never became part of Jewish ritual.

CELEBRATION OF A NEWBORN SON

Circumcision

> Such shall be the covenant between Me and you and your offspring to follow which you shall keep. Every male among you shall be circumcised . . . and that shall be the sign of the covenant between Me and you. And throughout the generations, every male among you shall be circumcised at the age of eight days. . . . And if any male who is uncircumcised fails to circumcise the flesh of his foreskin, that person shall be cut off from his kin; he has broken My covenant (Genesis 17:10–14).

The Covenant

The circumcision is the most important of all the religious ceremonies after birth. Jews circumcise their baby boys on the eighth day after delivery if the infant is in good health. Jews have imbued the rite of circumcision with great spiritual significance because it maintains the Covenant between God and Abraham, between God and the Jewish people. The Bible warns that one who does not fulfill this duty is "cut off" by God from the community; he receives the ultimate divine punishment, because God cuts off his soul from its spiritual source. Throughout the ages, rabbis have offered at least twenty different reasons for the importance of circumcision, revealing contemporary beliefs and tensions surrounding the ritual.[1]

Ritual circumcision involves the excision of the prepuce, the tearing of the mucous membrane to expose the glans penis, and suction of the wound, followed by its dressing. Father and circumciser recite blessings. The foreskin thus removed and the flow of the infant's blood are the Jew's offerings to God. In this way, a boy is given full membership in the Jewish community.

All Jewish parents who live according to halakhah circumcise their new-born son joyfully because this is a mitzvah, a divine commandment. This operation may stimulate complex emotions in a secular Jew, however. These emotions may include spiritual feelings and pride in Jewish continuity, but they may also include fear over a primitive sacrifice, confusion, distress, and even crisis over Jewish identity. Performance of this rite can make parents aware of the importance of continuing Jewish tradition, or it can become the focus of a conscious rejection of Jewish life. In addition, circumcision can be an occasion that cements family ties or an issue for family crisis. Thus, today, more than ever before, circumcision can have spiritual, religious, social, educational, and psychological significance.

Historical Perspective

Abraham and his Israelite descendants were likely not unique in circum-cising their sons: others in the ancient Near East probably did so, too. The Bible refers several times to mass circumcision of adult men, hardly an individual confirmation of a divine covenant, but more likely a result of social coercion to remove the disgrace of the foreskin—the Israelites clearly considered the foreskin contemptuously.[2] Even though the generation of the desert was uncircumcised, and the operation was some-times neglected during the Kingdoms of Israel and Judah, Genesis 17:10–14 elevated circumcision into a religious rite with individual religious significance.[3]

When the Greeks, and later the Romans, issued prohibitions against cir-cumcision, the religious ritual gained renewed importance in defining who was a Jew. Antiochus IV Epiphanes (c. 215–c. 163 B.C.E.) prohibited the rite, and mothers who had their sons circumcised were thrown off the city walls after being paraded de-meaningly around the city with their infants tied to their breasts. The Roman Emperor Hadrian (76–138 C.E.) similarly prohibited the rite and decapitated Jews who performed it on their sons. The early Christians in Jerusalem also rejected cir-cumcision, a step that had profound repercussions in later centuries.[4]

The Mishnah explains how and when to perform the operation. In the many volumes of Jewish law formulated during the first few centuries of the Christian Era, however, no tractate is devoted to circumcision. Circumcision was dis-cussed frequently at that time, but in the context of other Jewish laws, especially those pertaining to the Sabbath. In addition, during the talmudic period, the sages told many stories about the merits of circumcision, to stress its importance. They said that were it not for circumcision, heaven and earth would not exist. They taught that per-formance of this duty is proof of a Jew's acceptance of God, enables him to enter the Promised Land, and prevents him from entering Gehenna.[5] At that time, non-Jews in Palestine and in Babylon viewed circumcision as a mutilation and forbade it. In response, rabbis stressed that circumcision removes a blemish (the foreskin) and enables a man to achieve bodily perfection by fulfilling a divine commandment.[6]

The animosity toward circumcision of non-Jews continued into the Middle Ages, reinforced by the seventh-century Catholic Visigothic Code in Spain, which forced Jews to renounce the rite and further strengthened its importance for the Jewish people.[7] This Code influenced Spanish anti-Semitism for centuries.

Jews living among Moslems did not meet with the same hostility to circumcision as those living among Christians, because Islam recommends removal of the foreskin, although Islamic circumcision is not a covenant and does not have the religious significance that it has in Judaism. In Babylonia, in gaonic times, Jews introduced the custom of circumcising an infant who died before he was eight days old, at the grave before burial, so the infant's soul would not go to Gehenna.[8]

In the twelfth and thirteenth centuries, rabbis compiled a new chapter of halakhah headed "The Laws of Circumcision," sometimes still under the heading of the Laws of Shabbat, but increasingly as a legal topic in its own right. Here they collected all the laws pertaining to circumcision from earlier sources, discussed questions that had arisen in the practice of the ritual, and documented medieval customs for performing the ritual.[9]

At that time, new ideas emerged about circumcision. Maimonides pointed out that everyone who was circumcised bore the same sign that he believed in the unity of God. He also said that the ritual was not performed merely to achieve bodily perfection, but also to perfect man's moral shortcomings, because removal of the foreskin counteracted excessive lust, weakened the libido, and sometimes also reduced the pleasure of sexual relations. In the thirteenth century, a rabbi developed this idea to counter an anti-Semitic, Christian accusation that Jews were guilty of immoderate sexual behavior, enabled by their circumcision. The rabbi emphasized that the removal of the foreskin lessened a man's sexual desire and enabled him to concentrate on the Torah.[10]

At this time, Jews began to think of the ritual as a sacrifice, and the father who circumcises his son as a high priest. And mystics taught that circumcision enables one to find holiness in the Shekhinah, the divine presence.[11]

From the fifteenth to the eighteenth centuries, the Inquisition of the Roman Catholics to stamp out heresy on the Iberian peninsula and colonies (Goa in India, Central and South American colonies, the Philippine Islands, and the Canary Islands) condemned to death any Jew who had himself or his son circumcised. Jews were forced to convert to Christianity, yet some continued to practice Judaism secretly. Many of these "New Christians," known as *Marranos*, or *Conversos*, eventually found refuge in safe havens in the Ottoman Empire, in the Netherlands, and England, where they had themselves circumcised and circumcised their sons. For a Jew threatened with the Inquisition, and for an adult to undergo this ritual voluntarily, required a conscious awareness of its significance in Judaism. Thus, from the fifteenth to the eighteenth centuries, some of these Jews of Spanish and Portuguese origin contemplated the importance of this ritual; their thoughts reflected the society in which they lived and their familiarity with contemporary Christian views. One example is Isaac Cardoso, who noted that circumcision differentiated God's people from others. He repeated that circumcision enabled perfection of the body and the spirit, and the absence of a foreskin lessened a man's sexual impulses; however, in contrast to the rabbinic view, he wrote that Abraham's circumcision and sacrifice of Isaac took the place of crucifixion in satisfying Adam's original sin and that, without circumcision, a Jew could not be redeemed. He also gave a kabbalistic interpretation of the Hebrew word for circumcision, *milah*, which in *gematria* is equivalent to a Hebrew appellation of God, *Elohim*.

He also took a phrase in Deuteronomy 30:12 ("who among us can go up to the heavens . . . ?") and pointed out that the first letter of each Hebrew word in this phrase spells *milah*, whereas the last letter of each word spells the tetragrammaton.[12]

In the early modern period, rabbis continued to answer practical questions that arose in the fulfillment of the duty and to document local customs. Differences evolved in details of the ritual according to the locality and ethnic origins of the community. For example, small differences were noted in the blessings, in the choice of readings, and in the songs sung in a Yemenite community, in a Sephardic community, and in an Ashkenazi community. For this reason, each community had its own preferred publication of the Order of Circumcision.

Also in the early modern period, emancipation began to affect attitudes to circumcision within the Jewish community. Emancipation led directly to a movement of Reform Judaism away from ceremony and ritual, although reformists maintained Jewish ethics and morals. In 1843, leaders of Reformed Jewry in Frankfurt proposed abandoning circumcision, on the grounds that Mosaic law mentions only once the command to circumcise one's sons, and this command is not repeated in Deuteronomy. This proposal sparked an emotional controversy between reformists and traditionalists. The chief rabbis of Frankfurt and Hamburg each kept a notebook for a few years in which they blacklisted wayward parents who had not circumcised their newborn sons.[13] The dispute raged for many years, but it had no lasting effect on the continuing practice of circumcision among Jews.

In recent years, Reform Jews have returned to celebrating this and other religious rituals, maintaining certain major differences from the Orthodox. (One is the inclusion of women in the performance of the ritual and another is the recognition of patrilineal as well as matrilineal descent. Thus, Reform rabbis accept that the son of a Jewish father and non-Jewish mother can be considered Jewish if both parents are committed to raising him as a Jew, just like the son of a Jewish mother and non-Jewish father.) The Reform movement now recognizes the importance of circumcision to Jewish identity in a mixed society.

Jewish Identity

Circumcision was used in the past as a criterion by which Gentiles identified Jews. A tale from Galicia tells of just such a situation. It is about a wealthy Jew who was well respected by all the local Jews and Gentiles. He lived in a village where he owned an inn and a flour mill. He was pious, righteous, and generous, and he had married off all his children to good families. At sixty-five years of age, he had every reason to be proud and satisfied. One day, however, a village girl gave birth to a little boy who she claimed, without shame, was his. The scandal was horrific. On the one hand, his friends knew that such a man would never commit adultery; on the other hand, perhaps it was true after all.

The man's insistent denials were to no avail, his good name was under suspicion, and everyone avoided him. It was like the ninth of Av (a day of mourning). He fasted and even contemplated putting an end to his life, surely preferable to the frightful shame thrust on him.

The girl sued the Jew for child support, and the issue was taken to court. The Jew found a famous lawyer in another town who believed him innocent and agreed to take his case. The girl arrived for the hearing with her employer, the local priest, who was understandably concerned for her well-being. After the hearing, judgment was handed down: the Jew was sentenced to six months in prison and was ordered to make monthly payments to the girl until the boy reached the age of eighteen years.

As the judgment was handed down, the Jew's lawyer pulled out of his pocket a circumcision knife. If the court judged that the Jew was the father, the child must be circumcised, he said, and the lawyer commanded the girl to put the baby on the table so he could perform the operation on the spot. Terrified, the girl fell to her knees at the feet of the priest and looked up at him in despair: "Do you want your child to become a Jew and be circumcised?"

The Jew was thus acquitted and lived to a grand old age, enjoying the pleasures of his grandchildren and great-grandchildren.[14]

Nowadays many secular Jews, who otherwise do not observe tradition, recognize the importance of circumcision for Jewish identity and have a surgeon perform the operation on their newborn sons.

The Night before the Circumcision

Perhaps the arrival of the circumciser, *mohel*, on the night before a circumcision, to check that the baby was well enough for the next day's ritual, prompted the festivities that eventually became customary on this night in many Jewish communities. Unlike the celebrations on the first Shabbat after birth, which are religious and of ancient origin, rejoicing on the night before circumcision was primarily a secular celebration of life.[15]

Although the Zohar mentions that Jews stayed awake all night in Torah study on the night before a circumcision, this custom may not have been widespread until the eighteenth century.[16] In twelfth-century Europe, the night before a circumcision was more often spent in making music, dancing, eating, and drinking in the home of a newborn baby. In the early thirteenth century, rabbis in the Jewish communities of the Rhine issued rulings that limited feasting to religious celebrations, but allowed women to dine with a lying-in mother on this particular night.[17] The following century, in southern France, new parents offered their guests fruits on this special evening. In the fifteenth century, the Inquisition tried Spanish Jews celebrating a birth in this way.[18] After the expulsion of Jews from Spain in 1492, *Marrano* women continued the custom of visiting a friend or relative who was lying-in and celebrated the night before circumcision with music, singing, dancing, and feasting.

By the late fifteenth century the social gatherings on this night began to have protective purposes. A song written by an unknown author in Provence, as if for the baby to sing, mentioned the vigilance on this night.[19] In the late sixteenth century, a Galician rabbi wrote that the custom of remaining awake all night before the circumcision was to guard against Satan who resented that circumcision saved the Jews from Gehenna and therefore sought to kill the newborn before his circumcision. The noisy company all night in the well-lit room clearly helped parents overcome their fear of evil powers endangering the baby's life and soul until circumcision granted the child immunity.[20]

In the sixteenth century, Jews in Germany, France, and Italy spent this night at a feast with the baby's father, while the lying-in mother and her female visitors ate fruits. Guests came, often with a gift, to join the fun regardless of whether they had been invited. Some Italian community rulings from that time attest that dancing and gambling, which were not otherwise permitted, were tolerated on the night or nights preceding a circumcision.[21] In 1603, a Protestant German priest, who documented the social customs of Jews, reported that revelers on this night enjoyed a large feast, gambling, and drinking, to stay awake to guard against demons.[22] Whereas Rabbi Leone da Modena (1571–1648) confirmed that the celebration on this night was to watch over the child's well-being, he carefully omitted mention of gambling, for which he himself had a weakness.[23]

A German rabbi, Yair Bacharach (1638–1702), although well-read in the sciences, fueled parents' fears when he described the horrific case of a newborn who was bewitched and died on the night before his circumcision.[24] Such documentation by a respected, learned rabbi gave credibility to people's fears of sorcerers and demons and strengthened their desire to maintain vigilance on this night. Other accounts in the seventeenth and eighteenth centuries—by an Italian apostate, a rabbi of Rome, and travelers to Morocco and Rhodes (where some Spanish Jews had settled after their expulsion from the Iberian peninsula)—confirmed that Jews spent the night before a circumcision in merrymaking, dancing, and feasting on sweets, fruits, and wine, while maintaining their vigil against sorcery.[25]

Since the eighteenth century, hasidic Jews in Eastern Europe have told the story of how the Baal Shem Tov (c. 1700–1760) saved a baby's life on this night.[26] They told the story in flickering candlelight as people sat together, tired, yet trying to keep awake throughout the long night, and the tale's happy ending offered strength and hope.

One version of this tale concerns a squire whose home was surrounded by tall trees not far from a village. He could afford all the pleasures of life, but he lacked one pleasure—the joy of fatherhood. The farmers who lived nearby feared that evil spirits consorted in his house, because at sundown dogs barked and cats howled, and at times the farmers heard strange cries.

A Jew rented an inn from this man. Sadly, the innkeeper's babies had all died. His wife had borne him three sons, and each time, on the night before the circumcision, the innkeeper had found the baby strangled. Their grief was beyond imagining. He was a good and devout man, and in his prayers he asked God to grant him a son who would survive.

One night, the innkeeper walked past the home of the landowner. With his own ears, he heard the cries and wails that the farmers had gossiped about over their drinks. With his own eyes, he saw the spirits dancing and howling and barking. He watched the spectacle continue until midnight, and only then did the house grow quiet.

The Jew returned home, shaken, checked his mezuzzot, and went to bed, but he could not sleep the whole night. The next day, he and his wife, who was pregnant again, went to the city to tell the rabbi their fears. The rabbi told them to pretend to know nothing about the goings-on at the squire's house and to return to see him when the baby was born.

When the innkeeper's wife gave birth to another son, the innkeeper brought a quorum of Jews from a nearby village to keep vigilance over his wife and baby while he went back to see the rabbi. The rabbi instructed him to maintain strict vigilance throughout the first eight days, and particularly on the night before the circumcision, when everyone was to stay awake and on guard. As midnight approached, they were to look for a black cat stealing into the room; they were to catch it, put it in a sack, and beat it, but be sure that it remained alive. They were to keep the cat in the bag until dawn and only then release it.

"When you have done this," concluded the rabbi, "you will be blessed with the survival of your son."

The innkeeper returned home and carried out the rabbi's instructions. Indeed, on the night before the circumcision, as midnight approached, a black cat left the squire's house and made its way to the inn. No one at the inn had ever seen such a cat. They caught it, threw it in a sack, and beat it severely. In the morning, they released it, and, with difficulty, the cat dragged itself away.

The circumcision ceremony took place as planned, the baby was blessed, and the guests lacked nothing. The following day, the squire called for the innkeeper. When the Jew arrived, he found the squire dying.

"I want you to know that I am dying," the landowner told the Jew. "Your rabbi has beaten me. Your three sons died because I strangled them out of jealousy. The black cat you beat was no other than I. I am leaving you half of my property to console you for the sorrow I caused you. Please forgive me." With these words, his soul left him.[27]

Religious Study. The name used in many communities for the night before a circumcision is in the vernacular, not in Hebrew, confirming the essentially secular nature of the occasion. These names—*Wachnacht* among Ashkenazi Jews, *La Veglia* among Italian Jews, *La Viola* among Sephardic Jews, *Bilada* in parts of North Africa, *Lilat Elzaba* in Yemen—refer to the vigilance that had become customary on this night.[28] Now it is also called *Brit Itzhak*, Isaac's covenant.

From the thirteenth to the eighteenth centuries, the trend in Europe was to distance secular celebration from religion. This was evident in the rabbinic establishment, as well as in the Church. Thus, rabbis attempted to reinforce piety and to limit ostentatious jollity on the night before a circumcision. For example, they taught that the vigilance should be spent in Torah study. They tried to limit the company at the gathering to family members, under the spiritual guidance of a rabbi, and they encouraged songs with religious content (*piyyutim*).[29]

At the same time, community enactments meted out punishments to Jews who played cards and dice, "even at the bed of a woman confined in childbirth."[30] Such an announcement, in Moravia in 1708, implied that gambling was still not unusual on this night. In Ancona, Italy, in 1716, the rabbinate decreed that only women were allowed to dance—only on the night before a circumcision, and without masks, a statement implying that masked carnivals were the custom.[31] Yet rabbis remained unsuccessful in preventing women from playing cards and making merry when they visited the mother of a newborn. Moreover, men were not quick to desist from secular pastimes during the precircumcision vigil. A German etching of a lying-in scene dating from this period shows the new mother playing cards with her lady friends; the men are sitting feasting, and only one man is studying a book, in acknowledgment of the desires of the religious establishment.[32]

The rabbis continued to fight the secular nature of this celebration and vigil. In the early eighteenth century, selections of biblical and rabbinic texts for study on this night were published in Italy and Amsterdam.[33] By the close of that century, the attempt to convert the celebration into a religious occasion had succeeded, and the secular origins of the evening were soon forgotten. Jews of Tunisia tell that the custom of studying the night before a circumcision originated with a rabbi who was seriously ill and was advised that he would recover only if he studied that night in a home where a baby was to be circumcised the next day. After the night of study, he indeed recovered.[34]

Nineteenth-century accounts state that, in the homes of Sephardic Jews, rabbis led guests in prayer, and musicians sang and entertained with their instruments. Men read psalms and verses from the Book of Zohar and sang *piyyutim* and joyful ballads about Elijah the prophet (who is expected at every circumcision) and the birth of Abraham.[35] When the visitors had feasted and left, the child's maternal grandmother sat vigil the entire night, singing to her lying-in daughter and grandson.

In Eastern Europe, this night remained a night of vigilance, and men studied Torah and rabbinic texts, to create an atmosphere of holiness around the baby and to protect it from harm.[36]

Preparations for the Circumcision.   In addition to the vigilance against evil powers, Sephardic, North African, Middle Eastern, and Asian Jews in the twentieth century have made preparations on the night before a circumcision. In Iraq, Iran, Kurdistan, India, and Yemen, and among Sephardic Jews in the Holy Land and Morocco, men have read from the Bible and Zohar and then prepared the Chair of Elijah (discussed separately later in this chapter).[37] Traditionally, women sang biblical verses or traditional welcoming songs as they decorated this special chair and laid out a tray with many candles and a bowl of water on it. The lying-in woman lit the largest candle and put a coin in the bowl. The tray then passed to each guest, first to the men, then to the women. Each lit a candle and added a coin. When everyone had lit a candle, the tray was auctioned; the baby's family traditionally made the highest bid to keep the tray and, of course, the bowl of coins. When the father was poor, he often received the money collected, and no auction was held. When the father was wealthy, he sometimes gave the money to charity or the synagogue. In Morocco, Jews sometimes auctioned the honor of holding the baby during the circumcision and gave the money to charity. In Jerusalem and Hebron, the father sometimes gave the money collected in the bowl, "Elijah's Cup," to the midwife instead. In Syria, India, and parts of Yemen, Jews similarly passed around "the tray of Elijah," which was auctioned after the circumcision.

Most North African Jews have read the Zohar and have prepared Elijah's chair on the night before circumcision. Traditionally, the women in these communities made Elijah's chair by covering a table with a carpet or covering a chair with a prayer shawl and placing a Torah mantle over it. They hung colored scarves, usually red, on or near the doorposts of the room where the circumcision was to be held. This custom is said to have originated with the *Marranos* when circumcision was forbidden. The *Marranos* hung a scarf on the doorpost to inform other Jews that the circumcision was taking place. The women also prepared candles and aromatic herbs. In Morocco, on this night the father had his hair cut next to Elijah's Chair and rewarded the barber with silver.[38] Libyan Jewish women, and those in Djerba (an island off Tunisia where Jews have lived since ancient times), still sing on this night as they crush spices and dried flowers to make perfumed water for the guests after the circumcision.[39]

By the late nineteenth century, festivity on this night was abandoned in some communities, especially those influenced by enlightenment and reform. The celebration lost popularity in traditional communities as well, because it was not a religious obligation, it was a strain on the new mother, who needed to rest, and it disturbed non-Jewish neighbors. Today, those who still gather on the night before the circumcision read the Zohar and Psalms, invite yeshivah boys to recite the *Shema* in the baby's home, and enjoy sweets.

Circumcision Rite

As we have seen, circumcision is more than a surgical procedure; it is a religious duty, and Jews worldwide perform the rite according to an age-old pattern. Traditionally, the circumciser, *mohel*, is a pious man trained in surgical hygiene as well as the rabbinic laws pertaining to circumcision.[40]

A quorum of at least ten men attends the circumcision, although to make it a joyous event, many guests are usually invited. Sometimes the mother does not attend the rite itself. The father may honor certain guests by giving them roles in the ceremony. Thus, a woman guest (*kvatterin*, in Ashkenazi communities) may bring the baby from his mother to the door of the room where the ceremony takes place, and another (her husband, *kvatter*, in Ashkenazi communities) may carry the baby to the *sandek*, the person who holds the baby during the circumcision.[41]

Lit candles enhance the festivity. In some communities, spices or perfumes prepared by women on the preceding day lend fragrance to the atmosphere. The baby is clean and is dressed in beautiful clothes. The ceremonial objects used in the ritual are often artistically crafted and engraved. A decorated chair, the Chair of Elijah, plays a symbolic role in the ceremony and is prepared for the prophet, who is expected to attend.

Guests stand at the beginning of the ceremony to welcome the invisible prophet and to greet the arrival of the baby with a blessing. The father declares his intention to fulfill the biblical commandment, and the *mohel* recites blessings before and after the surgical procedure. The blessings delineate the fulfillment of the religious duty and include the hope that the newborn will grow up to fulfill the precepts of Torah, to marry, and to perform good deeds. The ceremony closes as the boy is named and a prayer is said for the parents' well-being.

After the circumcision is a celebratory feast.[42] Whenever possible, Jews have invited the whole community to a circumcision feast, because they have considered this a great mitzvah. Sometimes rabbis have limited the number of people invited to such a feast, however, to preserve the dignity of those who cannot afford to host gatherings, and also perhaps because large and joyous celebrations aggravated tensions with local Gentiles.[43]

In many communities, special songs, *piyyutim* and *z'mirot*, composed by Jewish poets and musicians, precede or follow the ritual and the meal.

For the wealthy, circumcision is a time to think of others less fortunate. As discussed earlier, sometimes a donation is made publicly on the eve of the circumcision, or such a donation takes the form of food distributed to poor people. Sometimes a father donates money to a charitable society, a local yeshivah where the boy may eventually study, or directly to the poor. For those who have little, local customs or charitable societies have provided funds to cover the celebration of circumcision without a father's loss of dignity.[44]

The Mohel

The Bible tells that Abraham circumcised his sons, and Moses' wife, Zipporah, circumcised one of their two sons. Thus, a precedent was set for a father to be a *mohel* and also for a woman to do this job. The *mohel* is usually a man, but Italy, in the Renaissance, had women circumcisers, as well as women doctors and women ritual slaughterers. Today, there are women circumcisers only in the Reform Jewish community.

Expertise and care are necessary for this delicate task, and no one untrained would undertake this job in modern times. The Talmud says that scholars were encouraged to learn this skill. If they did not, they took residence in a town with a *mohel*. Through the ages, most communities have engaged the services of a trained *mohel*, just as they have employed a ritual slaughterer to provide their kosher meat.

A *mohel* is pious, knowledgeable in all medical matters pertaining to circumcision, and a skilled and accurate worker. Often the circumciser does not charge a fee, because he considers the job to be a mitzvah.[45]

At least since 1700, a *mohel* often kept a record of the boys he circumcised, noting the name of the child and his father, the date and place of circumcision, and sometimes the name of the godfather. Because the job of circumcision was often taught by a father to his son, such a record book was sometimes kept in the same family for several generations, providing a comprehensive birth register of boys born in a certain area. (For example, the Turlach family of Baden maintained such records from 1703 until 1861 in a series of notebooks.)

The Prophet Elijah

According to tradition, Elijah the prophet is invited to every circumcision to see that Jews fulfill the covenant. Elijah had complained to God: "I am moved by zeal for the Lord . . . for the Israelites have forsaken Your covenant" (I Kings 19:10,14). Some commentators have said that Elijah's invitation is a reward for his piety. Others have said it is a punishment for his excessive zeal and his charge against the Israelites; these commentators have reasoned that if Elijah attends every circumcision, he will see that his accusation is wrong. This tradition, and the associated custom of preparing a chair for the prophet, apparently date from the gaonic period; they are not mentioned in the Talmud.[46]

The first Book of Kings tells that Elijah helped to ward off the Angel of Death.[47] Elijah's ability to ward off the Angel of Death, even from newborns, is a frequent theme in Jewish folktales. His legendary success in repelling Lilith is discussed in Chapter 10. Legend tells that Elijah attended the circumcisions of the famous Safed kabbalist, Isaac ben Solomon Luria, the "Ari," in 1534, and of Israel ben Eliezer, the Baal Shem Tov, around the year 1700.[48] Jews have believed that the prophet is visible only to a select few, whom God blesses specially. Thus, Elijah's attendance at these circumcisions presaged that the boys would be unusually blessed.

In ancient times, Elijah was called "The Angel of the Covenant."[49] He eventually became the guardian angel of the circumcision ceremony. As circumcision became increasingly ritualized, the seat of honor was dedicated to this guardian angel. This practice may be an adaptation of a local non-Jewish custom of setting aside a chair or table in the house for a god of fortune who was thought to bring luck. Talmudic sages forbade the custom, but they may not have succeeded, and in the eighth or ninth centuries it was legitimized by connecting the chair to Elijah in the manner just described. Conversely, the dedication of the special chair may be a carryover from the ancient custom of resting the Torah on a special chair when not in use. That chair was called the "Cathedra of Moses."[50]

As discussed earlier, when the circumcision takes place at home, the chair is usually prepared on the night before the ceremony by decorating a piece of furniture with beautiful cloth, silk, or embroidered brocade and sometimes with the Torah mantle or the crowns of the Torah scroll. In communities where the ritual is performed in the synagogue, however, a special chair is dedicated for this purpose. Regional differences are apparent in the chair's structural style, size, and decoration. However, a chair designated to be used as a Chair of Elijah is usually much finer than chairs used in daily life: ornately carved, painted, or upholstered in especially beautiful fabric, it sometimes bears a dedication signifying its special purpose.

Still today, the baby is placed on the Chair of Elijah at the beginning of the circumcision ritual, and then on the knees of the *sandek*. In some communities, the *sandek* sits on the Chair during the ritual, whereas in others, this chair is left empty for the Prophet.[51]

In the eighteenth and nineteenth centuries, synagogue congregations in England, Alsace, parts of Germany and Austria, and Safed in the Holy Land acquired large, benchlike double chairs in which the *sandek* could sit on one half, leaving the other half free for the prophet. In contrast, at that time some synagogues in Provence had a small, fancy, symbolic Chair of Elijah installed on the wall. There have been recent reports of such small, symbolic chairs on the walls of synagogues in Sefrou (Morocco), Kurdistan, and Yemen. In Italy two centuries ago, the community charitable society that helped with circumcision expenses sometimes commissioned the making of a beautiful Chair of Elijah.[52] In Morocco in the early twentieth century, childless couples sometimes commissioned such a chair, in the hope of meriting a child by this deed. Alternatively, they commissioned the chair when a first son was born after a long period of barrenness. In both instances, the chair was made available for the use of all the Jews in the community.[53]

Jews of Herat, Afghanistan, who are now living in Israel, prepare a chair with a beautiful covering on which Elijah could sit, and also a stick on which he could lean when standing. They tell that parents have kept the stick in the baby's room for two days after the circumcision as a protective charm for the boy's well-being. They have attributed healing properties to the stick.[54]

Redemption of the First-Born Son

A first child has special significance for both parents, and this was as true in biblical times as today, but then only when the child was male. A mother's first-born boy was consecrated to divine service, and a father gave his first-born son a double portion of his possessions as his birthright inheritance.[55] In medieval times, it was customary for a father to vow his first-born son to the study of Torah. In later centuries, too, it was not uncommon for an eldest son to study while his younger brothers learned a trade.[56]

The Book of Exodus tells that God spared the Israelite first-born sons when casting the tenth plague on the ancient Egyptians, because first-borns were divinely consecrated.[57] The Israelites raised their first-born sons to a life of priesthood. After the incident of the Golden Calf, however, only the tribe of Levi proved themselves worthy of priesthood.[58] Ever since, an observant Jewish father who is not of levitic or of priestly lineage (a *cohen*) has redeemed his wife's first-born son from lifelong service to God (provided his wife is not of a levitic or priestly family). The father redeems his baby when the child is one month old, by paying the money equivalent of five shekels "by the sanctuary weight."[59]

Additional details regarding this ritual were laid down in the Mishnah, in a tractate entitled *Bekhorot*, "first-borns," and in the later Codes. The blessings and statements recited during the ritual were formalized and included in the first true prayer book, in the ninth century.[60]

Unlike the circumcision ritual, the redemption of the first-born is postponed for a Sabbath or Jewish festival. It is not performed if the mother had aborted a formed fetus previously, because the miscarriage preceded the newborn in opening the womb, nor is it done if the baby was born by caesarean section, because in this case the womb was opened artificially.[61] If a mother had one or more babies by caesarean section and then eventually gave birth vaginally to a son, she would redeem this baby, the first to open her womb naturally.

In fifteenth-century Germany, if the father died without having redeemed his son, a little medallion with the words *ben cohen* was hung on a lace around the baby's neck to remind him to redeem himself when he reached maturity.[62] It soon became customary, however, to inscribe the medallion with the Hebrew letter *heh*, numerically equivalent to five, representing the five-shekel redemption fee.[63] Many collections of Judaica have preserved a *heyalakh*, a little *heh* medallion. To prevent the loss of such a necklace in the wear and tear of childhood, the medallion was sometimes kept instead in a safe place in the local synagogue: a medallion from Ianina,

Greece, tells that a baby born in 1865 was not redeemed, and a later inscription adds that the boy redeemed himself.[64] Nowadays, in traditional communities, when a father cannot redeem his first-born son, a relative or even a community dignitary may do this, instead of waiting for the child to do so himself when he is old enough.

Redemption Price

When it was no longer known what exact weight the five shekel coins should be, Jews used five silver pieces or five local coins as redemption money, or even a ring, a silver or pewter tray, or an item of clothing. A poor Jewish father could borrow some coins to present to the *cohen*, who returned them after the ceremony.

Once, in medieval times in the Rhineland, a tray (or in another account, a ring) was given to the *cohen* by way of redemption for a newborn son. The *cohen* later discovered the item was a fake and declared the boy unredeemed. An argument ensued between the father, who was willing to replace the tray with five coins, and the *cohen*, who wanted to keep the fake item and insisted the father pay the sum still outstanding. The rabbis ruled in favor of the *cohen's* demand.[65]

Sometimes the redemption money was put on a silver tray, thereby increasing the value of the father's contribution. A beautifully crafted tray from Danzig in the eighteenth century, of hammered copper with repoussé, shows the *cohen's* hands blessing the swaddled baby. It was a community possession, rather like the Chair of Elijah.[66] Ashkenazi communities in Europe and Eastern Europe in the nineteenth century commissioned skilled Jewish craftsmen to make such trays, which were heavily decorated with a biblical scene, usually the sacrifice of Isaac. The father placed the baby on the tray and decked him out in his mother's jewelry; he returned the tray and the jewels at the end of the ritual and paid the *cohen* in cash. The tray, the jewelry, and the baby's fancy clothing enhanced the beauty of the occasion. Like the medallions, these beautiful trays also feature in most Judaica collections.

Today, the Bank of Israel has minted special coins for use in this ritual. Jews still improvise, however: some Jews in Turkey use five silver spoons when redeeming their first-born son, and in Morocco, seven gold bracelets, which the *cohen* returns later, receiving a money gift instead.[67]

Regional Variations

Over the centuries, regional variations have occurred in the embellishment of the ceremony. In some Jewish communities in the early twentieth century, the redemption ceremony was dramatic. In Rabat-Salé, Morocco, for example, Jews created a festive atmosphere in the home with perfume and flowers and invited guests for the occasion. After prayers, the *cohen* asked the mother in the presence of the midwife to swear that this was indeed her first child and the child of her husband. He would then suddenly rise and pretend to leave with the baby. The mother's wails of despair prompted the father to negotiate the ransom of five jewels or silver coins. The *cohen* returned the baby only when they all reached an agreement. A few days later, the father visited the *cohen* and exchanged the jewels for money, which he distributed to the poor of the community.[68] In other Moroccan communities, the drama involved the mother's surrendering the jewelry she was wearing, piece by piece, until the *cohen* agreed to perform the ceremony.

Jews from some Sephardic and Syrian communities recall that a first-time mother dressed in her bridal gown; in Persian communities, she wore the veil from her wedding.[69] The new mother formally begged the *cohen* to return her baby. He would refuse, and she would persist in her pleas until the *cohen* reluctantly consented. The happy outcome was celebrated. In Salonika in the early twentieth century, the mother pretended to yearn for the return of her baby while the father avowed that he would prefer to sleep undisturbed at night, and guests teased and joked. A wealthy father offered a valuable gold or silver bracelet instead of the five biblical shekels; a poor father offered a new item of clothing.[70] Iraqi Jews report that when it was performed, the ceremony was a dramatic game between the *cohen* and the baby's father, using a kiddush cup instead of jewelry, and eventually ending when the father gave the *cohen* a symbolic sum of money.[71]

The redemption ritual is not mentioned in ethnographic accounts of Jewish life in India, Yemen, and Aden. Often these communities had no *cohen* to carry out the redemption, and therefore the ritual was not performed; when it was done, there was apparently little ceremony.[72] In Egypt, in the nineteenth century, the redemption was sometimes done on the eighteenth day (eighteen is the numerical equivalent of *hai*, the Hebrew word for life).[73]

In the late twentieth century, this ritual remains picturesque among those who practice it. Some Ashkenazi Jews still put the baby on a silver tray, surround him with sugar lumps (in the hope of good things to come) and garlic cloves (against evil spirits), and drape him with his mother's gold jewelry. Persian Jewish first-time mothers and Jewish women in Turkey still wear their bridal veil for the redemption ceremony.

Some Orthodox Jews see the redemption of a first-born son as a symbolic act of acknowledging God's supremacy and man's subservience.[74] Others see in it acknowledgement of the great significance for parents of the arrival of their first male heir, because the ritual's blessings express the feelings expected of first-time Jewish parents: gratitude to God for the first fruit of the mother's womb. Performance of this duty implies dedication to raise the infant within the Jewish faith.

In the last twenty years, some parents have created unorthodox variations of the traditional ritual, such as a redemption ceremony for a first-born daughter or a special kiddush for the opening of the womb.[75] Through these innovations, some Jews in the United States have sought to celebrate childbirth, to suit their spiritual needs. By modeling a new ceremony on the ancient redemption ritual, they acknowledge the psychological significance of a first child in a way that highlights Jewish continuity and has religious meaning for them.

CELEBRATION OF A NEWBORN DAUGHTER

Jews have welcomed the birth of a daughter according to local customs, and differently from the welcome accorded a son. Often they have done this on a Sabbath morning in the synagogue. Some communities, however, have held special home celebrations that date from medieval times and bear influences from local, non-Jewish naming ceremonies. Yet other communities have no ceremony at all.

Nowadays, a naming ceremony may stress a daughter's family continuity and her link with the biblical matriarchs, as well as introduce her to the Jewish community. This ceremony is not a covenant, however, and it does not have the same spiritual significance as circumcision. Nothing marks the baby physically or symbolically in the manner of circumcision.

Among Sephardim

The celebration for a newborn daughter among Jews in medieval Spain may have paralleled an old Spanish custom in which parents had their newborns blessed by good fairies, *hadas* in Spanish. This celebration was probably not in any way a religious ceremony. In the late fifteenth century, Jews in Spain performed the *hadas* celebration on the night before the circumcision, and the Inquisition considered this a Jewish custom. Spanish Jews probably celebrated the night leading into the eighth day in the same manner after the birth of a boy or a girl.[76]

In more recent times, some Sephardic Jews in Italy, Holland, the Balkans, and Turkey, as well as in parts of Morocco have invited relatives, friends, and the elders of the community on the thirtieth day for a festive naming celebration. This celebration has been called *fados*, or *hatas* (reminiscent of the celebration in medieval Spain), or *piadamento*, "the day of the gifts."[77] The rabbi picks up the baby's cradle, places a coin on the sheet, and passes the cradle to another person, who does the same. In the days of home birth, the collected money was given to the midwife. The rabbi announces the baby's name and blesses the infant and parents with *mi-shebeirakh* ("may the One who blessed") benedictions, such as the following:

> May the One who blessed Sarah, Rebekah, Rachel and Leah, Miriam the prophetess, Abigail, and queen Esther, daughter of Avihail, bless this beloved girl, whose name in Israel is . . . , with good luck, to grow up in health and peace. . . . give to her parents the joy of seeing her happily married, a radiant mother of children, rich in honor and joy and may she live to a ripe old age. May this be the will of God, and let us say, Amen.[78]

The rabbi blesses the little girl with the blessing of Rebekah, "May you grow into thousands of myriads . . ." (Genesis 24:60) and verses from Song of Songs.[79] A kiddush and festive meal follow the ceremony.

Among Ashkenazim

Ceremonial naming of girls also has a long history among Ashkenazi Jews in South Germany, the Rhineland, and Alsace. The custom appears to go back to a cradle ceremony in eleventh-century northeastern France, performed in the presence of a quorum, for a male infant, some time after his circumcision. The father placed a

Bible in the cradle with the baby, who was dressed in fancy clothes for the occasion. The men blessed the infant with "may he fulfill what is written in this book," recited many blessings, and helped to place an inkwell and feather pen in the baby's tiny hand so he would become a skilled Torah scribe.[80]

By the fifteenth century, the cradle ceremony had become known as *Hollekreisch* in Bavaria, where it was performed. The children of the community gathered around the cradle and raised it three times, chanting "Hollekreisch, Hollekreisch! What shall be this child's name?" After several passages were read from the Bible, the baby's name was announced, and the ceremony concluded with cakes and drinks. By the second half of the seventeenth century, urban Jews had abandoned this custom; it was practiced only in small towns and in rural areas. However, the custom spread to Alsace and the Rhineland, to southern Holland, and to the Jewish communities in what is now Switzerland. It has continued into modern times, no longer for boys, but only for the naming of girls.[81]

Several theories about the origin of *Hollekreisch* have been proposed.[82] In the fifteenth century, a scholar thought that the term possibly derived from the Hebrew word for "secular" (*hol*) combined with the German word "to shout" or "cry out" (*kreischen*): this explanation provided a fifteenth-century description of the custom of announcing the child's secular name. In the late nineteenth century, scholars elaborated new theories about the name. *Hollekreisch* was possibly a corruption of the French, *Haut la crèche*, "raise the cradle," and the German *Hohlgekreisch*, "an empty cry," suggesting the regret that the baby was only a girl and not a boy. Alternatively, it could have derived from the magical custom of drawing a circle around the cradle to protect the child from demons; *kreis* is German for "circle." Another plausible explanation is that the term derived from the fear of a demon-witch named Hulda, Holda, or Holle in old German mythology, who was believed to attack infants, like Lilith, but who could be frightened away by shouting the child's name and tossing the infant into the air three times. This ceremony may therefore have been a Jewish version of a ritual to fend off evil spirits.

In late sixteenth-century Poland, a couple visited the synagogue on the first Sabbath morning when the wife had risen from childbed, in token of the biblical duty to offer a sacrifice at the Temple after giving birth. This was the custom also in eighteenth-century Germany, and by the nineteenth century, most Ashkenazi Jews celebrated the birth of a daughter with a *kiddush* in the synagogue on a Shabbat morning, a month after birth, the custom still today.[83]

In Other Communities

In the twentieth century, Jews in India, Yemen, Syria, and Bukhara, and those living in the areas now known as Afghanistan, Iraq, and Iran, have welcomed and named a newborn daughter ceremoniously. Often, the ceremony has been called *zeved ha-bat*, "the gift of a [newborn] daughter."[84] The word *zeved* is biblical, meaning a gift. Arabic speakers enjoy the similarity between this Hebrew word and the Arabic for butter and cream; they say that a daughter should be smooth and rich like butter and cream.[85] In some parts of Yemen, Jewish women and children have celebrated the naming of a daughter on the third day after birth, by sharing together a special sweet dish. Persian Jews have named a baby girl at a joyous party on the seventh night. In Iraq and Kurdistan, and among the Baghdadi Jews in India, the midwife has announced the girl's name during a ceremony on the sixth night, during the *Shashah* celebration. When naming a newborn daughter, Jews in these communities, like the Sephardim, have also recited blessings, sometimes verses from Song of Songs, and a few other biblical verses. They have sung songs praising her beauty and have shared a festive meal.

Ethnographic accounts of Jewish life in Bombay and Calcutta at the beginning of the twentieth century reported that daughters were named on the sixth night after birth. The evening ceremony was reminiscent of that preceding a boy's circumcision, attended by a quorum of men and friends who read the Zohar or Song of Songs and blessed the baby. The guests feasted, accompanied by much singing and music. Indian Jews now living in Israel name their daughters in a ceremony attended only by women, and not necessarily on the sixth night after the child's birth.[86]

In many Jewish communities in North Africa and in the Caucasus in the early twentieth century, no ceremony was held for naming a girl; the mother or grandmother chose the name, which was not announced in the community.

Innovations

Nowadays, some Jews have incorporated a talmudic custom into a newborn girl's welcoming ceremony: they invite family and friends to join them when planting a tree, and they recite prayers of thanksgiving and blessings for the child's future.[87] In talmudic times, Jews planted a tree in honor of a baby's birth and later used branches from this tree to build the child's marriage canopy. When a boy was born, a cedar was planted, and after the birth of a girl, a pine, in the hope that the child would grow like the tree.[88] The planting of trees connects people to their land. As Jews were dispersed throughout the Diaspora, this custom was neglected. With the rise of Zionism, the return of Jews to the Holy Land, and the building of the Jewish state, tree planting has gained renewed significance, and the custom of planting a tree on the occasion of a birth has been revived. If, today, the tree is planted in the family's own garden, its branches can eventually be used for building the child's marriage canopy, as in ancient times. (Nowadays, some Jews plant trees in Israel, in the baby's name, for a boy or a girl.)

In the last twenty-five years, some Jews have wanted to create a ceremony for a newborn daughter in the style of a Jewish ritual with the weighty significance of the circumcision. The variety of new ceremonies for welcoming daughters in some communities reveals both a contemporary need for such a ceremony and the problems of creating a new Jewish ritual.

An initiation ritual should focus on the baby rather than on the parents, and it should change the baby's status in the community. To qualify as such a ritual, it must be done at a specific time and in a specific way. The timing is problematic; some opt for the eighth day after birth, like the circumcision, some choose Shabbat (the tradition in some communities), and yet others prefer the close of Shabbat, the day of the mother's postnatal purification, the day the baby achieves viability, or even the first day of the new moon.[89]

Some innovators have emulated the circumcision ceremony, but, obviously, without the surgery; some have emulated the redemption ceremony, to create a dedication ceremony. Some have ritually immersed the baby in a miniature *mikveh* or have just dipped her feet in water, symbolically. These ceremonies have various features in common: the welcoming of the baby, and then of the guests, prayers of thanksgiving and blessings, and the announcement of her name. Often parents select verses from the Torah and say a few words by way of interpretation. Sometimes they form an acrostic of the baby's name from verses from the psalms. They prepare a feast, as for other Jewish celebrations, sometimes with food symbolic of fertility.[90]

Various objects enhance a daughter's celebration. During the Ottoman period in Turkey, a newborn girl was named while wrapped in an embroidered veil that was eventually used again in her wedding ceremony. Today, in Reform communities, parents wrap their baby girl in a prayer shawl during the ceremony. This shawl, as well as candlesticks, a kiddush cup, and a Bible or prayer book, may be kept for her to use later at her Bat Mitzvah, and again still later at her wedding.

POSTNATAL PURIFICATION

The Bible depicts several situations that render a person "unclean" and instructs how a person can undergo purification. Thus, the Bible lists contact with dead bodies, leprosy, and issue from the sexual organs (including postnatal blood) as sources of "uncleanness." In biblical times, all these physical states were associated with the loss of life or the loss of potential life. The Bible says that this "uncleanness" is hateful to God and forbids sexual relations when a person is in this state. After a specified time, however, a person can immerse in flowing water, to reaffirm life, and offer a sacrifice, to rededicate himself or herself to God.[91] Jews have performed their ritual ablution in a ritual bath, *mikveh*, but their sacrificial offerings ceased when the Temple was destroyed.

Some ancient peoples of Asia Minor performed ritual purification to cleanse themselves from a state of impurity including after childbirth. Moreover, in the early twentieth century, anthropologists reported that the ancestral taboo over the blood of menstruation and childbirth had survived the ages also in non-Jewish societies as far flung as Polynesia and Alaska. Although physical reasons for the impurity exist, the Jewish concept of ritual purification is spiritual. A Jew performs this ritual only when he or she is already physically clean and accompanies the immersion with a blessing. Purity is a religious ideal and is a necessary step to achieving holiness.[92]

In the case of childbirth, the Bible considers a woman "unclean" for seven days after the birth of a boy and for two weeks after the birth of a girl. However, a woman purifies herself forty days after giving birth to a boy and eighty days after having a girl. Through the ages, rabbis have placed great emphasis on this and other biblical laws relating to a woman's ritual purity: a whole tractate of Mishnah and Talmud is devoted to this topic, with a chapter that deals explicitly with purification after childbirth. As practical questions arose, there was considerable discussion of this topic in all the codes of Jewish law and in the responsa literature.[93]

Although the Talmud permits sexual relations between a husband and wife as long as the woman is not "unclean," the gaonic sages forbade sexual relations until after postnatal purification. Therefore, in some Eastern communities, such as in Kurdistan, Yemen, and India, it was the custom until recently to separate a husband and wife after the birth of their child by removing the wife to another house or room where the husband would not sleep near her or touch her. The custom among some Ashkenazim of burying a woman who died in childbirth unwashed, in a well-sealed coffin, or in a separate part of the graveyard (discussed in Chapter 9), may have resulted from this ancient taboo over contact with the woman's "uncleanness." Such stringent interpretations of the biblical laws on a woman's postnatal impurity have led some people to conclude that those who have advocated them have had a primitive fear of blood and a disgust for women's natural issues.[94]

Reform Jews abandoned the laws relating to a woman's purity on the grounds that these were archaic and irrelevant to the modern world. Yet increasing numbers of women today in all streams of Judaism find positive meaning in these ancient laws, in terms of the physical and spiritual rebirth that they signal. Those who observe them enjoy temporary abstinence from sexual relations and the focus on nonsexual forms of marital communication at this time.[95]

Some scholars have tried to rationalize why the "unclean" period is doubly long after a girl's birth. One reason, proposed in ancient times, was that Adam was created after one week, whereas Eve was made in the second week, and Adam was brought by the angels to the Garden of Eden forty days after he was created, whereas Eve was brought eighty days after her creation. Perhaps there is a parallel with the talmudic idea (discussed in Chapter 4) that a male fetus is formed forty days after conception, whereas a female is formed after eighty days. Maimonides hypothesized that the uterus was larger after the birth of a girl than after a boy's birth and therefore required longer to contract to its nonpregnant size. The Zohar suggested that a baby's soul takes a longer period to settle into the body of a girl than a boy.[96] Some scholars have said that the longer period of impurity may accommodate a husband's displeasure with his wife when she has been delivered of a daughter. Yet another idea is that the double time for a girl takes into account the mother's loss of the extra life within her body, or the daughter's potential to give birth.[97]

Regional Practices

Jews who recently immigrated to Israel from rural Ethiopia gave birth in a special hut a short distance from the outskirts of the village. This "hut of malediction," or "hut of blood," was used also by menstruating women for seven days. A low stone wall surrounded the hut, to mark the limits of the "unclean" area. Food and drink were passed over the wall in a way that no one touched the "unclean" woman. At the onset of labor, two midwives accompanied the pregnant woman to this hut, delivered the baby, and then washed themselves and their clothing before returning home. The mother remained in the hut until the day of the circumcision, or for fourteen days after the birth of a girl. During this time, the family built another hut, the "hut of childbed." On leaving the first hut, the mother washed herself and her clothing and moved to the new hut, where she again remained segregated for another thirty-three or sixty-six days, just as the Bible dictated. While she was segregated, female relatives or neighbors undertook her housework and brought her food. On the last day of this period, she again washed thoroughly, shaved her head, put on clean clothes, and joined her family at sunset for a feast with family and neighbors. The childbed hut was then burned.[98]

Jews in some parts of Kurdistan observed a similar custom until the middle of the nineteenth century. Eight days after giving birth, the woman was transferred to a specially designated hut outside the town used only by "unclean" women, including those menstruating. Kurdistani Jews counted a woman "unclean" for forty days after delivery, regardless of the baby's sex.[99]

Until recently, a woman of the Bene Israel community in Bombay customarily delivered her first child in the home of her parents and remained there for the entire purification period. On the morning of the fortieth day after delivery of a son, or the eightieth if a daughter was born, the mother purified herself and washed her baby. That evening, a special dish of poultry was laid on a white sheet to symbolize a sacrificial offering. The family recited blessings and ate from this dish, and they sent a message to the husband telling him his wife and child were ready to return to him. Both dressed in new clothes and were sent off with gifts of jewelry. The father then gave a feast for friends and relatives to celebrate the homecoming. When a woman was confined in her husband's home, as was customary for subsequent deliveries, her parents took her to their home on the twelfth day after the birth and looked after her until her ritual purification.[100]

Yemenite Jews in Israel recall that, in Yemen and Aden, a woman remained in her own house until her purification. After this ritual, mother, baby, and friends went into the street with bundles of rue leaves, ululating, and the procession headed out of the village. After a distance they stopped, and turning around they symbolically threw away the leaves as they shouted, "come back in three years" (referring to pregnancy, of course) before making their way back again.[101]

Until the middle of the twentieth century, some North African Jews celebrated the end of this period with a ceremony at which all the woman's female friends and relatives gathered in their best clothes. A baby boy was presented with phylacteries, and a baby girl was presented with a needle and thimble.[102]

Burnt Offering and Sin Offering

The Bible tells that when a woman completes her period of postnatal purification, she must bring a "burnt offering" and a "sin offering" to the Temple for the priest to offer to God as an expiation.[103] The burnt offering symbolized a woman's rededication to God after her period of abstinence from the Sanctuary. Why was a sin offering necessary, however? What was the sin? The Talmud suggests that, while giving birth, a woman swears that she will never again have sexual intercourse with her husband: she regrets her vow in the joyous wake of the arrival of a baby boy after seven days, but the regret lasts a fortnight after the birth of a girl.[104] It is true that in moments of extreme suffering during labor some women vow never to become pregnant again, only to change their minds later, but perhaps the offering is to atone for Eve's sin in the Garden of Eden.[105] Whatever the reason, women ceased to observe this duty after the Temple was destroyed.

Syrian Jews have performed an atonement ceremony before the birth lest the woman die in childbirth. The few who still observe this custom today no longer are sure whether it is performed to absolve the woman of her sins should she die or whether the reason is that, as the Talmud suggests, she is sure to utter words in labor that she will regret later.[106]

WEANING CEREMONY

Abraham made a great feast on the day that Isaac was weaned, and Hannah offered a prayer of thanksgiving after weaning Samuel, but these customs never became part of Jewish ritual, although they were practiced in some communities.[107] An infant was weaned only when he or she was strong enough to cope with ordinary food, and not if the child was sickly. When a mother weaned her infant, she often expected another pregnancy soon afterward. Although Sarah was too old to conceive again, Abraham's feast may have been a celebration of his son's good health and his ability to leave his mother's arms and spend time with his father. In contrast, Samuel's weaning meant that Hannah had to fulfill her promise to dedicate him to lifelong service to God. She brought Samuel to the priest, uttered her emotional prayer of thanksgiving and praise to God, and left her son with the priest. For Hannah, weaning meant more than giving up the warm bodily contact she had with her son; it meant total separation.

Until the middle of the twentieth century, Syrian and Iraqi Jews celebrated weaning with a large festive party and served wheat cooked in sugar and cinnamon. Wheat is symbolic of fertility, and the celebration clearly greeted the possibility of a new pregnancy.[108]

In the early twentieth century, Jewish mothers in Eastern Europe celebrated weaning in a different way; the baby's first food was taken from a neighbor. When the baby accepted the offering, the mother said, "may this be the last time you will be supported by others." Sometimes a tiny bag of coins was hung around the baby's neck, symbolizing the receipt of his last donation.[109]

Infant survival, contraception, and paternal involvement in child care have all contributed to make weaning less significant for men than it was in the past. With nursing no longer a necessity for an infant's survival, the significance of weaning for a woman has changed, too.

In recent years, some non-Orthodox Jews have celebrated weaning as a life-cycle ritual. They have created a new ceremony and have linked it to Abraham's ancient banquet. This ceremony focuses on the nurturing roles of the parents and the joys of the child's independence. Some mark the occasion by giving charity to the hungry.[110]

In their joyous celebration of these ancient rituals, Jews maintain age-old traditions to affirm the Jewish identity of newborns and to mark a milestone in a woman's life cycle. They have found ways of adapting these traditions to suit modern conditions, for example, by reviving old customs or writing a new blessing, song, or poem to express the spirituality a parent may feel on the occasion of the ceremony. Secular Jews who find no meaning in such ceremonies may nevertheless perform a nonreligious circumcision. Although Orthodox Jews continue to redeem their first-born sons and to observe the biblical laws regarding a woman's purity, secular Jews often do not know of these duties or have consciously rejected them. As modern Jews rediscover their roots, some are now finding joy and meaning in these old traditions.

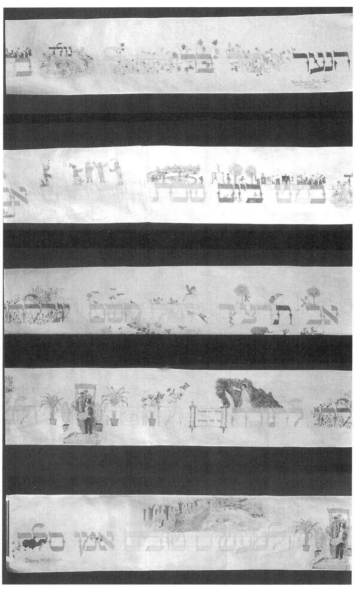

Plate 18. Torah binder (*wimpl*) bearing the following birth inscription: "The boy Asher, son of R. Raphael, born with good luck on Shabbat, new moon of Av (5)694 (14 July 1934). May the Lord raise him up to Torah, to the marriage canopy, and to good deeds, Amen, Selah." Lyon, France, 1934.
Undyed linen and silk, 4000 × 210 mm.
Gross Family Collection, Tel Aviv.

Chapter Thirteen

Blessings and Hopes

In addition to the traditional blessings recited when first greeting a newborn, Jews have recited a blessing when naming the infant and have noted the same blessing when reporting a birth in a letter to relatives, or on an endpaper of a book owned and valued by the family: "May the child [name inserted] grow up to Torah, to the wedding canopy and good deeds."[1] They have often added the hope that the baby was born under a lucky star—*be-mazal tov*. The same words have been embroidered and painted on Torah binders donated to the synagogue on the occasion of a baby's birth. These hopes and others have also been expressed in lullabies.

NAMING: HISTORICAL PERSPECTIVE

In the Bible, Jacob blessed his son and grandchildren, not when they were named (an occasion without ceremony), but when he was on his deathbed, with the hope that the children would remember their forefathers, Abraham, Isaac, and Jacob. In biblical times, family lineage was very important: genealogies were written down, and these rarely mentioned the same name twice.

In biblical times, a parent sometimes chose a baby's name from circumstances associated with the conception (as in the case of Isaac) or the delivery (as with Jacob and Benjamin), sometimes from divine acts or attributes (all those including as prefix or suffix "el," "eli," "ya," and "yahu") and sometimes from nature (for example, Deborah [bee] and Jonah [dove]).[2]

During the period of the Second Temple (516 B.C.E.–70 C.E.), Jews began naming their children after grandparents instead of after events and circumstances. This change in naming custom was due partly to the difficulty of maintaining genealogies in the Diaspora and partly to the influence of non-Jewish practices, especially Greek and Egyptian customs.

Since talmudic times, when naming his son at the baby's circumcision, a father has expressed the hope that his child will grow up to a life of Torah, to marry, and to perform good deeds.[3] This blessing has become part of the circumcision ritual, and centuries later, Jews have included it in girl-naming ceremonies, too.

Talmudic rabbis believed that, in biblical times, there had been divine inspiration for naming a baby, but when this ceased, parents chose names known to give good fortune, because a person's name was thought to determine his or her fate and destiny. A further consideration was that the Angel of Death, who was prone to make mistakes, could neglect a person who had the same name as one already dead. These two considerations have affected how Jews chose names for their newborns.[4]

In medieval times, Jews took great care when choosing a name, because they feared that a soul with the same name could transmigrate into the infant's body. They were also aware that the name chosen could determine the child's character.[5]

Traditionally, Ashkenazi Jews have not named a baby after a living relative, but after one who has died, to honor his or her memory. In contrast, Sephardic, North African, and Middle Eastern and Asian Jews have called their children after living relatives. Sephardic Jews have sometimes derived names from the circumstances of birth, as in biblical times; for example, they have named a son born during Hanukkah Nissim, meaning "miracles." Orthodox Jews still favor the traditional naming patterns, in which family names are passed from generation to generation, fostering a sense of family continuity and tradition. When a baby is named after a well-loved relative, the child may grow up identifying with this ancestor and may be proud to continue in family footsteps.

Jewish parents have never given a newborn the name of a baby who had died previously. Until the middle of the twentieth century, such parents gave the new infant a name believed to have protective charm in the hope that tragedy would not strike again. For example, the new baby in an Ashkenazi family was called Alter (if a boy) or Alte (if a girl) meaning "the old one," in the hope that the Angel of Death would not recognize or identify a baby without a real name. The child would receive a real name only on reaching a marriageable age. Sephardic parents gave a newborn the protective name of Marcado or Marcada, meaning "one that is sold," and Judeo-Arabic speakers named the infant Makhlouf, meaning "substitute" or "compensation," when previous babies in the family had died. Such a baby was symbolically sold at birth and was cared for by the "buyers" for the first three days. Sometimes parents named the baby Zion, son or daughter of the Jewish people, in the hope that this appellation was too general for the feared Angel of Death to recognize, or they named him Hayyim, meaning "life." In Yemen, parents named a baby with one of their own names if previous children had died, believing that this offered protection against evil forces or the Angel of Death.[6]

In recent times, some Jewish parents in the United States have discussed the significance of their baby's name and have spelled out their hopes for their child at the naming ceremony. For example, a couple named their daughter Rachel Tzipora and chose to read at the naming ceremony biblical verses beginning with the letters in these two names. Taken from Proverbs, Psalms, and the Book of Ruth, the chosen verses referred to qualities traditionally valued in Jewish women—virtue, wisdom, and love—as well as their hope for longevity and for their daughter to become like Leah and Rachel who, through their sons, built the community of Israel.[7]

RECORDING A BIRTH

Birth Records in Genealogies

In antiquity, the day a person was born was not of particular interest, but Jacob's blessing shows that it was important to know a person's parentage, and this became a reason for keeping birth records.

When the Temple was standing, attempts were made to safeguard the purity of descent of the priests who served there by keeping genealogical records, such as those in the Book of Chronicles. During the period of the second Temple, however, power struggles were based on false genealogical claims. Herod, for example, destroyed the birth records in the Temple and then forged his own family tree to establish his descent from King David.

In mishnaic and talmudic times, Jewish society was stratified according to birth; records may have been kept of who was of priestly lineage, who was a child of a disqualified *cohen*, a convert, a freed slave, a bastard (*mamzer*), or someone whose ancestral conversion to Judaism was considered incomplete. When a baby's father was unknown, or when the child was a foundling of unknown parentage, this too was important to record, because such information affected a person's marriage prospects on reaching maturity.[8] Here again, the necessary records were of lineage and circumstances of birth, not the date of birth. However, the date and time of birth may sometimes have been noticed in talmudic times for possible omens.

Genealogies have been maintained by proud families throughout Jewish history. (*Yiḥus* is the biblical word for genealogy, and a family with *yiḥus* is one with a record of high status in society.) Although in talmudic times rabbis stressed that it was more important to earn a good name through one's actions than to inherit it from birth into a good family, an impressive genealogy has undeniable privileges.[9]

Mazel Tov: A Lucky Star

Throughout the ages, reports of a birth have often included the hope that the baby had been born *be-mazal tov*, or *be-siman tov*, followed by the traditional blessing that the child grow up to a life of Torah, to marry, and perform good deeds. The announcement of a birth in a Jewish family today is greeted customarily by family and friends with the same Hebrew words, expressing hope that the infant was born with good luck—under a good sign, *siman*, or star, *mazal*. The Talmud uses *mazal* to mean "star" or "constellation"; this word has come to mean "luck" through the historical popularity of astrology.[10]

Talmudic sages discussed the effects of the celestial configuration on the night of birth on a person later in life and expected similarities between two people born under the same star. For example, one sage proposed that a person born on Sunday would be distinguished; on Monday, wrathful; on Tuesday, wealthy and sensual; on Wednesday, intelligent and enlightened; on Thursday, benevolent; on Friday, pious. If born on the Sabbath, he was destined to die on a Sabbath. Astrologers estimated that the influence of the ruling planet at the hour of birth could be decisive in determining character, health, and longevity. For example, someone born under the influence of Venus could become rich and adulterous, whereas someone born under Jupiter was more likely to become a righteous observer of commandments. The manner in which the celestial configuration governed behavior remained controversial among Jews for many centuries, however. Nevertheless, someone born under a favorable constellation was considered lucky, whereas if the ruling planet was likely to have unpleasant influences, a person would have to use intelligence and judgment to overcome expected ill effects.[11]

Many eminent medieval astrologers were Jews, who studied, among other things, the influences of the heavenly constellation at a client's birth. Thus, for example, in the twelfth century, Abraham ibn Ezra devoted a whole chapter of his book, *The Beginning of Wisdom*, to explain how the dominance of the planets and zodiac at the hour of birth affects a person's future personality and health. He put this theory to practice, and one horoscope that he cast (in 1160, in Narbonne) on the occasion of the birth of a child has survived the ages.[12]

Several other twelfth-century birth horoscopes calculated by Jewish astrologers in Egypt for Jewish clients are preserved in the Cairo *Geniza*. These horoscopes record the astrological coordinates of a birth in tabular form, giving the positions of the planets and the corresponding zodiac signs as well as a verbal account. Jewish astrologers noted the date according to the Islamic, Christian, or Jewish calendar, all accepted notation of the time.[13]

Another horoscope, calculated on the occasion of someone's birth, was bound into the manuscript book of a Jewish astrologer from Bari, southern Italy—David ben Yacov Meir of the Kalonymos family. A page of extensive calculations documented the night sky at 19 hours 02 minutes, on 28 March 1458.[14]

Some medieval Jews rationalized that the stars affecting people's behavior were themselves controlled by God's will. They taught that a person's pious behavior could possibly influence God to modify the fate determined for that person by the stars. The verses of a medieval Italian Jewish poet reflected his belief that the stars at one's birth influence one's fate; the autobiography of a seventeenth-century rabbi and astronomer from Candia (Crete), and a mystical text, *Sefer Razi'el*, which became popular in the eighteenth century, reveal the same belief.[15]

A popular medieval legend, which has been retold in a ballad sung at Jewish birth celebrations in the Balkans and which recounts the birth of Abraham, reflects the age-old importance attributed to celestial activity at the time of birth, as well as the medieval custom whereby kings employed astrologers to help them make strategic decisions. According to the legend, one evening King Nimrod summoned all his courtiers, councilors, and astrologers to make merry with him. Late at night, as they returned to their homes, they gazed up at the sky, and an enormous comet coursed across the horizon from the east and swallowed four stars, each in a different quarter of the heavens. The astrologers stood aghast and whispered to one another: "Terah's son has just been born. He will be a mighty Emperor. His descendants will multiply and inherit the earth for all eternity, dethroning kings and possessing their lands." Nimrod ordered the baby to be put to death and relaxed only when he was told that this had been done. The murdered infant was not in fact Terah's child, however; his baby, who grew up to be Abraham, was well hidden in a cave, where he was fed by the angel Gabriel.[16]

The astronomical discoveries of Copernicus in the sixteenth century dealt a severe blow to the practice of astrology. Even if some people take astrology columns in newspapers seriously, the study of the stars on the night of birth is usually far from the thoughts of a new father, and the only remnant of these customs is the blessing of *mazal tov*.

Personal Records

Since the fourteenth century, a Jewish father sometimes recorded his children's dates of birth for his own safekeeping. He wrote this information on a page of parchment in his possession that he would be sure not to lose, such as on a valued book. Thus, a medieval kabbalistic treatise has the birth dates of the owner's eight children in the first half of the fourteenth century (as well as the date of their deaths in some cases) on one folio, and on another, the birth dates of another four children of an owner a century later.[17] In La Coruña, in northwestern Spain, a father inscribed on the endpaper of his Bible the birth of his son in 1375, with the hope that he would grow up to a life of Torah, to marry, and to have many sons. The same Bible has a notation on the birth of a son of another owner, sixty-four years later, inscribed on the same page, and the birth of the son of yet another owner, in Turkey, in 1517, after the expulsion of the Jews from Spain.[18] Similarly, a prayer book (*mahzor*), completed in Rome in 1391, has a list of births between 1503 and 1574 recorded on an inside folio. In addition, a fifteenth-century copy of the Roman *mahzor* has a birth record inscribed in Hebrew verse, revealing the parents' hope that the baby was born *be-siman tov* and rejoicing over his birth.[19] Prayer books from Germany, from the same period, also include birth records.[20]

A page of Talmud, dating from the thirteenth or fourteenth centuries, whose calligraphy suggests that it originated in Spain or Italy, had handwritten records of several births between 1620 and 1646 inscribed, with appropriate blessings, in the margin. For example, "Under a good sign, at a good and successful hour, my son Solomon was born, at the third hour after midnight, may he be blessed under the sign of a good year (1640). May he be blessed with many good and pleasant years of Torah study and work and may he been seen at his wedding canopy, Amen." Other entries record infant births as well as an infant death a few months later. The reverse side of the page has the record of a daughter's birth, "*be-mazel tov* and with success, [named] Simha. . . ." The year of birth was given in the form of a pleasant word or phrase, such as "the heavens will rejoice," whose Hebrew letters add up to the correct date.[21]

The custom of maintaining such birth records was not limited to European Jewry. Yemenite manuscripts, too, especially Bibles, have birth records inscribed on their leaves. A Haggadah owned by a Jewish family from Morocco records the birth of a son on the first page.[22]

The custom continued once books were printed, too, in many families for as long as children were born at home.[23] Even when births were systematically registered by municipal authorities, a father registered the baby officially only some time after the birth. He kept his own notes to make sure that he did not forget the details.

Some immigrant Jewish artists who arrived in the United States in the late nineteenth century crafted and sold artistic baptismal certificates, making birth records for their own families, too. For example, Joseph Zelig Glick fashioned his own family record in a painted papercut, which was accepted as proof of his son Samuel's birth when Samuel eventually applied for Social Security benefits.[24]

A Baby in a Basket

A document preserved by Venetian magistrates tells of an unusual birth record in the seventeenth century. The mother recorded the day and time of birth in the hope that her newborn son, whom she abandoned in a Jewish neighborhood, would be circumcised on the eighth day, according to Jewish law, and raised as a Jew.

On the afternoon of July 5, 1691, a middle-aged woman, who had gone out for a moment to buy bread, noticed a basket covered with cloth as she passed through the gates of the Old Ghetto (the Jewish neighborhood) of Venice. She cried out in surprise, and a neighbor came running. Suspiciously, they lifted the cloth together and discovered a newborn baby.

They quickly found a wet nurse so the baby would not suffer. When they unwrapped the infant, they found a paper with the time of birth on the previous day, and a mezuzzah parchment for protection. If the father had been Christian, he would have taken the baby to the foundling home, and if the mother had been of that faith, the child would not be Jewish and would not have been left to be circumcised and raised in the Jewish Ghetto. Furthermore, it was soon ascertained that the baby had to be Jewish because he had been deposited inside the gates after the Ghetto had been locked.

The Ghetto rabbis wanted to know the baby's parentage and therefore posted notices of excommunication against anyone who knew of the baby's origin and did not testify. A few days later, a Jew came to the chief rabbi of Padua and admitted that the baby was born in the house of Ercole Zaccaria Rieti, a Jew from Castelfranco, and that the mother was Corona Levi. Rieti was duly summoned to Venice: he explained that, in April, his stepbrother had asked him to take in, as a servant, Corona Levi, a Jewish girl who was pregnant by him. Rieti and his wife felt they could not refuse the request and agreed to protect Corona's virtue. The baby's father promised to pay all expenses and stated that, after the birth, he would arrange for the baby to be taken to the house of a woman in the Venice Ghetto to be wet-nursed.

Finally, Corona Levi herself was brought to testify. She had worked for the baby's father as a servant for eight years, when she discovered that she was pregnant, and she had gone to the Rieti home, to prevent her family from finding out about the pregnancy. When the child was born, Corona was told that the baby was a girl. That evening, the baby's father came. He refused to tell her what he would do with the baby and took the child with him when he left the next morning. Since his departure, Corona had been praying to discover the baby's whereabouts. She had been crying and hoping for God's justice. She was relieved to have found her child at last, for she recognized her baby's bonnet and swaddling cloth, which she had sewn herself out of a white striped cloth with a little string on the end of the band.

We do not know whether Corona was able to keep her baby after all, or whether, for the sake of her respectability, or by the father's decision, the baby was given to another Jewish family for adoption. The child was permitted to remain in the Ghetto, however, and he was brought up as a Jew.[25]

The Wimpl

Jews have also noted births, with accompanying blessings, on gifts they have donated to the synagogue. For over four hundred years, some Ashkenazi Jewish women transformed the swaddling cloth used at a boy's circumcision into a Torah binder, in Hebrew a *mappah*, in Yiddish a *mape* or *wimpl*, and then donated this to the synagogue. Traditionally, the binder on the Torah scroll is a reminder of the belt worn by the High Priest of the Temple, which was woven with colorful threads and decorated. The binder made from swaddling cloth was decorated, too, with colored threads or paint, noting the name of the child and the name of the father, with the blessing "may God guard and protect him, [may he have been] born under a good constellation on [day of week, date, month, year] and grow up to Torah, the marriage canopy and good deeds."

This custom is said to have originated in an incident that happened in the early fifteenth century. Rabbi Jacob Segal Moellin, (known as the "Maharil"), was serving as *sandek* at a circumcision in a synagogue in Mainz, when it became apparent that the baby's family had forgotten to prepare a clean cloth in which to swaddle the baby after the ritual was performed. The rabbi looked around him and declared that the Torah binder could be used for this purpose. In response to the parents' worries about what they should do with the blood-stained cloth, he told them to launder it well and then return it to the synagogue, where it could again be used to bind the Torah. In addition, he suggested that the family should make a donation to the synagogue.[26]

By the seventeenth century, the custom of painting or embroidering Torah binders was common among the Ashkenazi Jews of western and southern Germany, as well as Switzerland, Denmark, and Bohemia, but it never spread to eastern Germany, Poland, or Russia. The swaddling cloth, usually linen, was laundered and then cut into four strips of about nine inches wide and three feet long that were sewn together, neatly hemmed, and beautifully decorated with the foregoing inscription and colorful motifs such as the signs of the zodiac (relating to the constellation at the time of the baby's birth, a vestige of astrology), fowl, fish, serpents, the marriage canopy, and a Torah scroll. In the late nineteenth and early twentieth centuries, patriotic themes were sometimes depicted on the binder, such as the flag of the nation in which the family resided.[27]

In southern Germany in the seventeenth century, a new mother embroidered the binder during the three weeks after the circumcision when she was housebound, and her husband donated the binder to the synagogue on her first visit there, a month after the birth of the child. A non-Jewish observer reported a few decades later that the custom was for a little boy to deliver the binder himself when he was a year old. If he was happy and eager when he gave it over, the women exclaimed at his wonderfully happy personality: if he gave it reluctantly, or tearfully, they predicted his deep attachment to Torah.[28] The child's binder was used again at his Bar Mitzvah when he was thirteen years old. Some white, undecorated binders and partially decorated (clearly unfinished) items that survived the ages indicate that either the mother or the baby died soon after the birth.[29]

Embroidered binders were stored in the synagogue and, like the book belonging to the *mohel*, formed a birth register for boys only. In Westhoffen, in 1794, these binders were successfully reclaimed after anti-Semitic pillaging, after the Jews claimed that these cloths were a form of community birth register and were not religious items.[30] In 1905, more than six hundred decorated binders were found in the attic of a synagogue in Worms, some dating back to 1570. Tragically, these were all burned when the synagogue was torched in 1938.

Jewish women in Italy also made Torah binders, which they themselves donated to the synagogue, to show their gratitude for safe deliveries. They sewed and embroidered these binders from new silk or fine linen and not from swaddling cloths.[31] In the Ottoman Empire, too, in Rhodes, Salonika, Bursa, and Izmir, women donated Torah binders to the synagogue after birth (although sometimes also before a birth, in the hope of safe delivery). Many of these binders carried inscribed dedications.[32]

The custom of making beautiful Torah binders out of swaddling cloths dwindled in the twentieth century and nearly disappeared during the Holocaust. Some German Jews who reached New York, Israel, and Argentina just before World War II continued this art, which has revived in recent times.[33]

Congratulatory Letters

Letters announcing and congratulating the arrival of a newborn are yet another source of birth records, which have often included blessings and hopes. Letters written by Jews in North Africa in the eleventh century included blessings for a newborn son, but not for a daughter. Verses from the Psalms were quoted to reveal the hope that the son would grow up to be the pride and strength of his father. Medieval letter-writing instructions recommended a formula for replying to the news that a girl had been born—"make her grow [like a plant] in bliss and happiness"—but this blessing has not been found in an actual letter from that time.[34]

Letter-writing manuals were used by scribes who wrote for clients who could not do so themselves. A scribe picked out the necessary formula from the handbook. In addition, for those who could write, it was often easier to copy out a congratulatory letter than to compose it oneself. Since the early seventeenth century, such letter-writing manuals have been printed, some in bilingual or trilingual editions with formulas for announcing the birth of a baby and appropriate congratulations and blessings. Sometimes they have included a letter to a *mohel*, to ask him to come in time to perform the circumcision.[35]

In the early twentieth century, a lying-in scene, a circumcision, or even a redemption of the first-born ritual was printed on a postcard and used as a greeting card, but not as a birth announcement. Printed birth announcements in newspapers and commercial greeting cards soon followed.[36]

LULLABIES

Lullabies have soothing melodies and relax the singer while calming the baby. In the early twentieth century, the mother (or nurse) expressed in her song her desire to hush the baby to sleep, her hopes for the baby's future, her fears, and her frustrations, or she let her tune drift into a dream or a familiar ballad. Some Yiddish lullabies were actually written by men and expressed archetypal hopes and fears—the national dreams of the Jewish people as well as their communal fear and insecurity in this harsh world. Some Judeo-Spanish lullabies were ballads that told well-known tales. These ballads may have been sung originally by men.

The welcoming songs of those who kept company with a lying-in woman in the first week after birth also served as lullabies. These songs often mentioned the circumcision, Elijah the Prophet, the angel who looked after the baby in the womb, local protective behaviors, and traditional gifts or foods offered during birth celebrations. The legend of the birth of Abraham, told earlier, has long been a favorite lullaby among Sephardic Jews.[37]

Lullabies were usually sung in the local vernacular, in Judeo-Spanish, Judeo-Arabic, Yiddish, Aramaic, and other languages spoken by Jews in daily life. It is difficult to know the age of a lullaby, because these songs were rarely recorded. The wide dispersion of similar versions of some Judeo-Spanish lullabies suggests early origins, before the expulsion of Jews from Spain. Many of the Yiddish lullabies known today date only from the nineteenth and early twentieth centuries.

Blessings and Hopes

Moroccan Jews have included their hopes for their son's intellectual future in the verses of a lullaby "with the help of God, the baby will grow up, to interpret the Talmud."[38] A traditional song for the first week, before a circumcision, includes hopes that the infant was born under a good sign, would grow and flourish like a moist garden, succeed, and escape all distress.[39] A Judeo-Arabic lullaby predicts that the boy will be a lawyer or perhaps a doctor. A Judeo-Spanish version, especially popular among Bulgarian Jews, predicts that the infant will soon go to school, then into business, and eventually study medicine.[40]

Ashkenazi Jews sang variations on the same theme; for example, Moishele will study Torah and write holy books, and (God willing) will be good and pious.[41] One pictures the infant as a Talmud scholar, a successful businessman, and a clever bridegroom, but then the mother snaps out of her reverie and notices that the baby is soaking wet.[42] Another lullaby acknowledges that the baby's father has gone to America, where there is food to eat every day, and hopes that one day he will send money to enable mother and baby to join him there. The singer imagines the tears of happiness as the family is united.[43] In yet another song, the mother imagines that the father will burn in the next world (for all his sins), but their son will redeem him with his piety, whereas she herself will go straight to heaven by virtue of her wonderful son.[44]

Perhaps the most famous Yiddish lullaby is *Rozhinkes mit Mandlen* ("raisins and almonds"), composed in 1880 for an operetta by Abraham Goldfaden (1840–1908). It tells of a lonely mother, a daughter of Zion who sits in the Temple, rocking the cradle of her only son. She dreams of a baby goat under the cradle, who went off to trade raisins and almonds, just as her son would one day trade successfully and become wealthy, or better still, become a Torah scholar. A version for a daughter, sung in a Romanian shtetl early in the twentieth century, repeats the scene of the baby goat and insists that the best trade of all is Torah scholarship; this will be the occupation of the baby girl's bridegroom.[45] The "daughter of Zion" is an expression for Jerusalem, where the Temple once stood, but stands no more. Thus, this lullaby expresses not merely a mother's hopes for the future of her child, but also her hopes for the nation, for national deliverance and redemption.

Lullabies composed for baby girls generally focused on the righteous man she would one day marry, or on her beauty. A lullaby for a newborn daughter, from Kurdistan, adopted a style more reminiscent of the Song of Songs, thanking God for her beauty—lips as delicate as thin paper, and a nose like a hazelnut.[46]

Outlet for Tension

Some lullabies expressed a mother's despair at her difficult circumstances, at hard times or at family tensions. For example, a Yiddish lullaby implied that a baby girl's crying irritated her father and implores the infant to go to sleep. A second tells the infant of the hardships of being poor: when he grows up, he will see the luxurious palaces that poor men build for the rich to live in, while the poor suffer sicknesses in their damp cellar homes. A third tearfully predicts that soon the child will leave home to travel across the distant seas; the mother begs in her song that she will receive a letter to ease her pain. Another Yiddish lullaby asks the infant to ignore mother's tears, shed for father who was dragged away and murdered. In one more, the mother notices that the sky is a cloudy gray, just like her heart. A Jewish servant girl in Bessarabia sang an even sadder tune, ending with the thought that it is better to be dead than alive in this ugly world.[47]

Lullabies have been a legitimate outlet for the tensions that arise when living with one's in-laws. The Sephardic story of the evil mother-in-law, mentioned in Chapter 7, was sung on the eve of a circumcision, if not also during the first week after birth, although it is not known whether this was a popular lullaby.[48] The hope that the new mother's own mother will come to help is expressed in a lullaby sung by Jews in Bombay.[49] Bulgarian Jews sang a lullaby of complaint, telling of the hunger of the lying-in woman, who longs for a chicken to eat. She would hide the bones under her bed (as offerings to evil spirits that might bother her).[50] Iraqi Jews sang of an evil sister-in-law who made the new mother's life a misery, and part of the lullaby is in the form of a dialogue between the young woman and her brother, asking for help. This lullaby was recorded in manuscript in the nineteenth century, and again recently by Jewish women who immigrated to Israel from Iraq.

Another lullaby sung by Iraqi Jews tells of the mother's climbing to the roof of her house on a hot and windy evening to look at the view. Up there, she escapes the burdens of her life to take a flight into fantasy. Her son appears in her dream, riding on a bright-eyed mare, while his enemy rides on a dog with clipped ears. The dream meanders through many verses, encompassing her hopes and fears for her son. Eight versions of this song are recorded, some in nineteenth-century manuscripts, others in recent times from Iraqi and Indian Jews. This lullaby is believed to be of Baghdadi origin.[51]

Although some Jews maintain traditional styles of naming their children after relatives, keeping alive the memories of grandparents and great grandparents, many Jews today prefer modern names for their newborns. Nevertheless, many parents still give their child a second name that belongs or belonged to a close relative, to maintain family continuity and a link with family history, or they choose a Hebrew name, to make clear the child's Jewish identity. Today, the name and date of birth of every child is registered by law, and parents keep their child's birth certificate in a safe place instead of writing the important information on a book's endpaper. Tradition is reviving, however, as some women return to the Jewish custom of making a *wimpl* and as artists today offer hand-made birth announcements and certificates with blessings in beautiful Hebrew calligraphy.[52]

Much more difficult is the revival of the traditional lullabies. Few young mothers nowadays understand the Jewish vernacular of the lullabies sung by their foremothers, and even if they know the tunes, which is unlikely, the words have lost their significance. Efforts are currently under way to preserve traditional Jewish lullabies before they are lost forever.[53] When a music box does not calm the baby's cries, a mother will make up a tune and some words to soothe the baby and herself. Many women sing to their newborns, even if they do not know a lullaby. The lullaby and the rocking motion that usually accompanies the song give a woman an active role in handling the baby's distress, by enabling her simultaneously to express or escape her frustrations and to soothe the baby.

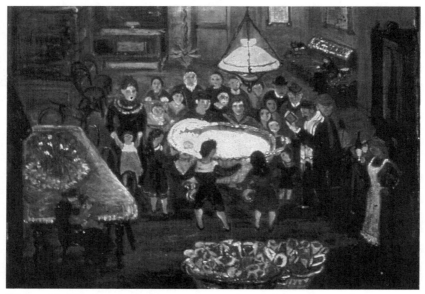

Plate 19. *Houlegraasch* (a ceremony for welcoming and naming a newborn daughter in Lengnau, Switzerland). c. 1950, Alice Guggenheim.
Oil on canvas, 45 × 54 cm. Collection and photo copyright, Israel Museum, Jerusalem.

Chapter Fourteen

Reflections

In the course of our study we have examined how individual Jews have viewed the creation, nurturing, delivery, and celebration of new life and have thereby set the experiences of childbirth today in their historical Jewish contexts—within the realm of personal Jewish experience, the Jewish family, the Jewish community, the secular society that envelops the community, the wider framework of humanity, and God's universe. We have noted how personal fears and pleasures have been given Jewish expression and have looked at the ceremonies, prayers, and blessings that Jewish parents have shared with the community. We have acknowledged that childbirth has sometimes elicited tensions between husband and wife, between daughter-in-law and mother-in-law, and even between a woman and her own mother. Such relationships have always been tested by childbirth, even more so in modern times. We have noted the social context in which childbirth has taken place. The Jewish community traditionally provided a midwifery service for the poor, a bed and food for a poor mother, and financial help in celebrating circumcision. In studying Jewish attitudes toward childbearing, we have also seen how high Jews have traditionally set moral and ethical standards for their communities. However, this aspect of Jewish tradition, like others, reflects patterns set long ago and that are fast disappearing outside Orthodox circles.

Looking around and ahead, what are the possibilities of Jewish expressions relating to childbirth today? Are traditional family roles no longer appropriate when it comes to bearing children? In what ways can or should the Jewish community help today? How do Jewish medical ethics adapt traditional values to modern situations occurring in today's secular world? Finally, what is the significance of childbearing for the Jewish people as a whole, now and in the future?

SPIRITUALITY IN CHILDBEARING

A Jew's beliefs and values mold his or her religious experiences. Thus, someone who accepts the yoke of Torah finds Torah in everyday life as well as in the special experience of bringing a child into the world. In addition, for such a person the prayers, the blessings, duties, and rituals associated with childbearing are all regarded as religious experiences. On the other hand, for many secular Jews, any spiritual feelings associated with childbearing remain amorphous, emotional, and difficult to verbalize. Secular Jews may acknowledge their Jewish feelings only when choosing a name for their newborn, or not at all.

Whether religious or secular, the many prayers, anecdotes, and memoirs in this study have demonstrated that childbearing is often a time when people become particularly sensitized to the spiritual dimension of their experiences.

Spirituality refers not to the institutionalized forms of religious experience, but rather to the existential dimension of faith, to the feeling of communion with God, to the inner consciousness of being Jewish.[1] This existential dimension emerges when a person feels the presence of God and realizes that there is a world or power beyond the earthly realm of everyday life. Such a feeling may also emerge when one's soul is roused—when it weeps or rejoices—or when one feels bound to the Jewish people and to the importance of continuing the tradition of previous generations. Any moment in the long process, stretching from conception through pregnancy and birth to the postnatal period, may have spiritual significance.

Jewish tradition has prescribed prayers, rituals, and duties for the process of childbearing, intended to help the individual transcend the ordinary and reach a higher dimension, to the sacred, to God. Through these prayers, rituals, and duties, Jews have stayed in touch with God. They have sought the transcendent through their offerings of praise and thanks, and through their petitions, alone or together with others. They have also meditated and introspected, repented, and atoned; they have fulfilled their duties, celebrated, and studied. In all these ways, Jews have acquired an appreciation of the meaning of their own lives, of humanity, and of the universe.

A person usually experiences this special awareness only when conducting prayers, duties, and rituals with "directed intention," that is, with a special mental concentration and devotion. Sometimes, however, a Jew cannot experience this devotion when reciting words formulated by ancient rabbis or when performing prescribed behaviors; the heart remains unmoved. For this reason, many Jews have sought new words and new ways of religious expression. Over the centuries, Jews have rewritten childbirth prayers, have added poems and songs, and have embellished rituals to express the spiritual feelings of the times. In the past, these changes came from within the Orthodox establishment; nowadays, they usually come from outside it.

Orthodox Jews today generally perform the accepted duties and rituals and recite prayers that have become "classic"; this is the tradition in their community. Other Jews, however, convinced that their feelings have been neglected in the existent devotional literature, have created new prayers or have changed existing ones, as some did in the past. Thus, new prayers and ceremonies for celebrating a first pregnancy, for mourning a pregnancy loss, for welcoming a newborn, and for naming a daughter reflect the reality that childbearing and Jewish identity today often result from conscious decision making, not from social expectations. These new prayers and rituals acknowledge the responsibility of creating new life and raising a child as a Jew, as well as the need for religious expression at these unique moments in life.

Although the Hebrew language of these prayers and rituals connects today's Jews to previous generations and to other Jews worldwide, it may exclude those who have no access to the language. For this reason, some Jews today, as in the last few hundred years, write many of their prayers in the vernacular.

As we have seen, some Jews have written new poems and songs to express their feelings relating to childbirth. Examples are the *piyyutim* added to Sabbath services when a new father was in the congregation, those added to the circumcision ritual, and the welcoming songs sung by the various Jewish communities. As in the past, poetry and song today find their place, together with new prayers and traditional blessings, in modern Jewish expressions of childbearing experiences.

The mystics, in particular, found new ways to "direct intention" and to achieve mental concentration to sanctify a unique moment. Sometimes they used these skills to help others with childbearing (as in the case of the hasidic tales described in earlier chapters). For the many Jewish women who could not read the holy language and master these methods, mystics inscribed parchment with powerful prayers for childbirth. Such a parchment, with the woman's own name inscribed on it, may have become her own personal petition for God's mercy and thus may have had spiritual significance.

Stories also express the spirituality of childbirth experiences. The incidents in the anecdotes related in earlier chapters and the stories embroidered around them are popular because they uplift the listener. Hearing a tale about the birth of a child after a long period of infertility, not only to Sarah in biblical times, but to a poor tailor more recently, may reassure us of God's continuing concern. How inspiring it is to learn that a Jewish midwife of Kurdistan, when called out in the middle of a stormy night, saw the fulfillment of her difficult task to be "like fulfilling all six hundred and thirteen commandments at once." Her faith in God helped her complete her task successfully. We also marvel at the prayer of the Moroccan midwife, a psychic journey from her individual experience to an appreciation of the needs of others, of her people, and of the Cosmos.

Religious rituals enable Jews to share with others both joyous and frightening experiences, so no one should have to face these alone. Prayer can also redeem a person's isolation, if someone else is praying for or with that person or if others in the same predicament have uttered the same prayer before.

Thus, prayer, ritual, and duty mark special moments and connect a Jew with other Jews and with God, today as ever before. These expressions can have special meaning during childbirth.

RELATIONSHIPS AND EXPECTATIONS

We have seen that, traditionally, a Jewish father prayed for his wife's well-being during childbearing and ensured that his son was circumcised, and, if necessary, redeemed. Today, many wives expect much more from their husbands; they expect their husbands to help in the way their own mothers would have done a generation or two ago.

Similarly, we have seen that a woman pregnant for the first time traditionally moved back to her mother's house or stayed in her mother-in-law's house to give birth, and the older woman provided and cared for the younger one. Young mothers often still expect help from the older generation and are disappointed when it does not materialize. The converse may also occur: the new grandmother may expect to help and is disappointed when her help is not called for or is actually rejected by her daughter or her daughter-in-law.

Thus, the traditional division of labor and the types of emotional and physical support offered a woman during childbirth by her husband and mother are often no longer what they were in the past.

Fathers

In Judaism, paternity, whether or not the parents are married, carries responsibilities. Traditionally, the Jewish father has circumcised and educated his sons, provided for the daily care of his children, and inspired their respect, but he has often done much more. A father's educational duty has been emphasized in Jewish writings through the ages; this duty has included teaching Jewish law, skills necessary for survival, and discipline. His educational role has already begun when the child is weaned and learns to speak. Thus, traditionally, a father has taught his child to be independent and to find a place in the outside world, while the child has learned emotional security and love from its mother.[2]

Although the tender bond between Jacob and his youngest son, Benjamin, is an example of a father's love for his son, in biblical times fathers (especially Jacob) often indulged in favoritism, incurring jealousy among siblings. In mishnaic times, Jewish men had little serious contact with children beyond religious matters, and, in the middle ages, Maimonides pointed out that the feeling and love of a father for his newborn is weak compared with when the child is two or three years old. The Zohar deduced that a man appreciates the love of his grandchildren more than that of his children. Even today, many older men find that they have more time for their grandchildren than they had for their own children.[3]

Most men today want to involve themselves with their children much more than their own fathers did, and they consider themselves better fathers as a result. However, usually only in legal cases of disputes about child care, paternity, or abortion are a father's duties, roles, and expectations defined. A couple may begin by sharing the daily chores and responsibility for the child, but soon one ends up doing more than the other, and sometimes resentment develops.[4]

Grandparents

"May you live to see your children's children" (Psalm 128:6) has been a favorite Jewish blessing since antiquity. It expresses the hope that a person will live a long life, long enough to welcome the arrival of grandchildren; Jewish tradition regards this as a blessing. The role of a grandparent has always carried a certain status and respect. Grandparents have offered advice and help; they have been consulted about religious affairs, business deals, marital conflicts, children's behavior problems, and even sticky questions concerning the Evil Eye. Grandfathers have been respected for their intellectual, spiritual, and legal wisdom, whereas grandmothers have been skilled in managing their households and sometimes in business, too, in curing ills and advising about childbearing.

Today's stereotypical "smother-mother" and depressed middle-aged "empty-nester" have resulted from an overemphasis on a woman's childbearing functions and a lack of other sources of fulfillment. In modern times, however, more and more people are discovering that in middle age one can find a new direction in life, through study or a change in career, and grandparents have other interests than to continue in their roles as mother and father. Thus, the sages taught that one is blessed with old age to live on meaningfully, creatively, and productively.[5]

Many middle-aged parents yearn for a grandchild and may feel bitterly disappointed that their children have not provided them with this expected source of happiness. Because grandparenting is a stage in the human life cycle that cannot be reached by willing, the older generation depends on their children's fertility and desires. When the children comply, family bonds are strengthened, but no Jewish ritual celebrates becoming a grandparent, and no rules about grandparents' responsibilities exist.

Many Jews still name their newborns after a grandparent. Grandparents have traditionally played an important role in the lives of their grandchildren. Just as grandchildren provide continuity into the future, so grandparents provide continuity with the past, with family history, with Jewish tradition, and with the history of the Jewish people as a whole.

In many families, social mobility has loosened the bonds of the extended family and has necessitated a reappraisal of the traditional roles of the elder generation and of mutual expectations. The extended family needs to make a conscious effort to maintain relationships. The birth of a child and family gatherings for subsequent birthday celebrations and Jewish holidays can help to maintain these relationships. Perhaps the elderly who live far from their children can, if they want, revive traditional roles by interacting with and helping younger members of their community, for example by helping a lonely new mother with cooking, shopping, and even babysitting or by reading to and teaching youngsters.

COMMUNITY INVOLVEMENT

The Jewish community's involvement in the process of childbearing has also changed in modern times. Today, when a couple cannot conceive, it is no longer regarded as a community problem or the business of relatives; it is the couple's private affair. When a woman gives birth, she is no longer delivered by her female relatives and neighboring women; she expects privacy, and she shares the experience with at most one or two persons of her choice. In the week after birth, new parents no longer need to cope with a flood of well-meaning visitors day and night; they are given time to recover and regain a sense of normality in their lives. At the circumcision or welcoming ceremony for a girl, the parents usually choose whom to invite, possibly the whole community if the ceremony is held on a Shabbat at synagogue, but probably not if at another time and place. In previous times, the entire community was involved because the birth of children was important to the continuity of that community, and everyone was relieved and grateful that the child had arrived safely and the mother had survived. Nowadays, the physical dangers are diminished, and the threat to continuity stems from assimilation, not infant mortality. We still celebrate birth, but not to the extent that it was celebrated in the past.

Although events that were shared before are now often privatized, events that were private before are often shared today. For example, in the past, a woman kept the news of her pregnancy to herself, for the first few months at least, and then probably shared it only with her husband and mother, whereas some women today want to share their joy of pregnancy with a wider group as soon as possible and celebrate in some way. In addition, the birth of a daughter is no longer a quiet family affair; the event has been upgraded in recent years, often to the same status as a circumcision. Now parents want to welcome a daughter ceremoniously and celebrate her arrival with the extended family and in the community as joyously as they welcome a boy. Moreover, weaning, which once was a private experience, is occasionally celebrated more openly, too, as Abraham and Sarah did in antiquity.

Traditionally, the Jewish mourning ritual, which encourages the sharing of grief, was not observed after miscarriage or stillbirth; each was a private tragedy (even if gossip soon made it common knowledge), more common in the past than in modern times. Nowadays, some Jews want social recognition of their grief when pregnancy ends in tragedy and observe all or part of the mourning cycle, or they create their own mourning ceremony.

The extent to which a Jewish community offers help with childbearing depends on the emphasis placed on birth within the community and its attitudes toward communal responsibility. Orthodox Jewish communities, where the birth rate is high, generally offer more help than other communities. Some of these communities still provide new mothers with financial support, home help or cooked meals, and even a bed in a rest home. Children have also been a first priority in the Israeli kibbutz, a society organized from the very beginning to ease the burden of new parents. The birth rate in secular kibbutz families is still higher than in secular families elsewhere in Israel.

Local Jewish Family Services sometimes offer advice about genetic counseling centers, childbirth preparation classes, mother–toddler groups (which can also serve as postnatal support groups), and day-care centers (which allow a mother to return to work). These last two are particularly important when the nuclear family has disintegrated, and even when it has not, when no extended family is available to help.[6] "Stars of David" is a national nonprofit support network for Jewish adoptive families. The National Council of Jewish Women, headquartered in New York, has set up a pregnancy loss counseling service for coping with miscarriage, stillbirth, and neonatal death. Yad Elisha offers similar support in Jerusalem.[7]

Few local Jewish communities offer care or any form of extra help for families with a child who needs special attention. Parents can contact their local Jewish Family Service to see what help is available. Such specialized support services are usually undertaken by nonsectarian organizations that work nationwide to help children with special needs and provide support groups to help parents cope with a specific problem, such as The National Tay-Sachs and Allied Diseases Association, which works from a base in Newton, Massachusetts. In some areas, non-Jewish services of this sort cater adequately to Jews, and the community may regard it as unnecessary to offer parallel services.[8] Parents with special needs may feel that the Jewish community should take a more active supportive role.

If childbearing is important to the community, then the community has to consider seriously what help its members require, such as information services, physical help, financial assistance, emotional support, and educational guidance.[9] Rabbis and Jewish social workers must be sensitized to the needs of infertile couples, young parents, single parents, families with special-needs children, and those who have lost a pregnancy or an infant. Moreover, the Jewish community must offer professional genetic counseling, abortion counseling, adoption counseling, marriage counseling, education for childbirth, and postnatal support.

ETHICAL CONCERNS

Jewish tradition has established certain ideals regarding childbearing. It has recommended that sexual intercourse take place in love and joy, in purity of mind and body. It has stressed the sanctity of human life and has dictated under what circumstances contraception and abortion should be practiced. It has also emphasized the importance of righteous, moral, and ethical behavior at all times, as well as parental responsibility to raise the child in the spirit of Torah.

In the modern secular world today, however, advances in medical technology now give people unprecedented power to intervene in the natural process of bringing a child into the world. Thus, with professional help from doctors, we can destroy a fetus in the womb, we can destroy our fertility or make ourselves temporarily infertile, we can conceive outside the womb, and we can engineer the sex of the baby we conceive. Local legislation and consensus are setting new standards about whether it is moral and ethical for people to use this new knowledge.

How do Jewish medical ethics adapt to such modern situations? Jewish medical ethics are guided by Jewish tradition and strive to uphold the high Jewish moral standards. Jews who use halakhah as the basis for decisions of what is moral and ethical judge each new situation in a thoroughly scholarly fashion and reach a decision on the basis of halakhic precedents and interpretations. Others, however, have abandoned halakhah as their basis, ascribing instead to a rights ethic based on the protection of individual liberties as long as these do not disturb the community. Many liberal rabbis have been influenced by public opinion, by politicians, and by secular lawyers in forming their views on, for example, the legality of abortion, contraception, and infertility treatments. In addition, some secular Jews argue that a traditional framework is unnecessary, that each person can make an individual decision of what is moral and correct. They contend that traditional Jewish attitudes have become archaic and irrelevant. Thus, they would say that if a Jew wants a vasectomy to render himself infertile (a sin according to halakhah), he can decide for himself that this is right for him.[10] Problems arise, however, when the people involved disagree, when, for example, a mother wants to abort a fetus but the father does not want to lose his child. Who should decide what course to follow? On what basis will the decision be reached? Jewish medical ethics would give the baby's life priority over parental whims, whereas in the secular world, a woman could abort the child regardless of the father's desire. Without an ethical framework, it is not always easy to know the right path.

Because Jewish medical ethics differ from secular medical ethics, decision makers do not always reach the same conclusion about what is moral and ethical. For instance, if a child is conceived by rape, not in love and joy, and not in purity of mind and body, that is, when a woman's sanctity has been violently abused, the consensus of secular opinion would back the woman's demand for an early abortion, professionally performed, and would deem this neither unethical nor immoral. In contrast, Jewish medical ethics require a scholarly opinion that takes into account the rights to life of both mother and fetus, and the anticipated grave psychological or physical hazard to the mother of bearing the unwanted baby. The final decision could be the same in both systems, but often it is not.

The modern possibilities and potential abuses of vasectomy and female sterilization, contraception, abortion, artificial insemination by a donor, the freezing of embryos, surrogate motherhood, and genetic engineering raise problems not only for halakhah and Jewish medical ethics, but also for humanity in general. For this reason, it is important that there be some sort of ethical framework that limits the practice of these behaviors, especially when more than one party is involved. This is not solely the concern of Orthodox rabbis; today, interdisciplinary teams made up of theologians, lawyers, doctors, and scientists are continually working on this problem.[11]

SIGNIFICANCE OF CHILDBEARING FOR THE JEWISH PEOPLE

Jewish tradition teaches that people's behavior affects the society in which they live, the world at large, and even the coming of the Messiah. Thus, the arrival of a newborn is important not just for the baby's family, but also for Jews as a people. That is why there is social pressure in many Jewish communities to have children—pressure from prospective grandparents, from those who already have children, from the family, and from Jewish leaders.

Rabbis teach that having children is an act of faith. Ultimately, the reward for having children, like the reward from the fulfillment of other religious commandments, is great, stretching beyond the limits of one's life on earth and benefiting the Jewish people as a whole. This abstract idea is an essential element in a Jew's acceptance of "the yoke of Torah."[12] Thus, Orthodox Jewish couples generally have large families, if they can, at the expense of many of today's luxuries, because they believe that their enrichment and their future lies in their children.

In our own time, the experience and memory of the Holocaust have affected the size of Jewish families: many survivors and their children want to restore families that were decimated. Jewish leaders often urge people to have larger families, to bring the Jewish population back to where it was before the Holocaust.[13]

Jewish leaders who are not Orthodox have also encouraged Jewish parents to have more children, to counteract the threat to Jewish survival posed by the declining rate of marriage, by family planning, and by postponement of childbearing, as well as by assimilation and secularization. Jewish communities that have modernized have had little or no natural population increase. Furthermore, statistics warn that the overall Jewish population is on the decline. Some Jewish feminists protest that these calls for increased Jewish birth rates turn women into baby-making machines. They also point out the double standard in Jews' advocating zero population growth for the over-populated world but not for the Jews.[14]

The significance of childbearing for the Jewish people is not just a question of numbers, however. Rather, it is a qualitative issue that involves Jewish identity and Jewish education because if Jewish children are raised in an environment lacking any Jewish content, an increase in birth rate among Jewish mothers will not contribute to the continuity of the Jewish people. Only children who develop Jewish identity and who have Jewish education will contribute to that continuity.

May we laugh with delight, like Sarah, when we discover that we are going to have a child, and may our children be born with *mazel tov*, healthy and strong. May they grow up inspired by their Jewish heritage, to live up to the ideals of Torah, and to perform good deeds, and may we ourselves live to enjoy our children's children.

NOTES

1. Fertility

1. Genesis 8:17, 9:1, 9:7.

2. Genesis 12:2, 13:16, 15:5, 17:2–6, 21:13, 22:17, 26:4, 26:24, 28:14, 32:12.

3. Exodus 32:13; Leviticus 26:9; Deuteronomy 1:10–11, 7:13; Isaiah 45:18; Jeremiah 3:16, 23:3; Ezekiel 16:7, 36:9–11; Hosea 1:10; Psalms 45:17, 127:3–5, 128:3.

4. Deuteronomy 28:4, 18, 62.

5. Hosea 9:14.

6. *B. Avodah Zarah* 5a; *B. Yevamot* 62a, 63b; *B. Niddah* 13b; *Genesis Rabbah* 24:4. This view is also found in the early kabbalistic text of *Sefer ha-bahir*. For an overview of this literature and more sources, see Cohen, J., *"Be Fertile and Increase, Fill the Earth and Master It": The Ancient and Medieval Career of a Biblical Text* (Ithaca: Cornell University Press, 1989), 115–119, 201–202.

7. *B. Berakhot* 10a; *Song of Songs Rabbah* 1:4. Maimonides, M., *The Code of Maimonides: Mishneh Torah*, translated by I. Klein (New Haven: Yale University Press, 1972), The Book of Women, 15, 16.

8. *B. Berakhot* 31b; in a midrash from the early Middle Ages, *Midrash tadshe*, edited by A. Epstein, in *Mi-kadmoniyot ha-yehudim: mehkarim u-reshimot*, edited by A.M. Habermann (Jerusalem: 1957), vol. 9, pp. 152–153; and in a midrash from the late Middle Ages, *Midrash ha-gadol*, edited by M. Margoliyot (Jerusalem: Mossad ha-rav Kook, 1956), vol. 1, p. 435.

9. *Genesis Rabbah* 34:14; Zohar I, 12b–13a.

10. Ruth 4:15; *B. Yevamot* 65b; *J. Kiddushin* 1:7:9. Caro, J., *Shulhan arukh*, edited by Z.H. Preisler and S. Havlin (Jerusalem: Ketuvim, 1993), *Even ha-ezer*, 154:6.

11. Abrahams, B.Z., *The Life of Glückel of Hameln*, (London: Horovitz, 1962), 104. The imagery of children "like olive plants" comes from Psalm 128.

12. Zohar I, 115b.

13. Friedenwald, H., *The Jews and Medicine* (Baltimore: Johns Hopkins University Press, 1944), vol. 1, p. 382, quoting Amatus Lusitanus (1511–1568), *Centuria*; he was an outstanding physician, born to *Marrano* parents, but was only able to practice Judaism openly in the last decade of his life. Many of the early Reform communities abandoned this custom, but some are now reinstating it, allowing daughters also to recite the *Kaddish*, not only sons.

14. Genesis 18:11–14; *Genesis Rabbah* 94:9.

15. Zborowski, M., and E. Herzog, *Life Is with People* (New York: Schocken, 1962), 308–309, quote the "scooped-up" one, without giving the original Yiddish word. Scholars of Yiddish at Bar Ilan University, Tel Aviv, did not know of this custom, or the Yiddish word that Zborowski and Herzog had in mind. Hayyat, S., "Ha-mishpahah be-pitgamim shel yehudei Bavel," *Folklore Research Center Studies*, 3 (1973): no. 216. My thanks to Zvi Yehudah, at the Babylonian Jewry Museum, for his comments.

16. *Yevamot* 6:6; *Shulhan arukh, op. cit.*, sign. 1.

17. Ecclesiastes 11:6; *B. Yevamot* 62b. Cohen, J., 1989, *op. cit.*, pp. 130–131 reviews rabbinic attitudes to the acceptance of a *mamzer* as fulfillment of the duty to procreate: most post-talmudic rabbinic sources followed the Palestinian Talmud and accepted a *mamzer* as fulfillment of the duty, although Judah ben Samuel of Regensburg (Judah the Pious), *Sefer Hasidim*, edited by R. Margoliyot (Jerusalem: 1957), sign. 500, ruled to the contrary.

18. *Yevamot* 6:6; *B. Yevamot* 61b and 65b. For more detailed discussion, see Cohen, J., 1989, *op. cit.*, pp. 140ff.

19. "Should life prisoners 'be fruitful and multiply'," *The Jerusalem Post*, Dec. 20, 1985.

20. Genesis 48:16, 49:22; Ruth 4:11–12.

21. Patai, R., *On Jewish Folklore* (Detroit: Wayne State University Press, 1983), 294.

22. Attias, M., *Romancot ve-shirei am be-yahadut Sepharadit* (Jerusalem: Ben Zvi Institute, 1961), 44. Hacohen, M., *Hagid Mordekhai: korot Luv ve-yehudeiah* (Jerusalem: Ben Zvi Institute, 1979), 275.

23. Ben-Ami, I., "Le mariage traditionel chez les Juifs Marocains," *Israel Folklore Research Center* 4 (1974): 52ff.

24. Rashi's exegesis on this verse makes the link between fish and fertility: see Rashi on Genesis 48:16 in *Chumash with Targum Onkelos, Haphtaroth and Rashi's Commentary*, translated by A.M. Silbermann and M. Rosenbaum (Jerusalem: Silbermann, 1985). Also *Exodus Rabbah* 1:17.

25. The biblical promise and comparison with the seeds of the field are quoted at the beginning of this chapter: Ezekiel 16:7. This practice in talmudic times is found in *B. Berakhot* 50b; the *Tosafot* commentary to this passage reports that the custom was observed in medieval Europe. Ethnographic documentation of this tradition has been reviewed by Shtal, A., *Mishpaḥah ve-giddul yeladim be-yahadut ha-mizraḥ* (Jerusalem: Academon, 1993), 283.

26. A documentary film on the *mikveh* celebration before the wedding has been made recently in Jerusalem, by Arlene Edelman, for Emunah. *Encyclopedia Judaica* (Jerusalem: Keter, 1972), vol. 5, p. 1265 reports the custom of the *Koilich Tanz*. Debbi Cooper recently photographed this tradition at a hasidic wedding in Jerusalem. Lamm, N., *A Hedge of Roses* (New York: Feldheim, 1977), 100–103 revives the bride's prayer that the marriage will result in children; this dates from c. 1800, Italy.

27. *B. Baba Batra* 16b; *B. Berakhot* 59b–60a; *B. Niddah* 31b; *B. Sanhedrin* 100b; *B. Yevamot* 62b.

28. *B. Gittin* 57a.

29. *B. Baba Batra* 141a. This idea is evident in Jewish proverbs from many communities, for example in Yiddish, Judeo-Spanish, and Judeo-Arabic proverbs; see sources quoted in notes 35, 36, and 38 below.

30. *B. Niddah* 31b.

31. Jacob ben Asher, *Arba'ah turim* (Vilna: 1900), *Va-yikra* 12:2.

32. *Numbers Rabbah* 11:13.

33. Goitein, S.D., *A Mediterranean Society* (Berkeley: University of California, 1978), vol. 3, p. 226. Also Friedman, M.A., *Ribui nashim be-Israel* (Tel Aviv: Bialik Institute and Tel Aviv University, 1986), 202–203.

34. Shtal, A., 1993, *op. cit.*, pp. 331ff. The strong preference for sons was reported, for example, by Isaac, I.A., *A Short Account of the Calcutta Jews* (Calcutta: 1917), 9; Chorny, J.J., *Sefer ha-massa'ot be-eretz Kavkaz* (St. Petersburg: 1887), 195–196; Brauer, E., *The Jews of Kurdistan*, edited by R. Patai (Detroit: Wayne State University Press, 1993), 160–161; Molkho, M., "Leidah ve-yaldut bein yehudei Saloniki," *Edot* 2 (1947): 256.

35. Zborowski, M., and Herzog E., 1962, *op. cit.*, p. 310.

36. Alkali, A., *Emrot ve-pitgamim shel yehudei Sefarad* (Jerusalem: 1984), 187, 193.

37. "*Caucasioni*," The Organ of the Caucasiological Center and the Gapmor Literary Society, V (1980).

38. Dahan, H., *Otzar ha-pitgamim shel yehudei Marocco* (Tel Aviv: Stavit, 1983), nos. 36ff. and notes.

39. Alexander, T., and Noy, D., *Otzaro shel abba* (Jerusalem: Center for Research of Sephardi and Oriental Culture, 1989), 135–136.

40. *B. Berakhot* 60a. In the first two days after the couple's union, the husband should pray that the seed should not putrefy and die.

41. Epstein, Y.M., *Kitzur shnei luḥot ha-brit* (Jerusalem: 1984), *Inyanei zivvug*, p. 75. The first part of this prayer is attributed to Nahmanides. The first printing of this book was in Fürth in 1683, although it was based on an earlier book by Isaiah ben Avraham Horowitz, *Shnei luḥot ha-brit*, which was first published in Amsterdam, 1649. Epstein, Y.M., *Seder tefillah derekh yesharah* (Frankfurt an der Oder: 1703), 24a–b includes prayers for sons. Hannover, Nathan Nata, *Sha'arei tziyyon* (Prague: 1662), *Sha'ar* 5, *Tikkun*, repeats the same prayer in Epstein's *Kitzur* and similarly attributed it to Nahmanides. This same bedside prayer for a son was copied by David Tevle Ashkenazi, *Beth David* (Williamsdorf: 1704), 22a.

42. *Seyder tkhines* (Amsterdam: 1752), 9b, translated from Yiddish by C. Weissler and quoted in Weissler, C., "The traditional piety of Ashkenazic women," in *Jewish Spirituality from the Sixteenth Century to the Present*, edited by A. Green. (New York: Crossroad, 1987), 260–261. This prayer is also

found in the Yiddish *Seyder tkhines u-vakoshes* (Fürth: 1762), 93, and in at least two early nineteenth-century Italian prayer books, *The Voice of Supplication* (Trieste, 1824), in the collection of the Sir Isaac Wolfson Museum in Heikhal Shlomo, in Jerusalem, and in a leather-bound volume in the collection of Mr. Itzhak Einhorn, Tel Aviv.

43. An example of such a prayer book is in the collection of Mr. Itzhak Einhorn, Tel Aviv.

44. A Hebrew version of the Yiddish prayer exists in a handwritten, leather-bound book of prayers for the *mikveh* belonging to an Italian Jewish woman and dating from the early nineteenth century; the book is now owned by Mr. Itzhak Einhorn, Tel Aviv. Another earlier (late eighteenth century) manuscript version has recently been printed in Hebrew and English translation: Cardin, N.B. *Out of the Depths I Call to You* (Northvale, NJ: Jason Aronson, 1992), 36–37, 42–43, 70–71. Also personal communication from Prof. Meir Benayahu.

45. Neuda, F., *Hours of Devotion*, translated by R. Vulture (Vienna: Jos. Schlesinger, c. 1900), 110–111. The original German prayers were published under the title *Stunden der Andacht* (Prague: 1857), and in twenty-eight subsequent editions by the 1920s. Another English translation, by M. Maier, was published in New York.

46. Weiss, J., *Studies in Eastern European Jewish Mysticism* (Oxford: Oxford University Press, 1985), 126–130. The talmudic reference is *B. Baba Kamma* 92a.

47. An example of the prayer on an amulet is given in Davis, E., and D.E. Frenkel, *Ha-kame'a ha-ivri* (Jerusalem: Institute for Jewish Studies, 1995), 126. An early nineteenth-century popular Sephardic prayer book recommends that a man donate oil to the synagogue, in the name of Rabbi Meir Baal Ha-ness, in the hope of calling on the spirit of this worker of miracles to intercede that a son be born: Papo, Eliezer ben Itzhak, *Beit tefillah* (Jerusalem: 1968), 61. Also Ben-Ami, I., *Ha'aratzat ha-k'doshim* (Jerusalem: Magnes Press, 1984), 58–59, 584.

48. *B. Niddah* 31a–b. See also Rosner, F., "Sex Determination as Described in the Bible and Talmud," in *Medicine in the Bible and Talmud* (New York: Ktav, 1977), 173–178.

49. Feldman, D.M., *Marital Relations, Birth Control and Abortion in Jewish Law* (New York: Schocken, 1978). Chapter 7 of Feldman's book is devoted to the rabbinic interpretation of this phrase.

50. *B. Niddah* 31b.

51. Cohen, S.J., ed., *The Holy Letter: A Study in Medieval Jewish Sexual Morality, Ascribed to Nahmanides* (New York: Ktav, 1976), 144ff. The Hebrew treatise, *Iggeret ha-kodesh*, was first published in Rome in 1546.

52. *B. Berakhot* 5b.

53. Ilem, I., *Seker ethnologi shel kehilla ha-gruzinit be-Ashkelon* (Hebrew University, Sociology and Anthropology Department, 1974), 389. Brauer, E., 1993, *op. cit.*, p. 168. Ben Simhon, R., *Yahadut Marocco* (Lod: Orot Yahadut Magreb, 1994), 14, 100. Ohana, R., *Mareh ha-yeladim* (Jerusalem: 1990), 37: this remedy book, which contains many talmudic remedies and citations as well as many folk potions that are not kosher, was first published in Jerusalem in 1901.

54. Zunser, M.S., *Yesterday—A Memoir of a Russian Jewish Family* (New York: Harper & Row, 1978), 100–101.

55. *Sefer Hasidim*, 1957, *op. cit.*, sign. 452–453. See also *Encyclopedia Judaica*, vol. 8, pp. 1027–1028.

56. *Segullot ve-refu'ot* no. 143, requires the testes of a donkey: this is an Ashkenazi remedy book of the sixteenth or seventeenth century that is in the Jesselson Collection in New York. Luntz, Elijah ben Moshe, *Toldot Adam*, (Zolkiew: 1720), items 13, 14, 96 provide recipes for sons including the testes of a rabbit. Badehev, Itzhak b. Michael, *Segullah zahav*, (Jerusalem: 1894), 34–35, offers ten items of advice for those desiring a son, repeating some of the advice in *Toldot Adam*. Other recipes using parts of a male animal for a son and parts of a female animal in a potion for when a daughter was desired were offered in the medieval remedy book attributed to Abraham Ibn Ezra: Leibowits, J.O., and S. Marcus, *Sefer ha-nisyonot* (Jerusalem: Magnes Press, 1984), 225. The brain of a male swallow was recommended by Joseph Tirshom in *Shoshan yesod olam*, (Damascus: c. 1550); Sassoon ms. 290, item 440. See also Patai, R., 1983, *op. cit.*, p. 348 ff. for many magical remedies involving animal parts, used by Jews in the early twentieth century in North Africa, Turkey, and Jerusalem.

2. Barrenness

1. Genesis 16:2; I Samuel 1:10.

2. Genesis 38; Deuteronomy 25:5–10.

3. The *akarah* is distinguished from the *aylonit* ("ram-like," "barren woman"), who had never menstruated. See Rashi on Genesis 15:2 concerning a man without an heir, in *Chumash with Targum Onkelos, Haphtaroth and Rashi's Commentary*, translated by A.M. Silbermann and M. Rosenbaum (Jerusalem: Silbermann, 1985).

4. Isaiah 54:1.

5. Genesis 16:5; 30:2.

6. Judges 13; *B. Yevamot* 64a.

7. *B. Avodah Zarah* 5a; *B. Nedarim* 64b.

8. *B. Sanhedrin* 36b.

9. *Yevamot* 6:5–6, 64b. The tale comes from *Song of Songs Rabbah* 1:4:2.

10. Maimonides, M., *The Code of Maimonides: Mishneh Torah*, translated by H. Klein (New Haven: Yale University Press, 1964), The Book of Women: The Levirate, 1:2, and Jacob ben Asher, *Arba'ah turim* (Vilna: 1900), *Even ha-ezer* 165.

11. Zunser, M.S., *Yesterday—A Memoir of a Russian Jewish Family* (New York: Harper & Row, 1978), 76ff.

12. Allouch-Benayoun, J., and D. Bensimon, *Les Juifs d'Algerie* (Toulouse: Privat, 1989), 144. For the talmudic view that infertility is established only after the second marriage proves childless, see *Yevamot* 6:6 and *B. Yevamot* 64b.

13. Patai, R., *Gates to the Old City* (New York: Avon, 1980), 548–552, an English translation of a tale found in a collection of minor midrashim published in the original Hebrew and Aramaic in *Otzar Midrashim*, edited by J.D. Eisenstein (New York: 1915), vol. 2, pp. 350–351. Also in medieval times, Judah the Pious warned that a childless man is lost both from this world and the World to Come; Judah ben Samuel of Regensburg (Judah the Pious), *Sefer Hasidim*, edited by R. Margoliyot (Jerusalem: Mossad harav Kook, 1957), sign. 517.

14. Hacohen, Eliyahu ben Shlomo Avraham, *Shevet mussar* (Jerusalem: Y. Rubinstein, 1963), part 2, chap. 24, p. 193. This book was first published in Constantinople in 1712. The author lived in Smyrna (Izmir) and died in 1729.

15. Friedman, M.A., *Ribui nashim be-Israel* (Tel Aviv: Bialik Institute and Tel Aviv University, 1986), 175–178, 202–203: these are transcripts of medieval letters, preserved in the Cairo *Geniza*, written by childless married men requesting remarriage for the sake of having offspring. See also Feldman, D.M., *Marital Relations, Birth Control and Abortion in Jewish Law* (New York: Schocken, 1978), 38 nn. 90–91, and 39, quoting from the Responsa of Solomon ben Adret (d. 1310). Maimonides's ruling accepting bigamy is in *The Code of Maimonides: Mishneh Torah*, translated by H. Klein (New Haven: Yale University Press, 1964), The Book of Women: Marriage, 3:9.

16. I interviewed the great-grandmother in Rehovot, Israel, in 1985. See also Deutsch, G., "All My Wives," *Jerusalem Post Magazine*, Nov. 20, 1992, pp. 6–7.

17. Shenhar, A., and H. Bar-Itzhak, *Sippurei am me-Beit She'an* (Haifa: Haifa University Press, 1981), 174.

18. Ben Simhon, R., *Yahadut Marocco* (Lod: Orot Yahadut Magreb, 1994), 13, 17, offers remedies to "wake" the baby in the womb.

19. Katznelson-Shazar, R., ed., *Memoirs of the Pioneer Women of Palestine*, translated by M. Samuel (New York: Herzl Press, 1975), 224.

20. Genesis 18:14; 25:21.

21. I Samuel 1; Judges 13:3, 24.

22. *B. Yevamot* 64a; *Genesis Rabbah* 45.4; *Song of Songs Rabbah* 11.14.8.

23. *Genesis Rabbah* 73.4, *Deuteronomy Rabbah* 7:6.

24. Genesis 25:21.

25. I Samuel 1:11.

26. Binesh, Binyamin, *Sefer amtahat Binyamin* (Wilmersdorf: 1716), 17b. Also *Seder tehinot* (Prague: 1712), sect. 12.

27. Neuda, F., *Hours of Devotion*, translated by R. Vulture (Vienna: Jos. Schlesinger, c. 1900), 110; my adaptation.

28. Weissler, C., "The traditional piety of Ashkenazic women," in *Jewish Spirituality from the Sixteenth Century to the Present*, edited by A. Green. (New York: Crossroad, 1987), 245–275. Weissler quotes other such prayers for reciting at the *mikveh*: *Seyder tkhines* (Amsterdam: 1742), 9b; *Seder tkhines u-vakoshes* (Fürth: 1762), no. 93; *Shloyshe she'orim*, attributed to Sore Bas-Toyvim, also eighteenth century. See also Cardin, N.B., *Out of the Depths I Call You* (Northvale, NJ: Jason Aronson, 1992), 20ff., for prayers recited by an Italian Jewish woman in the late eighteenth century when lighting the Sabbath candles, at the *mikveh*, before sexual intercourse. The same prayer for reciting when lighting candles, that includes the plea that God not count this woman as one of the barren, and that she should be worthy of having outstandingly gifted and devout children and grandchildren, is found in another Italian prayer book for women, *The Voice of Supplication* (Trieste: 1824), 4, in the collection of the Sir Isaac Wolfson Museum, at Heikhal Shlomo, Jerusalem. This book also includes the same prayer (as in Cardin's book), for a woman to recite before sexual intercourse, with the request for pure seed and pregnancy (p. 8b). *The Merit of Our Mothers: A Bilingual Anthology of Jewish Women's Prayers*, compiled and introduced by T. Guren Klirs, translated by T. Guren Klirs, I. Cohen, and G. Schweid Fishman (Cincinnati: Hebrew Union College Press, 1993), 112–113, includes an English translation and Yiddish original of a "*Tkhine* for when a Woman Goes to Observe the Mitsve of Immersion in the Mikve," taken from *Rokhl Weeps for Her Children* (Vilna: 1910).

29. Hannover, Nathan Nata, *Sha'arei tziyyon* (Amsterdam: 1662), *Sha'ar* 5, *Tikkun Kiryat Shema*. See also Epstein, Yehiel Michl, *Seder tefillah derekh yesharah* (Frankfurt an der Oder: 1703), 24–25. Both these sources included a prayer attributed to Nahmanides. The Aramaic incantation against Lilith was taken from Zohar III, 19a. For an explanation of the incantation and formula, see Scholem, G., *On the Kabbalah and Its Symbolism* (New York: Schocken, 1995), 108–109, 157. My thanks to Prof. Hava Turniansky for calling to my attention also the prayers in *Tefillah derekh si'ah ha-sadeh*, Bodleian Library, Oxford, Opp. Octo 732, p. 30, which I was unable to consult.

30. *The Merit of Our Mothers, op. cit.*, 1993, includes an English translation and the Yiddish original of a "*Tkhine* for Having Children," for a woman who has no children, taken from *Rokhl Weeps for Her Children* (Vilna: 1910), 114–115.

31. *Neue tehinos u-vakoshes* (Hamburg: 1729), sect. 23.

32. Elisha enabled the barren Shunammite woman to have a son: II Kings 4:9ff. See Fraser, J.G., *The Golden Bough* (New York: Macmillan, 1927), 48ff. on the easy confusion between magic and intercessors: Jews, like other peoples, assign supernatural powers to an intercessor; if this person achieves his goal through divine insight this is religion, but otherwise, some magic may be involved.

33. The quotation is from *Song of Songs Rabbah* 1:4:2. See also *B. Berakhot* 34b, where Ḥanina ben Dosa is called upon to intercede with prayer for the sons of Gamaliel and Johanan ben Zakkai.

34. Poll, S., *The Hasidic Community of Williamsburg* (New York: Schocken, 1969), 118.

35. Buber, M., *Tales of the Hasidim: Later Masters* (New York: Schocken, 1948), 204 tells of the visit of a barren woman to Rabbi Isaskhar Baer of Radoshitz (d. 1843); p. 310 tells that childless couples would visit Rabbi Yitzhak Meir of Ger (d. 1866), in the hope of his help in conception. Sabar, Y., *The Folk Literature of the Kurdistani Jews* (New Haven: Yale University Press, 1982), 172, relates a Kurdistani folktale that tells of the custom of a barren woman visiting a great rabbi for a blessing to conceive. Alexander, T., and D. Noy, *Otzaro shel abba* (Jerusalem: Center for Research of Sephardi and Oriental Culture, 1989), nos. 4, 8, and 24 are Sephardic tales about Jewish women who went to the rabbi to ask him to pray for them to conceive. Tales no. 26 and 69 are also Sephardic tales about childless couples, whom Elijah the Prophet helps to fulfill their desire to have children. See also Band, A.J., *Nahman of Bratslav: The Tales* (New York: Paulist Press, 1978), 109–111. Bar Itzhak, H., and A. Shenhar, *Jewish Moroccan Folk Narratives from Israel* (Detroit: Wayne State University Press, 1993), 55, 116 quote two folk narratives about barren women seeking help from a rabbi to conceive. In both these stories, the childless couple had to decide whether they wanted a girl or a boy, and in both cases the rabbi predicted the child's fate to be unhappy. This is a common motif in Jewish folktales from Morocco, Tunisia, Turkey, Iraq, Persia, and India.

36. Buber, M., *Legends of the Ba'al Shem Tov* (New York: Schocken, 1969), 121ff. tells that many childless women visited the Baal Shem Tov. See also Ben-Amos, D., and J.R. Mintz, *In Praise of the Baal Shem Tov* (Bloomington: Indiana University Press, 1972), 132, 214, 224–226. Patai, R., 1980, *op. cit.*, pp. 743–745, regarding the Maggid of Koznitz.

37. Buber, M., *Tales of the Hasidim: Early Masters* (New York: Schocken, 1972), 292.

38. Trachtenberg, J., *Jewish Magic and Superstition* (New York: Atheneum, 1982), 64. For an example of such prayers, see Zelig, Shmuel ben Yehoshua, *Sha'arei dim'ah* (Jerusalem: 1884). The author, rabbi of Dalhinov, died in 1858.

39. Ben-Ami, I., *Ha'aratzat ha-k'doshim* (Jerusalem: Magnes Press, 1984), 58, n. 16.

40. *Ibid.*, pp. 243, 246, 247, 446, 522, 539, 584. Noy, D., *Moroccan Jewish Folktales* (New York: Herzl Press, 1966), 39–40. Also Patai, R., *On Jewish Folklore* (Detroit: Wayne State University Press, 1983), 36ff.

41. Solomon, Jacob ben Abraham, *Ma'aneh lashon* (Tel Aviv: Sinai, 1965), 65–66, my translation. This book was first printed in Prague in 1615. Many later editions were published in Central and Eastern Europe, including some in Yiddish, Hebrew, German, and Hungarian.

42. Ben Simhon, R., 1994, *op. cit.*, p. 11 quotes two prayers, one in Judeo-Arabic, recited by Moroccan Jewish women, and another in Hebrew taken from a book by Baghdadi rabbi Yosef Hayyim (b. 1834), *Hukkei ha-nashim*.

43. Genesis 20:17–18; Leviticus 20:20–21; II Samuel 6:23; *J. Sukkah* 5:4:4. *Sefer Hasidim*, 1957, *op. cit.*, para. 476. See also note 30 above and note 44 below.

44. Sadeh, P., *Jewish Folktales* (New York: Doubleday, 1989), 337–338. Sadeh took this story from the Hebrew version in Bar Hayyim, Z.A., *Sippurim nifla'im* (Jerusalem: Ravid ha-zahav, 1964).

45. Buber, M., 1969, *op. cit.*, pp. 179–184. In another tale, the Baal Shem Tov explains that a man's childlessness was due to his having committed adultery; Ben-Amos, D., and J.R. Mintz, 1972, *op. cit.*, pp. 185–186.

46. *B. Yevamot* 64b; *B. Gittin* 70a. Jastrow, M. ed., *A Dictionary of the Targumim, the Talmud Babli and Yerushalmi, and the Midrashic Literature* (New York: Verlag Choreb, 1926), vol. 1, under *aylonit*. For advice on foods that increase sexual potency, see *B. Berakhot* 40a; *B. Baba Kamma* 82a; *B. Gittin* 70a; *B. Sotah* 11b; *B. Yoma* 18a–b. The frequent reference to this problem reveals its importance.

47. Rosner, F., ed., *Sex Ethics in the Writings of Moses Maimonides* (New York: Bloch, 1974), chap. 20, pp. 69–72; chap. 22, pp. 50, 65. Rosner, F., *Maimonides' Commentary on the Aphorisms of Hippocrates: Maimonides' Medical Writings* (Haifa: Maimonides Research Institute, 1987), 152.

48. Bodleian Library, Neub. ms. 2142, col. 741 f. 250a(1). My thanks to Dr. R. Barkai for the transcript; my translation.

49. *Zikaron ha-holayim*, Montefiore ms. 440, f. 15v; my translation. My thanks to Dr. R. Barkai for the Hebrew transcript.

50. *Sefer ha-toledet*, Jews College ms. 253, now British Library, London, Montefiore ms. 420. This is a medieval Hebrew adaptation of Muscio's (sixth century) Latin text, *Gynecia*, which in turn was a translated version of Soranus's treatise on this topic, written four centuries earlier. Two other manuscripts of *Sefer ha-toledet* are preserved in Rome (Casanatense Library, J.IV.5), and in the Vatican (ms. Heb. 366 no. 5). A French translation has been published: Barkai, R., *Les infortunes de Dinah: Le livre de la génération* (Paris: Editions du Cerf, 1991).

51. Zahalon, J., *Otzar ha-hayyim* (Venice: 1683), book ix, 90c.

52. Lampronti, I., ed., *Pahad Itzhak* (Livorno: 1834). See entry *akar, akarah*.

53. Cohn, T., *Ma'aseh Tuvya* (Venice: 1708), part 6, chaps. 3, 7, 13. Remedy books often offered sterility tests, which usually applied to women only. Urine was tested with bran for its generative powers (if the bran germinated she was fertile, but if it rotted she was sterile), or garlic was put in her womb to see whether the smell would pervade her (if it pervaded, she was sterile).

54. Leibowitz, J.O., and S. Marcus, *Sefer ha-nisyonot, the Book of Medical Experiences Attributed to Abraham ibn Ezra* (Jerusalem: Magnes Press, 1984), 63. Maimonides explained that suffocation of the uterus occurs when the woman loses her breath and is helped by sneezing: Rosner, F., 1987, *op. cit.*, pp. 140–141.

55. The ancient urine test is translated in Betz, H.D., ed., *The Greek Magical Papyri in Translation* (Chicago: University of Chicago, 1986), PDM xiv 956–960. This papyrus dates any time between the second century B.C.E. and the fifth century C.E. Also see Luntz, Eliahu ben Moshe, *Toldot Adam* (Zolkiew: 1720), sects. 30 (for the same urine test), 3 (for the bugloss infusion), and 10 (another suggestion for enabling conception).

56. Blondheim, S.H., and D.E. Blondheim, "Matriarchal Infertility, and Adoption as a Prelude to Conception," *Koroth* 9 (1985): 90–91, quoting the views on this subject of Rashi, Levi ben Gershon, Rabenu Nissim, and Ovadia S'forno. Gold, M. *And Hannah Wept* (Philadelphia: Jewish Publication Society, 1988), chap. 7, "Adoption as a Jewish Option."

57. *B. Yevamot* 34b.

58. *J. Nedarim* 11:12.

59. Trachtenberg, J., 1982, *op. cit.*, p. 34. The story was taken from *Sefer Hasidim*. Nowadays, some psychotherapists have encouraged patients to experience a symbolic birth as a form of treatment: Verny, T., and J. Kelly, *The Secret Life of the Unborn Child* (London: Sphere, 1982), 193–195, tells how psychotherapists enact birth with pediatric patients to cure physical ills. Estes, C.P., *Women Who Run With the Wolves* (London: Rider, 1995), 431, 441 discusses the importance of birth symbolism in the psyche, for mental health. Infertility doctors today usually look for physical causes first, before examining the possibility of psychological causes and referring patients to a psychotherapist.

60. Buber, M., 1948, *op. cit.*, p. 204.

61. Shenhar, A., Beth Hatefutsoth video documentary.

62. *Shabbat* 6:10.

63. *J. Sanhedrin* 7:13:4a–r. Retold as a folktale in Schwartz, H., *Miriam's Tambourine* (Oxford: Oxford University Press, 1988), 35–38.

64. For example, Eleazar of Worms, Elijah of Chelm, Isaac Luria (the Ari), Judah Loew of Prague, and Israel ben Eliezer (the Baal Shem Tov) all allegedly performed magical deeds. See tales in Sadeh, P. 1989, *op. cit.*

65. *B. Gittin* 68a–b.

66. *The Testament of Solomon*, para. 22–25. This text was originally written in Greek and has strong Jewish elements, although it may or may not have been written by a Jew. Sixteen manuscripts have survived the ages, in four different recensions. An English translation, by F.C. Conybeare, of one manuscript, is found in *Jewish Quarterly Review* 11 (1899): 20–21.

67. Luntz, Eliahu ben Moshe, 1720, *op. cit.*, sect. 1.

68. Zohar V, 43a, 194b. Another remedy from Solomon's magic book, to stop a baby's crying, is recorded in a Yiddish remedy book, dating from the sixteenth or seventeenth century, attesting to the continued popularity of this magic book. This remedy book is in the collection of Mrs. L. Jesselson, New York; see item 65.

69. *Sefer Hasidim*, 1957, para. 391, 447, 476, 517. These beliefs were not limited to Germany. Also Jews in Mediterranean lands attributed a man's impotence to his wife's casting a spell on him; see Friedman, M.A., 1986, *op. cit.*, pp. 166–168.

70. Ulmer, R., *The Evil Eye in the Bible and Rabbinic Literature* (Hoboken, NJ: Ktav, 1994), 158ff. Deshen, S., and M. Shokked, *Yehudei ha-mizrah* (Jerusalem: Shocken, 1984), 65–66.

71. Naveh, J., and S. Shaked, *Magic Spells and Formulae* (Jerusalem: Magnes Press, 1993), 160–161, quoting from the *Geniza* fragment T.S. K.1.19 in the Taylor-Shechter collection of Cambridge University Library. Also Luntz, E., 1720, *op. cit.*, sects. 108–111, 130 and Itzhak ben Eliezer, *Refuah ve-hayyim me-Yerushalayim* (Jerusalem: Bakall, 1974), 26–27, which is a modern edition of an earlier kabbalistic text.

72. *B. Shabbat* 66b and Rashi; *Genesis Rabbah* 45:2. For the rabbinic position regarding the general use of amulets, *Shabbat* 6:2 and 61a.

73. Such amulets can be found in some collections of Jewish amulets, such as in the Israel Museum in Jerusalem (for example, Feuchtwanger no.788), in the collection of the Glazer Institute of the History of Medicine, Jerusalem (XXB, 12), in the Jewish Museum in Basel (JMS 513), in the

Wellcome Institute in London (Heb. 28), and in the collection of Itzhak Einhorn in Tel Aviv. Some folktales tell of barren women visiting a rabbi for an amulet, that they might conceive: for example, there are two in Bar Itzhak, H., and A. Shenhar, 1993, *op. cit.*, pp. 55, 116.

74. *B. Shabbat* 66b and commentary. Trachtenberg, J., 1982, *op. cit.*, p. 134 and p. 295 n. 3. A picture of an eagle stone used by non-Jews for protection in difficult labor, in Bavaria in the late nineteenth century, is reproduced in Ploss, H.H., and M. and P. Bartels, *Woman*, edited by E.J. Dingwall (London: Heinemann, 1935), vol. 3, p. 23.

75. Miriam Katz-Russo, of the Israel Museum, personal communication.

76. Ashkenazi, David Tevle b. Yacov, *Beit David* (Williamsdorf: 1704), 22b. Elzet, Y. (J.L. Zlotnik), "Me-minhagei Israel," *Reshumot* 1 (1918): 363, quoting from *Sha'ar ha-shamayim*, chap. 5.

77. Rosner, F., 1987, *op. cit.*, p. 151 cites an oft-quoted fumigation test of Hippocrates for ascertaining whether a woman is capable of conceiving. Maimonides explained which sharp subtances should be used for the fumigation. If the scent of the fumigation passes through her from its source below her and reaches her nostrils and mouth, there is no reason why she should not conceive. See also Patai, R., 1983, *op. cit.*, pp. 339–362. Patai cites the pig's testicles remedy on pp. 353–354.

78. Josephus, *The Jewish War* (Harmondsworth: Penguin, 1959), 397–398. This is a translation, by G.A. Williamson, of the book by Joseph ben Matithyahu, later called Josephus Flavius.

79. Krispil, N., "Eggs of the Witch," *Israelal* 41 (1992), 8–12. Krispil N., *Yalkut ha-tzemahim* (Jerusalem: Cana, 1983), 115–121. Both of these publications have many illustrations, historical and modern, of the mandrake plant.

80. Bodleian Library, Neub. 2142, col. 741, f. 252a.

81. Bahya ben Asher, *Bi'ur al ha-Torah*, edited by H.D. Shawal (Jerusalem: Mossad ha-rav Kook, 1967), vol. 2; Exodus 28:17.

82. Bibliothèque Nationale, Paris, ms. Heb. 1199, f. 22v.

83. Basnage, J., *République des Hébreux* (Amsterdam: 1713), vol. 2, pp. 339–340; my translation.

84. Krispil, N., 1983, *op. cit.*, p. 121, and 1992, *op. cit.* Hamoi, A., *Ha'ah nafshenu* (Jerusalem: Bakall, 1981), 68: this is a reprint of a remedy book first printed in 1871. Pallache, H., *Sefer refuah ve-hayyim* (Izmir: 1873), and O'Hana, R., *Mareh ha-yeladim* (Jerusalem: 1990): this is a reprint of the remedy book first printed in 1901.

85. Zohary, M., *The Plants of the Bible* (Cambridge: Cambridge University Press, 1982), 188. The reference to *duda'im* in Song of Songs 7:13 describes them as fragrant. Rashi and Nahmanides, in their commentary to Genesis, also suggested that the plant referred to is jasmine.

86. Exodus 28:17–21. *Numbers Rabbah* 2:7 explains that Reuben's stone was *odem* (a red stone), and the color of his flag was red, on which were embroidered *duda'im*.

87. In the seventh century B.C.E., the ancient Babylonians used carnelians to revive the dead and believed that red stones symbolize life: Pritchard, J.B., *The Ancient Near East: An Anthology of Texts* (Princeton: Princeton University Press, 1958), 85, 88. *B. Baba Batra* 16b tells of Abraham having worn a precious stone that healed all those who looked at it.

88. See note 81.

89. Trachtenberg, J., 1982, *op. cit.*, pp. 137, 265. The manuscript is in the Jewish Theological Seminary Library, and the relevant entry is on f. 43a.

90. Itzhaki, I., *Lahash ve-kame'a* (Tel Aviv: Shakked, 1976), 135.

91. Sperling, A.I., *Ta'amei ha-minhagim ve-makor ha-dinim* (Jerusalem: Eshkol, 1961), 567. *Midrash talpiyot*, under the letter *aleph*, is quoted as his source.

92. Pallache, H., 1873, *op. cit.*, chap. 9. Another remedy book published in Izmir at that time, Hamoi, 1871, *op. cit.*, also refers to the use of rubies in this way, but quotes *Cahana Rabbah* as a source.

93. Miriam Katz-Russo, personal communication. There are many examples of these rings in the Israel Museum.

94. *B. Berakhot* 55b. The Sir Isaac Wolfson Museum in Jerusalem has several red stone amulets on display. Two of these are pieces of red coral, as described by Bahya ben Asher. Both are labeled as eighteenth century, one from Morocco (4 cm long), the other "from Eastern lands" (6 cm long). Another reddish

stone, no more than 1 cm in diameter, with a hole through the middle, must have also served barren women. It is labeled as being of Babylonian origin. Two others are elliptical carnelian (a form of chalcedony), with Hebrew inscriptions, one with a *Magen David* and incantations (labeled Iraq, nineteenth century), the other with Psalm 16:8 and all of Psalm 67 in the shape of a *menorah* (probably also of a similar provenance and date). Both would have been used to keep the Evil Eye from harming the woman. Another small red stone amulet, very similar to these, a pink carnelian with an inscription of Genesis 49:22 and Psalm 121, commonly used for fertility and childbirth, is in the Steiglitz Collection of the Israel Museum. Midwife Rachel Shalkowsky of Jerusalem and gynecologist Dr. Sara Daniel of Rehovot both reported to me the use of reddish stones today among hasidic Jews desiring to conceive.

95. Horowitz, H.M., ed., *Tosefta atikta* (Cracow: 1890), part 5, p. 19, footnote.

96. Layard, J., *The Lady of the Hare* (Boston: Shambhala, 1988).

97. *Sefer ha-toledet, op. cit.*, p. 53a.

98. Bodleian Library Neub. 2142, *op. cit.*, f. 250(2)b; my translation.

99. Luntz, Eliahu ben Moshe, 1720, *op. cit.*, sect. 2. Luntz was reputedly from Chelm, Poland.

100. Simner, Zekhariah ben Yacov, *Sefer zekhirah* (Wilmersdorf: 1729), 53b; my translation. This book of Jewish folk remedies was especially popular in Eastern Europe and was frequently reprinted in the eighteenth and nineteenth centuries. The same instructions were copied into other remedy books, such as Badehev, I.M., *Sefer segullah zahav* (Jerusalem: 1894), 32, and O'Hana, R., 1990, *op. cit.*, p. 81.

101. A. Hamoi, 1981, *op. cit.*, p. 74. *Sefer segullot ve-hiddot* (Damascus: 1870), 75a, a manuscript containing old recipes that Dr. R. Patai located, includes advice for conception: dry the stomach of a hare in a pan together with a fish within another fish, then powder the contents and consume with a drink. A remedy book published in Jerusalem favors a recipe using a hare's womb; O'Hana, R., 1990, *op. cit.*, p. 82, under *herayon*, and another using the burned skin of a hare can be found in Rozenberg, Y., *Rafael ha-malakh* (Pietrkov: 1911), under *herayon*.

102. *Refu'ah ve-ḥayyim me-yerushalayim* (Jerusalem: Bakall, 1974), 43. Sperling, A., 1891, *op. cit.*, p. 567. Rozenberg, Y., 1911, *op. cit.*, also offered a fertility potion made of willow, quoting the *gematria*; see *herayon*, last entry. Ovadiah, D., *Kehillat Sefrou* (Jerusalem: *Maḥon le-ḥeker toldot kehillot yehudei Marocco*, 1975), vol. 4, p. 47.

103. Raphael, F., and R. Weyl, *Les Juifs en Alsace* (Toulouse: 1977), 243.

104. Gold, M., 1988, *op. cit.*, p. 71.

3. Contraception and Abortion

1. A letter in the Cairo *Geniza* tells of a friend's warning to a young man whose first baby was a daughter: do not be too eager to have a child every year lest they all be girls: Goitein, S.D., *A Mediterranean Society* (Berkeley: University of California, 1978), vol. 3, p. 230.

2. For an in-depth study of the rabbinic approach to these issues, the reader is referred to Feldman, D.M., *Marital Relations, Birth Control and Abortion in Jewish Law* (New York: Schocken, 1978); Rosner, F., and J.D. Bleich, eds., *Jewish Bioethics* (New York: Sanhedrin Press, 1979); Rosner, F., ed. *Medicine and Jewish Law* (Northvale, NJ: Jason Aronson, 1993), vol. 1, pp. 105–222; Steinberg, A., *Jewish Medical Law, Compiled and Edited from Tzitz Eliezer*, translated by D.B. Simons (New York: Bet Shamai, 1989), part 4.

3. Mishnah and *B. Ketubbot* 63a–64b. *The Code of Maimonides: Mishneh Torah*, translated by I. Klein (New Haven: Yale University Press, 1972), The Book of Women, 15:1. A fragment preserved in the Cairo *Geniza* reveals that one married woman threatened to divorce her husband if he did not agree to complete abstinence; see note 1 above. Caro, J., *Shulḥan arukh*, edited by Z.H. Preisler and S. Havlin (Jerusalem: K'tuvim, 1993), *Even ha-ezer*, 77:1–2.

4. *B. Yevamot* 63b.

5. *B. Sotah* 12a; *Exodus Rabbah* 1:13.

6. *B. Baba Batra* 60b.

7. The laws limiting sexual relations during menstruation and before ritual immersion are Leviticus 20:18 and the tractate of *Niddah* in the Mishnah and Talmud. Maimonides, M., *The Code of Maimonides: Mishneh Torah*, translated by I. Klein (New Haven: Yale University Press, 1972), The Book of Women, 15:1, p. 93. *Shulḥan arukh*, 1993, *op. cit., Even ha-ezer*, 76:5.

8. For rabbinic discussion of the "safe period," see Feldman, D.M., 1978, *op. cit.*, pp. 247–248.

9. *B. Kiddushin* 30b; *B. Sotah* 44a. *Zohar Hadash* I, Genesis 4d warned that in the old days the sages were willing to let their wives and children go hungry while they devoted themselves to the study of Torah, but nowadays no one should marry until his livelihood is secured. See translation by D. Goldstein in *The Wisdom of the Zohar*, edited by F. Lachower and I. Tishby (Oxford: Oxford University Press, 1989), 1384. Feldman, D.M., 1978, *op. cit.*, pp. 27–28 nn. 34 and 35, documents the responsa on this topic. Jakobovits, I., *Jewish Medical Ethics* (New York: Bloch, 1975), 363 n. 6. In-depth demographic studies show that the pattern of early marriage changed as a function of non-Jewish legislation, urbanization, industrialization, and education. For example: Lowenstein, S.M., "Voluntary and Involuntary Limitation of Fertility in Nineteenth Century Bavarian Jewry," in *Modern Jewish Fertility*, edited by P. Ritterband and P. Hyman (Leiden: E.J. Brill, 1981), 94–111. Here the large majority of Jewish husbands married in their thirties and were professionals or had learned a trade. In comparison, a study of Eastern European Jews in the eighteenth century revealed that, in an unskilled population, more than half the Jewish men had married before the age of twenty: see Plakans, A., and J.M. Halpern, "An Historical Perspective on Eighteenth Century Jewish Family Households in Eastern Europe," *Ibid.*, 18ff.

10. Jakobovitz, I., 1975, *op. cit.*, chap. 13.

11. Genesis 38:9.

12. *B. Yevamot* 34b. See Feldman, D.M., 1978, *op. cit.*, chaps. 6 and 8 for full rabbinic discussions of the issue. For a slightly different interpretation of the same sources, see Satlow, M.L., *Tasting the Dish: Rabbinic Rhetorics of Sexuality* (Atlanta: Scholars Press, 1995), 236ff.

13. Maimonides, M., *The Code of Maimonides: Mishneh Torah*, translated by L.I. Rabinowitz and P. Grossman (New Haven: Yale University Press, 1965), The Book of Holiness: Laws Concerning Illicit Intercourse, 21:18. Judah ben Samuel of Regensburg, *Sefer Hasidim*, edited by R. Margoliyot (Jerusalem: 1957), sign. 499. The quotation is taken from Zohar I, 219b. See also the same ruling in Ganzfried, S., *Code of Jewish Law: Kitzur Shulḥan Arukh*, translated by H.E. Goldin (New York: Hebrew Publishing, 1961), vol. 4, chap. 151.

14. Leviticus 22:24; *B. Shabbat* 110b; *Tosefta Makkot* 5:6; *Tosefta Bekhorot* 3:24; Caro, J., *Shulḥan arukh*, edited by Z.H. Preisler and S. Havlin (Jerusalem: K'tuvim, 1993), *Even ha-ezer* 5:11.

15. Judah ben Samuel of Regensburg, *Sefer Hasidim* (Berlin: Hevrat Mekitzei Nirdamim, 1891), 2nd ed. (Frankfurt: J. Wistinetzki, 1924), sign. 18. Concerning the issue of vasectomy today, see Rosner, F., 1993, *op. cit.*, p. 106ff.

16. *B. Shabbat* 110a.

17. *B. Yevamot* 65b–66a. Rosner, F., *op. cit.*, pp. 111–115.

18. *B. Yevamot* 34a–b.

19. *Genesis Rabbah* 23.2; *J. Yevamot* 6:5; Rashi on Genesis 4:19, in *Chumash with Targum Onkelos, Haphtaroth and Rashi's Commentary*, translated by A.M. Silbermann and M. Rosenbaum (Jerusalem: Silbermann, 1985).

20. *Zikaron ha-ḥolayim*, Jews College London, Montefiore ms. 440, f. 24a.

21. Benveniste, S., *Ha-ma'amar be-toladah*. Bodleian Library Neub. ms. 2142: f. 254a.

22. Jakobovits, I., 1975, *op. cit.*, p. 164.

23. Feldman, D.M., 1978, *op. cit.*, p. 240 n. 35, citing Rabbi Solomon Luria, and p. 237, citing Rabbi Joshua Falk.

24. Lampronti, I., ed., *Paḥad Itzḥak* (Livorno: 1834), see entry *Kos shel ikkarin*.

25. Feldman, D.M., 1978, *op. cit.*, pp. 237–238.

26. *B. Yevamot* 12b, 100b; *B. Niddah* 45a; *B. Nedarim* 35b; *B. Ketubbot* 39a.

27. Soranus, *Gynecology*, translated by O. Temkin (Baltimore: Johns Hopkins University Press, 1956), book 1:19, no. 60.

28. *B. Ketubbot* 37a; *B.Yevamot* 35a.

29. *Sefer ha-toledet*, British Library, London, Montefiore ms. 420. Many recipes for a *mokh* are given on pages 49a–53a. For French translation and commentary, see Barkai, R., *Les infortunes de Dinah: Le livre de la génération* (Paris: Editions du Cerf, 1991).

30. He took this recipe from a book by the Persian physician, Rhazes (c. 865–c. 930), although the *Book of Medical Experiences* was copied from the work of an Arab physician, Abd-al Rahman ibn al-Haitham, who in turn attributed this recipe to Dioscorides, a Greek physician who lived in the first century. Dioscorides in fact gave few recipes for vaginal contraceptive pessaries, preferring oral contraceptives. Papyri from Greco-Roman Egypt include the recommendation for a vaginal contraceptive suppository with magical properties.

31. Exodus 22:17; *B. Sanhedrin* 67a–68a. For a summary of early magical remedy books, see Alexander, P.S., "Incantations and Books of Magic," in *The History of the Jewish People in the Age of Jesus Christ 175 B.C.–A.D. 135*, edited by E. Schürer, rev. ed. and translation by G.Vermes, F. Millar, and M. Goodman (Edinburgh: T. and T. Clark, 1986), vol. 3, pp. i, 342–379.

32. Leibowitz, J.O., and S. Marcus, *Sefer ha-nisyonot: The Book of Medical Experiences Attributed to Abraham ibn Ezra* (Jerusalem: Magnes Press, 1984), chap. 3, pp. 64–65, 228–229. The same advice—to hang on oneself the heart or foot of a hare—was offered by Meir Aldabi, in the fourteenth century, as well as the stool or the heart of a mouse: Aldabi, M., *Sh'vilei emunah* (Warsaw: 1887), part 5, sign. 1, p. 112. Aldabi also quoted advice from Hippocrates for a contraceptive suppository. Isaacs, H., *Medical and Paramedical Manuscripts in the Cambridge Geniza Collections* (Cambridge: Cambridge University Press, 1994), cites a medieval Judeo-Arabic pharmacopeia with advice for contraception in the Cambridge University Library: TS.AS. 169.150.

33. Benayahu, M., "Inyanei refu'ah be-katov-yad lo yadu'a shel Hayyim Vital," *Koroth* 9 (1987): 12.

34. Simner, Zekhariah ben Yacov, *Sefer zekhirah* (Wilmersdorf: 1729), 54a.

35. Patai, R., *On Jewish Folklore* (Detroit: Wayne State University Press, 1983), 366–369.

36. Hamoi, A., *Ha'aḥ nafshenu* (Jerusalem: Bakall, 1981), 64. See entries for *neged herayon*. This is a reprint of the 1870 edition published in Izmir. Gross YM 11.41, p. 2 in the Gross Family Collection, Ramat Aviv.

37. Shepherd, N., *A Price Below Rubies: Jewish Women as Rebels and Radicals* (Cambridge, MA: Harvard University Press, 1993), 216–221. Hyman, P.E., "The Immigrant Jewish Experience in the U.S.A.," in *Jewish Women in Historical Perspective*, edited by J.R. Baskin (Detroit: Wayne State University Press, 1991), 228.

38. *B. Sanhedrin* 72b; *J. Sanhedrin* 8:9:3. Maimonides, M., *The Code of Maimonides: Mishneh Torah*, translated by H. Klein (New Haven: Yale University Press, 1954), The Book of Torts: Murder and Preservation of Life, 1:9.

39. Aldabi, M., 1887, *op. cit.*, part 5, sign. 1, p. 112. Aldabi had studied the medical writings of the ancient Greeks and drew widely on these. However, he was clearly also familiar with contemporary medicine.

40. *Sefer ha-toledet, op. cit.*, f. 28r. Barkai, R., 1991, *op. cit.*, p. 141.

41. Feldman, D.M., 1978, *op. cit.*, pp. 277–283. A woman whose pregnancy threatened her with approaching deafness also qualified for abortion.

42. Glick, S., "A Comparison of the Oaths of Hippocrates and Asaph," *Koroth* 9 (1986): 297–302.

43. Quoted in Feldman, D.M., 1978, *op. cit.*, p. 288.

44. Bleich, J.D., "Abortion in Halakhic Literature," in Rosner, F., and J.D. Bleich, eds., 1979, *op. cit.*, pp. 152–153.

45. Genesis 34.

46. *Pirkei de Rabbi Eliezer*, edited and translated by G. Friedlander (New York: Hermon Press, 1981), chap. 38. See Graves, R., and R. Patai, *Hebrew Myths* (New York: Doubleday, 1964), 235ff. for various versions of the story, and for its recent formulation as a folktale, see "The Golden Amulet," in Schwartz, H., *Miriam's Tambourine* (Oxford: Oxford University Press, 1988), 158–162.

47. *B. Yevamot* 35a; *B. Ketubbot* 37a.

48. Bleich, J.D., 1979, *op. cit.*, p. 175, n. 92; and Feldman, D.M., 1978, *op. cit.*, p. 287, quoting Resp. *Or Gadol*, no. 31.

49. Jakobovits, I., "Jewish Views on Abortion," in Rosner, F., and J.D. Bleich, eds., 1979, *op. cit.*, p. 128.

50. *B. Ketubbot* 37a; *B. Yevamot* 35a.

51. *B. Niddah* 30b.

52. Gaster, M., "The Sword of Moses," in *Studies and Texts* (New York: Ktav, 1971), vol. 1, pp. 300, 326, no. 88.

53. Riddle, J.M., *Dioscorides on Pharmacy and Medicine* (Austin: University of Texas Press, 1985), 58. Soranus, 1956, *op. cit.*, book 1:19, no. 60.

54. Leibowitz, J.O., and S. Marcus, 1984, *op. cit.*, pp. 64–65, 228–229.

55. *Zikaron ha-ḥolayim, op. cit.*, f. 21b.

56. Benveniste, *op. cit.*, f. 254a. See Schäfer, P., "Jewish Magic Literature in Late Antiquity and Early Middle Ages," *Journal of Jewish Studies* 41 (1990): 88. Here the author reports that a medieval remedy book preserved in the Cairo *Geniza* also gives advice on how to abort a fetus: T-S. NS 322, 10, f.16, lines 27ff. and f. 2a lines 13ff. I was not able to study this manuscript.

57. Isaacs, H., 1994, *op. cit.*, cites Arabic and Judeo-Arabic pharmacopoeias, TS.Ar.43.47 (blue licorice to help expel the fetus), TS.Ar.45.30, and TS.AS. 181.83 include abortifacients and recipes for inducing menstruation. TS.Ar.42.151 has a recipe for an abortifacient for use when the fetus has died in the womb.

58. Marx, A., "The Scientific Work of Some Outstanding Medieval Jewish Scholars," in *Essays and Studies in Memory of Linda R. Miller*, edited by I. Davidson (New York: Jewish Theological Seminary of America, 1938), 145. A Jewish physician from Spain, who wrote a medical treatise in the fourteenth or fifteenth century, included a warning about a strongly astringent potion (for which he gave the recipe): "Beware lest you give it to a pregnant woman, for she would instantly miscarry." Patai, R., *The Alchemists* (Princeton: Princeton University Press, 1994), 214, quoting from Paris, Bibliothèque Nationale, heb. 1207, ff. 157r–158v.

59. Bernstein, M., ed., *Two Remedy Books in Yiddish from 1474 and 1508* (Bloomington: Indiana University Press, 1960), 289–305. The second manuscript mentioned is in the collection of Mrs. L. Jesselson, New York. I am grateful to Sharon Lieberman-Mintz for bringing it to my attention.

60. Bodleian Library, Oxford, ms. 2135, Opp. 181, f. 68b. This manuscript is dated 1594.

61. Quoted and referred to in Feldman, D.M., 1978, *op. cit.*, p. 236 n. 7.

62. Luntz, Eliahu ben Moshe, *Toldot Adam* (Zolkiew: 1720), no. 74.

63. Goldman, E., *Living My Life* (New York: Knopf, 1934), 185–186. Schneider, S.W., *Jewish and Female* (New York: Touchstone [Simon and Schuster], 1985), 232.

64. Friedenwald, H., *The Jews and Medicine* (Baltimore: Johns Hopkins University Press, 1944), vol. 1, p. 369, also reprinted in Marcus, J.R., *The Jew in the Medieval World* (New York: Atheneum, 1981), 318.

65. Simon, I., "La prière des médecins, de Jacob Zahalon," *Revue d'Histoire de la Médicine Hébraïque* 25 (1955): 44.

66. Goldman, E., 1934, *op. cit.*, p. 186.

67. Szwajger, A. Blady, *I Remember Nothing More* (New York: Pantheon, 1991), 148–149. Such a personal choice is quite different from the permanent damage that the Nazis inflicted on some Jews, purposely, to destroy their fertility. In one instance, they ordered Dr. Rosalie M. Wijnberg to sterilize Jewish women who had married non-Jewish men. Showing great courage, she refused, and the order was not carried out: Hes, H.S., "Wijnberg, R.M.," in *Jewish Physicians in the Netherlands, 1600–1940* (Assen: Van Gorcum, 1980); *Encyclopedia Judaica* (Jerusalem: Keter, 1972), vol. 2, p. 100 cites Rabbi Ephraim Oshry's ruling, *Mi-ma'amakim*, no. 20, permitting abortion in the Kovno ghetto.

68. Quoted in Schneider, S.W., 1985, *op. cit.*, p. 232.

69. Bleich, J.D., 1979, *op. cit.*, pp. 160–161. The ruling that enabled Jewish women to obtain abortion, when a severe handicap is diagnosed in the fetus in the womb, was made by Rabbi Eliezer Waldenberg in 1979.

70. From *Abortion—A Fundamental Right in Jeopardy* (New York: American Jewish Congress Commission on Law and Social Action, March 1981).

4. The Formation of the Embryo

1. Genesis 1:27, 20:17–18, 22:17, 25:21, 30:2; Leviticus 20:20–21; Deuteronomy 28:4, 18, and 62; I Samuel 1:5 and 19; II Samuel 6:23; Jeremiah 1:5; Ezekiel 16:7; Hosea 14:9; Psalms 127:3.
2. *Leviticus Rabbah* 14:9.
3. *B. Niddah* 31a.
4. *B. Sanhedrin* 91b; *Genesis Rabbah* 34:10.
5. Lachower, F., and I. Tishby, eds., *The Wisdom of the Zohar* (Oxford: Oxford University Press, 1989), vol. 2, p. 699.
6. Mansoor, M., ed., *The Book of Direction to the Duties of the Heart: Bahya ben Joseph ibn Paquda* (London: Routledge and Kegan Paul, 1973), 161–162. He also wrote a poem (now part of the morning service of Yom Kippur), in which he considers what happens to the soul once it enters the body, how it becomes fouled: the poem is an admonition for self-purification (pp. 448ff.).
7. Carmi, T., ed. and trans., *The Penguin Book of Hebrew Verse* (London: Penguin, 1981), 316: a translation by Carmi of Ibn Gabirol's poem "Before I Was," about the origins of his being. Here he refers to the imagery of Job and to the fact that God gave him breath and wisdom, but not his evil inclination.
8. David, Y., ed., *Shirei ibn Ghiyyat* (Jerusalem: Ahshav Publications, 1987), 99–100. This poem sticks closely to the talmudic ideas.
9. Levine, M.H., *Falaquera: The Book of the Seeker* (New York: Yeshiva University Press, 1976), 54.
10. Zohar II, 99b. This imagery comes from the *Sefer ha-bahir*, an earlier kabbalistic text.
11. This imagery is taken from the Talmud, *B. Shabbat* 152b, *B. Hagigah* 12b, and was developed by Moses de Leon in his earlier work, *Midrash ha-ne'elam*. Tishby describes the evolution of this theory in Lachower, F., and I. Tishby, 1989, *op. cit.*, pp. 704, 754ff.
12. Zohar I, 49b–50a and 85b; V, 43a–b; *Zohar Ḥadash* to Genesis 11a. See also Cohen, S.J., ed., *The Holy Letter: A Study in Medieval Jewish Sexual Morality, Ascribed to Nahmanides* (New York: Ktav, 1976), part 1. See Lachower, F., and I. Tishby, 1989, *op. cit.*, p. 702 for an explanation of the apparent self-contradiction in the views of the creation of the soul in the Zohar.
13. Scholem, G., *Kabbalah* (New York: Meridian, 1978), 347–348.
14. Levin, M., *Hasidic Stories* (Tel Aviv: Greenfield Press, 1975), 3–9. For other versions, see Hacohen, M., "Neshamot tzaddikim ve-leidatam," *Maḥanayim* 6 (1994): 224–229, which gives three versions of the special circumstances surrounding the birth of the Besht, as well as the legend that Rabbi Itzhak of Berdichev was born with the soul of Rabbi Akiva, and the legend that Rabbi Abraham Yehoshua Heschel was born with a soul that had transmigrated ten times and had belonged once to a high priest, a king, and various other notables.
15. Scholem, G. 1978 *op. cit.*, pp. 344–348. The doctrine of transmigration was rejected by Sa'adia Gaon and other medieval rationalist philosophers but became increasingly popular after the sixteenth century. Bin-Gorion, E., *Memakor Israel*, translated by I.M. Lask (Bloomington: Indiana University Press, 1976), 876, "Those who are cut off before their time . . ."
16. *B. Sanhedrin* 91b. A sage named Rabbi thought the soul enters at the time of conception, whereas Antonius taught him that it must be at birth. Feldman, D.M., *Marital Relations, Birth Control and Abortion in Jewish Law* (New York: Schocken, 1978), 271–275. The Jewish attitude is in marked contrast to the Catholic tradition in this respect. The Catholics were concerned to baptize an infant who died in the womb or an unborn child still in the womb of a deceased mother, or else the baby's soul would be destined to an eternity of perdition.
17. Zohar V, 43b.
18. Judah ben Samuel of Regensburg, *Sefer Hasidim*, edited by R. Margoliyot (Jerusalem: 1957), 28, sign. 51.
19. Lauterbach, J.Z., "The Naming of Children in Jewish Folklore, Ritual and Practice," in *Studies in Jewish Law, Custom and Folklore* (Hoboken, NJ: Ktav, 1970), 27, citing the beliefs of Hayyim Vital and Emanuel Riki. Also Bacharach, Naphtali ben Jacob Elhanan, *Emek ha-melekh* (Amsterdam: Banbanashti Press, 1648, reprinted B'nei Brak, 1973) chap. 11, p. 19b.

20. Buber, M., *Tales of the Hasidim: Early Masters* (New York: Schocken, 1972), 273–274.

21. Patai, R., *Gates to the Old City* (New York: Avon, 1980), 385; and Bin-Gurion, E., 1976, *op. cit.*, pp. 876–877.

22. For Jewish attitudes toward the soul, see also *Encyclopedia Judaica* (Jerusalem: Keter, 1978), vol. 15, pp. 172–181.

23. Aristotle, *De generatione animalium*, translated by A. Platt (Oxford: Oxford University Press, 1958), 739b. Needham, J., *A History of Embryology* (Cambridge: Cambridge University Press, 1959), 64; this book covers in some detail the ancient ideas on embryology. Many Jews lived in Alexandria, spoke and read Greek, and were familiar with the Greek views on embryology. Alexandria was a leading medical center: Soranus studied and worked there before eventually moving to Rome. His treatises "On the Seed" and "On Generation" were lost, but Galen wrote on these subjects a few decades later.

24. Reider, J., *The Book of Wisdom* (New York: Harper & Brothers, 1957), 109. This is a translation of Wisdom of Solomon 7:2.

25. Rosner, F., and S. Muntner, *Studies in Judaica: The Medical Aphorisms of Moses Maimonides* (New York: Bloch for Yeshiva University Press, 1973), chap. 1, p. 72.

26. Maimonides, M., *The Code of Maimonides: Mishneh Torah*, translated by L.I. Rabinowitz and P. Grossman (New Haven: Yale University Press, 1965), The Book of Holiness: Laws Concerning Illicit Intercourse, 5:4.

27. Feldman, D.M., 1978, *op. cit.*, chap. 7, "Excursus—On Female Seed."

28. Leviticus 12:2.

29. Quoted in Feldman, D.M., 1978, *op. cit.*, p. 138. Isaac Aboab (1433–1493) held the same view.

30. Barkai, R., *Les Infortunes de Dinah: Le livre de la génération* (Paris: Editions du Cerf, 1991), 70–75, quoting Gershom ben Shlomo (late thirteenth century), Joseph Colon (c. 1420–1480), and a medical manuscript, *Zikhron ha-ḥolayim* (Montefiore, Jews College ms. 440), as followers of the talmudic, Hippocratic view. Feldman, D.M., 1978, *op. cit.*, p. 137, quotes the views of Nahmanides (thirteenth century), Joshua ibn Shu'ab (early fourteenth century), and Isaac bar Sheshet (fourteenth century) on the controversy between the two differing positions.

31. Feldman, D.M., 1978, *op. cit.*, p. 138.

32. See *Ibid.*, pp. 136–137, for citation of Nahmanides's Commentary to Genesis 2:18 and Leviticus 12:2 and 18:19.

33. Cohen, S.J., ed., 1976 *op. cit.*, p. 78.

34. Duran, Simon ben Tzemah, *Magen avot* (Livorno: 1785), 40a–41a.

35. Quoted in Feldman, D.M., 1978, *op. cit.*, p. 141.

36. *Ibid.*, p. 142. The talmudic references are *B. Berakhot* 60a and *B. Niddah* 31a.

37. Genesis 30:31ff.

38. Kottek, S., "La force de l'imagination chez les femmes enceintes," *Revue d'Histoire de la Médicine Hébraïque* 107 (1974): 43–48. This is a documentation of a debate, held in the early eighteenth century, about the influence of the imagination on the baby's eventual characteristics. Rashi's grandson, Samuel ben Meir ("Rashbam," d. c. 1174), Abraham ibn Ezra (d. 1167), David Kimhi (d. 1235), and Obadiah ben Jacob S'forno (d. c. 1550) supported the interpretation that Jacob's action was due to his belief in the effect of maternal imagination on the fetus.

39. *Genesis Rabbah* 73:10, *Numbers Rabbah* 9.34. A similar version is found in book 1 of Soranus' treatise on obstetrics (second century).

40. *B. Berakhot* 20a.

41. Patai, R., 1980, *op. cit.*, pp. 381–382.

42. Zlotnik, Y. (Elzet, J.L.), "Me-minhagei Israel," *Reshumot* 1 (1918): 362–365. Also Shtal, A., *Mishpaḥah ve-giddul yeladim be-yahadut ha-mizraḥ* (Jerusalem: Academon, 1993), 310 n. 4, 313 n. 549.

43. Hadad, B., *Sefer Djerba yehudit* (Jerusalem: Beit Ha-otzer Ha-ivri, 1979), 57.

44. *B. Ketubbot* 60b; *B. Nedarim* 20b; *Zohar Ḥadash* to Genesis 11a–b.

45. *B. Eruvin* 100b; *B. Nedarim* 20b; *Genesis Rabbah* 26:7; *Numbers Rabbah* 9:1.

46. Simon, I., *Asaph Ha-iehudi: Medecin et astrologue du moyen age* (Paris: Librairie Lipschutz, 1933), 48–49.

47. *Aggadat bereshit*, tenth-century midrash, quoted by Patai, R., 1980, *op. cit.*, pp. 295–296. The gossip was that Sarah might have "obtained her seed elsewhere," from another man, since she and Abraham had been childless for so long.

48. Yasif, E., *Sippurei Ben Sira be-yamei ha-benayim* (Jerusalem: Magnes Press, 1984), 198–199.

49. *B. Hagigah* 15a.

50. *Pirkei de Rabbi Eliezer*, edited and translated by G. Friedlander (New York: Hermon Press, 1981), chap. 21, pp. 150–151. The talmudic references are *B. Avodah Zarah* 22b; *B. Shabbat* 146a; *B. Yevamot* 103a.

51. Shtal, A., 1993, *op. cit.*, pp. 317–318. The tale told by Iraqi Jews involving fertility acquired from magic apples is recorded in Agassi, E., *Ha-mikhtav she-nishlach im ha-ru'ah: Sippurei am shel yehudei Bavel* (Tel Aviv: Am Oved), 49–56. And another, told by Sephardic Jews, also involving magic apples is mentioned in Grunwald, M., "Tales, Songs, and Folkways of Sephardic Jews," *Folklore Research Center Studies* 6 (1982): xxxii, no. 54. The tale of the suspicious bone comes from Persia, and the tale of the powdered skull comes from Iraq; see Yasif, E., 1984, *op. cit.*, p. 37 n. 36.

52. Gold, M., *And Hannah Wept* (Philadelphia: Jewish Publication Society, 1988), 107–109.

53. Lilith's relations with Adam and Cain are related in Zohar I, 19b, 34b. *Genesis Rabbah* 20:11, 24:6.

54. Patai, R., *The Hebrew Goddess* (Detroit: Wayne State University Press, 1990), 225ff., quotes such bills of divorce and a medieval story where the demonic wife kills her husband when he divorces her.

55. This was a talmudic idea: *B. Eruvin* 18b.

56. Zohar I, 54b–55a.

57. Bacharach, N., 1648, *op. cit.*, chap. 11, p. 19c; my translation. Patai, R., 1990, *op. cit.*, p. 232ff., has pointed out that the velvet probably refers to the scarlet dress that harlots could have worn. The sea refers to Lilith's abode; the story of Lilith is related in my Chapter 10.

58. Nathan Nata Hannover, *Sha'arei tziyyon* (Prague: 1662). This was reprinted in Amsterdam in 1671 and in many other towns subsequently.

59. Kaidanover, Z.H., *Kav ha-yashar* (Frankfurt: 1706), chap. 29. Reprinted Jerusalem: Ha-ktav Institute, 1982, pp. 160–162. For an English rendering, see Sadeh, P., *Jewish Folktales* (New York: Doubleday, 1989), 77–79, or Trachtenberg, J., *Jewish Magic and Superstition* (New York: Atheneum, 1982), 52–54. Stories about demonic offspring were by no means limited to Eastern Europe. See, for example, the Kurdistani folktale about the midwife called on to deliver a demonic baby, in my Chapter 7.

60. *B. Niddah* 9a.

61. *Tosefta Niddah* 4:10. See also *B. Niddah* 25b.

62. *B. Niddah* 30b. Aristotle, *History of Animals*, translated by D. W. Thompson, in *The Works of Aristotle Translated into English*, edited by J. A. Smith and W. D. Ross (Oxford: Oxford University Press, 1967), 583b.

63. *B. Niddah* 30b–31a.

64. *B. Niddah* 38a; *J. Niddah* 1:3; *B. Yevamot* 80b.

65. Hippocrates proposed this, Aristotle accepted this theory, and Galen promoted it. *B. Yevamot* 42a; *J. Yevamot* 4:2; *B. Niddah* 8b; *Tosefta Shabbat* 15:5.

66. *Genesis Rabbah* 14:2, 20:6; *Numbers Rabbah* 4:3; *Tosefta Shabbat* 15:7.

67. *B. Shabbat* 135a, *B. Yevamot* 80a.

68. *B. Niddah* 27a.

69. *B. Niddah* 27a; *J. Niddah* 3:4. See comment in Feldman, D.M., 1978 *op. cit.*, p. 183 and n. 42. Aristotle, 1958, *op. cit.*, part I, book 4, chap. 5, p. 773b.

70. *B. Yevamot* 12b, *B. Niddah* 45a.

71. *Pirkei de Rabbi Eliezer*, 1981, *op. cit.*, chap. 36, p. 272; Patai, R., 1980, *op. cit.*, p. 312, quoting Margalioth, M., ed., *Midrash ha-gadol* (Jerusalem: 1956), Exodus p. 24. This midrash was compiled by David ben Amram Adani, in Yemen, in the thirteenth century.

72. Moellin, Jacob ben Moses, *Sefer Maharil* (Warsaw: 1834), 24b. See also Wasserstein, A., "Normal and abnormal gestation periods in humans," *Koroth* 9 (1985): 221–229.

73. Aldabi, Meir, *Sh'vilei emunah* (Warsaw: 1889), sign. 4, 40b. Meir Aldabi lived in the first half of the fourteenth century. Similar theories relating astrology to embryology were proposed by Shem Tov Falaquera (thirteenth century), Gershon ben Solomon (thirteenth century), and Simon ben Zemach

Duran (1361–1444): see Zimmels, H.J., *Magicians, Theologians and Doctors* (London: Edward Goldston & Sons, 1952), 62–64.

74. Barkai, R., 1989, *op. cit.*, pp. 101–104, 118, quoting and discussing a medieval medical manuscript in the Bibliothèque Nationale, Paris, ms. Héb. 1120 f. 67r.

75. Zimmels, H.J., *op. cit.*, pp. 70–71.

76. Castro, Rodrigo de, *Universa muliebrum Morborum* (Cologne: 1689), book 4, chaps. 5–6, pp. 190ff., reiterated the astrological ideas. This book was first published in Hamburg in 1603. Barkai, R., 1991 *op. cit.*, p. 82, quoting from Sa'adia Gaon, *Otzar ha-geonim*, vol. 8.

77. *Sefer Hasidim*, 1957, *op. cit.*, sign. 515.

78. Feldman, D.M., 1978, *op. cit.*, p. 183–184, quoting Rabbi Solomon ben Tzemah Duran (sixteenth century), a descendant of Simon ben Tzemah and Solomon ben Simon Duran.

79. Castro, Rodrigo de, 1689, *op. cit.*, book 3, chap. 13. Cardoso, I., *Philosophia libera* (Venice: 1678), book 6, chaps. 24 and 99.

5. The Experiences of Pregnancy

1. Genesis 38:24; *Genesis Rabbah* 85:10.

2. *B. Niddah* 8b–9a, 10b.

3. *B. Yevamot* 80b. Hippocrates offered a pregnancy test: the woman should drink honey water before going to sleep; she is pregnant if she develops pains in the abdomen. Maimonides explained why this worked: Rosner, F., *Maimonides' Commentary on the Aphorisms of Hippocrates* (Haifa: Maimonides Research Institute, 1987), 143.

4. A popular medieval pregnancy test relied on inducing nausea. A woman was given to eat pepper kernels that looked like a plant louse. If nausea followed, then pregnancy was established. This advice is offered in Bernstein, M., ed., *Two Remedy Books in Yiddish from 1474 and 1508* (Bloomington: Indiana University Press, 1960), 299, and in Ashkenazi, David Tevle ben Yacov, *Beit David* (Williamsdorf: 1704), 22a. Of course, nausea, without the aid of pepper kernels, would have reinforced a woman's suspicions of pregnancy.

5. Ghalioungui, P., *Magic and Medical Science in Ancient Egypt* (London: Hodder and Stoughton, 1963), chap. 8.

6. Zimmels, H.J., *Magicians, Theologians and Doctors* (London: Edward Goldston & Sons, 1952), 62, n. 21; his sources are Rabbi Joel Sirkes (1561–1640) and Rabbi Akiva Eger (1761–1837). It was also recommended by the physician Tobias Cohn, *Ma'aseh Tuvya* (Venice, 1708), chap. 13.

7. A sixteenth-century remedy book of Ashkenazi Jews includes such advice: Mrs. L. Jesselson collection, New York. Badehev, Itzhak ben Michael, *Sefer segullah zahav* (Jerusalem: 1894), 38. See Luntz, Eliahu ben Moshe, *Toldot Adam* (Zolkiew: 1720), no. 30, for urine test of barrenness.

8. *Sefer ha-goralot*, Etz Hayyim Collection of the Portuguese Israelite Seminary of Amsterdam, ms. 47E41 (eighteenth-century edition), "gemini," fourth item.

9. Schwarzbaum, H., *The Mishlei Shu'alim (Fox Fables), of Rabbi Berechiah Ha-nakdan* (Kiron: Institute for Jewish and Arabic Folklore, 1979), 417.

10. Zborowski, M., and E. Herzog, *Life Is with People* (New York: Schocken, 1962), 313. Buber, M., *Tales of the Hasidim: Later Masters* (New York: Schocken, 1948), 150.

11. Goshen-Gottstein, E., *Marriage and First Pregnancy* (London: Tavistock, 1966), 62.

12. Lorenzo and Ayse Salzmann, and Eti Alkanli of California, personal communications, 1990.

13. Ben Simhon, R., *Yahadut Marocco* (Lod: Orot Yahadut Magreb, 1994), 19, 28–29. Malka, E., *Essai d'ethnographie traditionelle des Mellah* (Rabat: 1946), 17. Mathieu, J., "Notes sur l'enfance juive du Mellah de Casablanca," *Bulletin de l'Institut d'Hygiene du Maroc*, 7 (1947): 19. Allouch-Benayoun, J., and D. Bensimon, *Les Juifs d'Algerie* (Toulouse: Privat, 1989), 146–147.

14. Ovadia, D., *Kehillot Zafro* (Jerusalem: 1975), vol. 1., p. 293.

15. Yehosha, Y., *Yaldut be-yerushalayim ha-yeshanah* (Jerusalem: R. Mass, 1966), 79–80.

16. Brauer, E., *The Jews of Kurdistan*, edited by R. Patai (Detroit: Wayne State University Press, 1993), 149.

17. Zadok, H., *Be-ohalei teiman* (Tel Aviv: David Ben Nun, 1981), 105. Amdor, M., "Orkhot Hayyeihem shel yehudei Aden," *Yeda Am*, 50–51 (1984): 120.

18. Patai, R., *Adam v'adamah* (Jerusalem: 1942), vol. 2, p. 198.

19. Diamant, A., *The Jewish Baby Book* (New York: Summit Books, 1988), 32–34. Schneider, S.W., *Jewish and Female* (New York: Touchstone [Simon and Schuster], 1985), 118ff.

20. Zonderman, S., "Spiritual Preparation for Parenthood," *Response* 1 (Spring 1985): 29ff.

21. Frymer-Kensky, T., "A Ritual for Affirming and Accepting Pregnancy," in *Daughters of the King*, edited by S. Grossman and R. Haut (Philadelphia: Jewish Publication Society, 1992), 290ff. The reference to the behavior of Manoah's wife is biblical: Judges 13:7ff. The *mi-shebeirakh* blessing dates back to gaonic times when it was recited in synagogue, to request that God hear the prayers of the person being blessed just as God heard those of the patriarchs in biblical times.

22. *B. Gittin* 23b; *B. Hullin* 58a.

23. *B. Hagigah* 12b: the Talmud makes several references to the pre-existence of a *guf*, or body, of souls, created by God, "at the beginning of time." See also *Genesis Rabbah* 8:7. *Midrash tanhuma* (Warsaw: 1902), *Pekudei*, 244 assumed that God created all souls in the first six days of Creation and stored them in the Garden of Eden. This work is of unknown date and origin, first published in Constantinople in 1522. See also the telling in Strassfeld, S., and M. Strassfeld, eds., *The Second Jewish Catalogue* (Philadelphia: Jewish Publication Society, 1976), 13–14.

24. *B. Niddah* 30b. *Midrash tanhuma, op. cit.*, pp. 244–246 and Jellinek, A., ed., *Beit ha-midrash* (Jerusalem: Bamberger & Wahrmann, 1938), *Seder yetzirat ha-vlad*, vol. 1., pp. 153–154. In a book by Schwartz, H., *Gabriel's Palace: Jewish Mystical Tales* (Oxford: Oxford University Press: 1993), the author retells (p. 57) a version of this story, taken from *Midrash tanhuma*. He dates it Babylonian, ninth century. The Zohar also depicts a version of these fetal experiences: Zohar II, 161b; III, 41b–42a; V, 43a. The midrashic version was reproduced by hand in an Italian woman's prayer book, dating from the first half of the nineteenth century. This is in the collection of Mr. I. Einhorn, Tel Aviv.

25. Patai, R., *Gates to the Old City* (New York: Avon, 1980), 378–381. Patai provides the full translation of the midrash. I have rendered it abridged. In antiquity, Plato (c. 400 B.C.E.) stressed the importance of prenatal knowledge in later life, and he may have provided the stimulus for this apparently Jewish legend. Israel Tishby proposed the Platonic origins of this legend; see Lachower, F., and I. Tishby, eds., *The Wisdom of the Zohar* (Oxford: Oxford University Press, 1989), vol. 2, pp. 751, 683.

26. Thus the battle between the two inclinations begins even before the child emerges into the world. For zoharic reference, see note 24 above.

27. Buber, M., *Ten Rungs: Hasidic Sayings* (New York: Schocken, 1970), 89.

28. Manger, I., *The Book of Paradise* (New York: Hill and Wang, 1965).

29. Judges 13:4.

30. *B. Ketubbot* 60b–61a.

31. Aldabi, M., *Sh'vilei emunah* (Warsaw: 1887), part 5, sign. 1, p. 112.

32. *Yoma* 8:5; *B. Yoma* 82a–b; and Rashi.

33. Rosner, F., and S. Muntner, *Studies in Judaica: The Medical Aphorisms of Moses Maimonides* (New York: Bloch for Yeshiva University Press, 1973), sixteenth treatise, nos. 23–24. Aldabi, M., 1887, *op. cit.*, pp. 111–112. Following the Greco-Roman "science," Aldabi also adhered to the talmudic view that the fetus craves food and that if the woman does not satisfy the craving, she will miscarry.

34. Barkai, R., *Les infortunes de Dinah: Le livre de la génération* (Paris: Editions du Cerf, 1991), 139. Thanks to Wendy Blumfield, president of the Israel Childbirth Education Center, for pointing out the hazards of fasting if cravings persist. Even pregnant ultra-Orthodox women today usually do not fast totally on Yom Kippur if they have not yet reached thirty-six weeks.

35. Cohn, Tobias, 1708, *op. cit.*, chap. 15. Zacuto Lusitanus, A., *Medici et philosophi, praxis historiarum* (Lyon: 1644), book 3, chap. 15 on diet and cravings and chap. 20 on loose bowels and stomachache in pregnancy. Warnings to pregnant women to indulge their cravings lest they miscarry were also issued in Simner, Zekhariah ben Yacov, *Sefer zekhirah* (Wilmersdorf: 1729).

36. Abrahams, B. Z., ed., *The Life of Gluckel of Hameln* (London: Horovitz, 1962), 100.

37. See, for example, Malka, E., 1976, *op. cit.*, p. 15.

38. See, for example, Zborowski, M., and E. Herzog, 1962, *op. cit.*, p. 33.

39. For example, Yehosha, Y., 1966, *op. cit.*, p. 79.

40. Brauer, E., 1993, *op. cit.*, p. 152.

41. Ploss, H.H., and M. and P. Bartels, in *Woman*, edited by J. Dingwall (London: Heinemann, 1935), vol. 2, p. 457.

42. Brauer, E., *Ethnologie der Jemenitischen Juden* (Heidelberg: 1934), 181.

43. Sternberg, G., *Stefanesti: Portrait of a Romanian Shtetl* (Oxford: Pergamon Press, 1984), 124.

44. *J. Yevamot* 1:6, 3a; Rashi to *Avot* 2:8.

45. G. Sternberg, private correspondence, 1987.

46. Rozenberg, Y.Y., *Rafael ha-malakh* (Piotrkow: 1911), under *me'uberet*.

47. Feldman, D.M., *Marital Relations, Birth Control and Abortion in Jewish Law* (New York: Schocken, 1978), 181 and n. 27.

48. *B. Niddah* 31a.

49. Feldman, D.M., 1978, *op. cit.*, pp. 69, 186, citing that this was codified in Jacob ben Asher's *Tur, Even ha-ezer*, 23, 25 and *Orhot hayyim* 240:1 and in Caro, J., *Shulhan arukh*, edited by Z.H. Preisler and S. Havlin (Jerusalem: Ketuvim, 1993). Also in Isaac of Corbeil, *Sefer mitzvot katan*, Positive Commandment no. 285 (Ladi, 1805). In recent times, Feinstein, M., *Iggrot Mosheh* (New York: 1961), *Even ha-ezer*, no. 102 specified the duty of sexual relations in pregnancy.

50. Jewish law insists that a husband should give his wife sexual happiness when he notices her desire, but a wife has no such obligation: Exodus 21:10; *B. Ketubbot* 61b–62a; *Shulhan arukh, op. cit., Even ha-ezer*, chap. 76. Although a woman is not duty-bound to consent to having sexual relations with her husband, if she persistently refuses him she may be fined or divorced: *B. Ketubbot* 61b, 64b; *Shulhan arukh, op. cit., Even ha-ezer*, chap. 77. For a full discussion of this topic and sources, see Feldman, 1978, *op. cit.*, chaps. 4 and 10.

51. Maimonides, M., *Mishneh Torah: The Book of Knowledge*, translated by M. Hyamson (Jerusalem: Boys Town, 1962), Laws Relating to Moral Disposition and Ethical Conduct, 4:19 (p. 52a).

52. Abraham ben David of Posquières (Ravad), *Ba'alei ha-nefesh* (Brooklyn: 1980), *Sha'ar ha-kedushah*, 81. The first edition of this work was published in Venice in 1602. This particular marital advice was handed down from generation to generation, copied by later rabbis and incorporated into the Tur code (early fourteenth century), the popular *Menorat ha-ma'or* of both Israel Al-Nakawa (late fourteenth century) and Isaac Aboab (late fifteenth century), and the *Siddur* of Jacob Emden (eighteenth century).

53. For example, *B. Kiddushin* 30b; *Genesis Rabbah* 9:7; *Zohar* I, 61a. For other rabbinic sources on the evil inclination, see Montefiore, C.G., and H. Loewe, *Rabbinic Anthology* (New York: Schocken, 1974), chap. 11.

54. Gefen, Y., and A. Katz, *Ha-sefer ha-tzahov* (Tel Aviv: Massada, 1973), 8–12, 27.

55. The matriarchs were barren, the rabbis suggested, so their husbands could derive pleasure from them, for "when a woman is with child she is disfigured and lacks grace"; *Genesis Rabbah* 45:4. The stories of Lamech and Er are found in *Genesis Rabbah* 23:3.

56. *B. Ketubbot* 17a, *B. Ta'anit* 31a.

57. We have already seen that in many Jewish communities women made as little change as possible in their dress so as not to reveal pregnancy, although some celebrated pregnancy sometime in the last few months, probably dressing up for the occasion. In contrast, Jewish women in Bombay treated pregnancy as a time when a woman should take extra care with her appearance; she dressed richly, and decorated her hair, since for a four- or five-month period after giving birth this was forbidden (Kehimkar, H.S., *The History of the Bnei Israel of India* [Tel Aviv: Dayag, 1937]). The married Jewesses of Cochin generally dressed in plain clothing without jewelry after the birth of their second child (Isaac, I.A., *A Short Account of the Calcutta Jews* [Calcutta: 1917]). For modesty as a feminist issue, see Schneider, S.W., *Jewish and Female* (New York: Touchstone [Simon and Schuster], 1985), 234–240.

58. *Maternité*, oil on canvas, Stedelijk Museum, Amsterdam. Chagall used a similar image in a lithograph, 1912. Amadeo Modigliani painted his wife when she was pregnant with their daughter, in 1918.

59. Meira Grossinger (b. 1950), living in Rehovot, Israel: artist's catalogue, 1994. Another Israeli artist,

Achiam, now living in Paris, has also sculpted stone on the theme of the ancient fertility goddesses. Moreover, Chana Orloff (1888–1968) sculpted pregnant women, changing her style from the well-polished, clearly delineated, idealistic, goddess-like pregnant woman depicted in 1916 to the more realistic portraits that she created toward the end of her life.

60. Carmi, T., ed. and trans., *The Penguin Book of Hebrew Verse* (London: Penguin, 1981), 463.

61. Colson, F.H. and G.H. Whitaker, *Philo* (Boston: Harvard University Press and W. Heinemann, 1949), vol. V, 285ff. *B. Berakhot* 57a.

62. Morag, E., ed., *Pitron ḥalomot lefi ha-yahadut* (Hod Hasharon: Astrolog, 1995), 103ff., 125ff. Eleazar ben Judah of Worms, *Hokhomat ha-nefesh* (Lemberg: 1876), 6, *pitron ḥalomot*.

63. Almoli, S., *Mefaresh ḥalomin* (Salonika: 1515), gate 3, chap. 3, part 2, *yonah, turim, tarnegol*, and gate 4, part 3, *yoledet*. This book was republished under the title *Pitron ḥalomot*, in Constantinople in 1518, in Cracow in 1576, and soon after in Venice, too. It was later translated into Yiddish (Amsterdam: 1694). It was in popular use in subsequent centuries. In 1902, a Yiddish edition was published in Brooklyn. For a study of this work by a Jungian analyst, see Covitz, J., *Visions of the Night* (Boston: Shambhala, 1990).

64. Ratzhabi, Y., "Pitronei ḥalomot," *Edot* 2 (1947): 121–125, items 3 and 28. The first omen appears unconnected with the talmudic interpretation that a dream of being gored by an ox portends that one's sons will fight each other, *B. Berakhot* 56b.

65. *B. Shabbat* 11a; *Berakhot* 55b; Trachtenberg, J., *Jewish Magic and Superstition* (New York: Atheneum, 1982), 244ff.

66. Bin-Gorion, E., *Me-makor Israel*, translated by I.M. Lask (Bloomington: Indiana University Press, 1976), 876, no. 297.

67. Nahman of Bratslav, *Sefer ha-middot* (Jerusalem: 1980), *ḥalom*. Buber, M., 1948, *op. cit.*, p. 179.

68. This conclusion was drawn from interviews with Moroccan Jewish pregnant women. The influence of their dreams in the choice of a baby's name has been documented: Abramovitch, H., and Y. Bilu, "Visitational Dreams and Naming Practices among Moroccan Jews in Israel," *Jewish Journal of Sociology* 27 (1985): 13–21.

69. *B. Sotah* 12a tells about Jochebed's premonitions, whereas *Genesis Rabbah* 63:6 and *B. Yoma* 82b tell of Rebekah's premonitions.

70. *B. Berakhot* 10a. Zimmels, H.J., 1952, *op. cit.*, p. 67.

71. Aristotle, *De generatione animalium*, translated by A. Platt (Oxford: Oxford University Press, 1958), book 4, chap. 1, 765b. Hippocrates said that if a woman is pregnant with a son, her appearance is good; if with a daughter, her facial appearance is bad. Maimonides commented that this applies "in most cases": Rosner, F., 1987, *op. cit.*, p. 143. *Sefer ha-toledet*, British Library, London, Montefiore ms. 420 f. 27b and Barkai, R., *Les infortunes de Dinah: Le livre de la génération* (Paris: Editions du Cerf, 1991), 138. In contrast, Aldabi, M., 1887, *op. cit.*, p. 112, cited Hippocrates as saying that a thicker left breast presaged a boy and that a male fetus caused a woman to be weaker than when she was carrying a female fetus.

72. Isaacs, H., *Medical and Paramedical Manuscripts in the Cambridge Geniza Collections* (Cambridge: Cambridge University Press, 1994), no. 1086, quoting TS.AS. 154.291. *Sefer ha-goralot*, eighteenth-century manuscript, Etz Hayyim Collection of the Portuguese Israelite Seminary of Amsterdam, Ms. 47E41, pp. 2–4. Maimonides, M., *Guide for the Perplexed* (New York: Dover, 1956), 337ff.

73. Trachtenberg, J., 1982, *op. cit.*, chap. 14. There is an illustration of a pregnant woman consulting a man with an open Bible in the Yehudah Haggada (Germany, fifteenth century), f. 31v, Israel Museum.

74. Aldabi, M., 1887, *op. cit.*, p. 112. Ashkenazi, D. T., 1704, *op. cit.*, pp. 22a, 23b. See also references in Trachtenberg, J., 1982, *op. cit.*, pp. 189, 303 n. 14.

75. Zimmels, H.J., 1952, *op. cit.*, p. 76.

76. Itzhaki, I., *Laḥash ve-kame'a* (Tel Aviv: Shakked, 1976), 81, 135.

77. Zunser, M.S., *Yesterday—A Memoir of a Russian Jewish Family* (New York: Harper & Row, 1978), 101–102.

78. *Genesis Rabbah* 65:12 says that no man knows what a woman is bearing. For Maimonides's view,

see Rosner, F., 1987, *op. cit.*, p. 146.

79. Rosner, F., "Tay-Sachs Disease: To Screen or Not to Screen," in *Jewish Bioethics*, edited by F. Rosner and J.D. Bleich. (New York: Sanhedrin Press, 1979), 178–190.

80. Wendy Blumfield, Israel Childbirth Education Center, private communication.

6. Pregnancy Loss

1. *Niddah* 3. See Chapter 12 for a discussion of postnatal purification.

2. *B. Niddah* 23a–25b. *Zikhron ha-holayim* (Montefiore, Jews College London, ms. 440), a medieval Hebrew manuscript on diseases of the generative organs reported a case of a live abortion resembling a snake.

3. *B. Shabbat* 32b; *Genesis Rabbah* 26:7. Hacohen, Eliyahu ben Shlomo Avraham, *Shevet mussar* (Jerusalem: Y. Rubinstein, 1963), 192. Hacohen (1650–1729), rabbi of Izmir, published this ethical text in Constantinople in 1712. Here he reminded his readers of the truth in these ancient ideas regarding the causes of miscarriage.

4. Exodus 21:22; *Avot* 5:5; *B. Gittin* 31b; *B. Niddah* 16b–17a; *B. Shabbat* 63b. Fear as a cause of miscarriage is also mentioned in a medieval manuscript, *Zikhron ha-holayim, op. cit.*, f. 20b.

5. Ginzberg, L., *The Legends of the Jews* (Philadelphia: Jewish Publication Society, 1947), vol. 2, pp. 109, 112; vol. 4, p. 419.

6. II Kings 2:19: this verse uses the Hebrew word for a woman who miscarries or loses a child, *maskelet*.

7. Naveh, J., and S. Shaked, *Magic Spells and Formulae* (Jerusalem: Magnes Press, 1993), See amulets nos. 27, 28, and 30, and *Geniza* document no. 10. See also Luntz, Eliahu ben Moshe, *Toldot Adam* (Zolkiew: 1720), sect. 56. For more examples of such amulets, see Ben Simhon, R., *Yahadut Marocco* (Lod: Orot Yahadut ha-magreb, 1994), 14, 21.

8. *B. Niddah* 25b–26a.

9. Rosner, F., *Maimonides' Commentary on the Aphorisms of Hippocrates, Maimonides' Medical Writings* (Haifa: Maimonides Research Institute, 1987), 139, 144, 145, 149. Zimmels, H.J., *Magicians, Theologians and Doctors* (London: Edward Goldston & Sons, 1952), 71–72. Here a few reasons and reports of still-birth and handicap are mentioned, gleaned from rabbinic (not medical) authors from the early fourteenth century and the nineteenth century. *Zikhron ha-holayim, op. cit.*, f. 20b and *Sefer ha-toledet*, both medieval medical manuscripts, mention a woman's deformities, fever, and gangrene as causes of miscarriage: See Barkai, R., *Les infortunes de Dinah: Le livre de la génération* (Paris: Editions du Cerf, 1991), 141, 192. Isaacs, H., *Medical and Paramedical Manuscripts in the Cambridge Geniza Collections* (Cambridge: Cambridge University Press, 1994), citing a Judeo-Arabic text TS.NS.90.58 on diseases of womb causing miscarriage.

10. Rosner, F., and S. Muntner, *Studies in Judaica: The Medical Aphorisms of Moses Maimonides* (New York: Bloch for Yeshiva University Press, 1973), 38–39. An ancient treatise on ritual purity also warns that steambathing can cause miscarriage and advises pregnant women to bathe infrequently: Horowitz, H.M., *Tosefta Atikta* (Frankfurt: 1890), part 5, p. 28. An English translation is offered in Patai, R., *On Jewish Folkore* (Detroit: Wayne State University Press, 1983), 366. Judah ben Samuel of Regensburg (Judah the Pious), *Sefer Hasidim*, edited by R. Margoliyot (Jerusalem: 1957), sign. 247.

11. Benayahu, M., "Inyanei refu'ah be-katov-yad lo yadu'a shel Hayyim Vital," *Koroth* 9 (1987): 3–17.

12. My interviews with Israeli women, 1984.

13. *B. Niddah* 8b–9a.

14. Conybeare, F.C., "The Testament of Solomon," *Jewish Quarterly Review* 11 (1899), 31, no. 61.

15. Aristotle, *De generatione animalium*, translated by E. Platt (Oxford: Oxford University Press, 1958), book 7, pp. 775b–776a. Meyerhoff, M., and D. Joannides, *La gynécologue et l'obstetrique chez Avicenne (ibn Sina), et leurs rapports avec celles des Grecs* (Cairo: R. Schindler, 1938), 41. *Sefer ha-toledet*, British Library, London, Montefiore ms. 420, f. 38r. Zacuto Lusitanus, A., *Medici et philosophi, praxis historiarum* (Lyon: 1644), book 3, chap. 16.

16. Cohn, Tobias, *Ma'aseh Tuvya* (Venice: 1708), *Gan na'ul*, chap. 14.

17. Ben-Amri, S., *Ha-shed Tintal* (Or Yehuda: Center for Babylonian Heritage, 1987), 88–89.

18. *B. Berakhot* 60a.

19. *B. Ta'anit* 27b.

20. Epstein, Y.M., *Kitzur shnei luḥot ha-brit* (Jerusalem: 1984), 136. This is an edition of *Shnei luḥot ha-brit*, by Isaiah ben Avraham Horowitz (1565?–1630), first published in Amsterdam, 1649. Epstein's edition was first published in Fürth, 1683 and 1696. Also *Kol T'khinah* (Trieste: 1824), 11b, in the collection of the Sir Isaac Wolfson Museum in Heikhal Shlomo, Jerusalem. Ben-Yaakov, A., *Otzar ha-segullot* (Jerusalem: 1991), 33 discussed the custom of reciting the *mi shebeirakh* prayer in this context, but did not give his sources. Epstein's prayer book, in Hebrew and Yiddish, for those who could not read the *Kitzur shnei luḥot ha-brit*, also includes a prayer for pregnancy and birth, but does not distinguish between the seventh and ninth month of pregnancy: *Seder tefillah derekh yesharah* (Frankfurt an der Oder: 1703), 26b.

21. Azulai, Y.D., *Sefer avodat ha-kodesh* (Pressburg: 1818), 101.

22. Papo, Eliezer ben Yitzhak, *Sefer beit tefillah* (Bilograd: 1860). This prayer has been reproduced in Hebrew with an English translation, by Rosenthal, D.S., "A Joyful Mother of Children" (Jerusalem: Feldheim, 1982), 36–39.

23. Yerushalmi, Moses ben Hanokh, *Brantspiegel* (Basel: 1602), 121.

24. The book from Mannheim and one Italian prayer book with these prayers are in the collection of Itzhak Einhorn, of Tel Aviv. Another small Italian prayer book with such prayers is in the collection of the Isaac Wolfson Museum, Heikhal Shlomo, Jerusalem. Page 11 of this volume carries a prayer to protect against miscarrying a flat-fish shaped miscarriage, *sandal*. There are surely many other such items among the rare books of many other collectors. Cardin, N.B., *Out of the Depths I Call to You* (Northvale, NJ: Jason Aronson, 1992), 70ff., transcribes and translates childbirth prayers, from a late eighteenth-century Italian Jewish woman's prayer book, for reciting during pregnancy: the prayer for reciting in the seventh month is a female version of the prayer in *Kitzur shnei luḥot ha-brit*, referred to earlier.

25. Isaac ben Abraham Ger was a circumciser in Leeuwarden, Holland. In 1829, he copied out some prayers for pregnancy and childbirth at the beginning of a large notebook that he used for registering all the circumcisions he performed. This is now preserved in the Etz Hayyim Collection of the Portuguese Israelite Seminary of Amsterdam, ms. 47D27. Page 3 has exhortations for a pregnant woman, in Hebrew and Yiddish, and p. 4 has a supplicatory prayer for a husband to pray for his pregnant wife, also in Hebrew and Yiddish.

26. *The Merit of our Mothers: A Bilingual Anthology of Jewish Women's Prayers*, compiled and introduced by T.G. Klirs (Cincinnati: Hebrew Union College Press, 1992), 124–125.

27. Diamant, A., *The Jewish Baby Book* (New York: Summit Books, 1988), 31, quotes this prayer, by Rabbi Judy Shanks.

28. Neuda, F., *Hours of Devotion*, translated by R. Vulture (Vienna: Jos. Schlesinger, c. 1900), 128; my editing.

29. Ben Simhon, R., *Yahadut Marocco* (Lod: Orot Yahadut ha-magreb, 1994), 27.

30. Wurfel, A., ed., *Historische Nachricht von der Judengemeinde in dem Hofmarkt* (Furth: 1754), 7–8, para. 24.

31. Solomon, Jacob ben Abraham, *Ma'aneh lashon* (Prague: 1615). Mr. Itzhak Einhorn, Tel Aviv, has a charm in his collection that is for a pregnant woman with a copy of this prayer, probably made for a Jewish woman who could not read Hebrew.

32. Naveh J., and S. Shaked, 1993, *op. cit.*, pp. 93, 102, 155.

33. Isaacs, H., 1994, *op. cit.*, citing TS. Ar.43.200. TS. Ar.1c.15 offers similar advice. *Shimmush tehillim* (Cracow: 1648), see Psalms 1 and 128; for an English translation, see *Jewish Encyclopedia* (London: 1903), "Bibliomancy."

34. Tirshom, Joseph, *Shoshan yesod olam*, Sassoon ms. 290, items 599, 657, 664, 707, 750, 757, 1208, 1554. Luntz, E., 1720, *op. cit.*, sects. 44 and 75 provide formulas for making amulets for protection of pregnancy. Rozenberg, Y.Y., *Rafael ha-malakh* (Piotrkow: 1911), see *me'uberet*, to be written in Assyrian letters. Davis, E., and Frenkel D.A., *Ha-kame'a ha-ivri* (Jerusalem: Institute for Jewish Studies, 1995), amulets no. 296, 340–342.

35. Gaster, M., *Studies and Texts: The Sword of Moses* (New York: Ktav, 1971), 322 (37), no. 42. Another incantation for the same purpose was recorded in Luntz, E., 1720, *op. cit.*, no. 149.
36. Gross YM 11.39, Collection Bill Gross, Tel Aviv; my translation. There are many manuscripts of remedy books in the collection. Two more nineteenth-century remedy book manuscripts from Yemen in Mr. Gross' collection have similar formulas for the protection of pregnancy, in Aramaic and in Hebrew, also with angel script and a magic square: Gross YM 11.33, p. 145, Gross YM 11.25, p. 68.
37. Grunwald, M., "Charms and Magic Recipes," *Edot* 1 (1945): 241ff., no. 50 (180).
38. Sternberg, G., *Stefanesti: Portrait of a Romanian Shtetl* (Oxford: Pergamon Press, 1984), 83.
39. *B. Shabbat* 66b and Rashi, *Genesis Rabbah* 45:2.
40. Marcus, J.R., *The Jew in the Medieval World* (New York: Atheneum, 1981), 195. Trachtenberg, J., *Jewish Magic and Superstition* (New York: Atheneum, 1982), 133–134, 137, 295 n. 3. Ashkenazi, David Tevle ben Yacov, *Beit David* (Williamsdorf: 1704), 23b. Binesh, Binyamin, *Sefer amtahat Binyamin* (Wilmersdorf: 1716), 19a. Also Itzhaki, I., *Laḥash ve-kame'a* (Tel Aviv: Shakked, 1976), a remedy book used by Syrian Jews in the nineteenth century. Rozenberg, Y.Y., 1911, *op. cit., me'uberet*, first item. Sperling, A.I., *Ta'amei ha-minhagim ve-makor ha-dinim* (Jerusalem: Eshkol, 1961), no. 574. *Otzarot Yerushalayim*, part 36. Ploss, H.H., and M. and P. Bartels, in *Woman*, edited by J. Dingwall (London: Heinemann, 1935), vol. 2, p. 489, and Fraser, J.G., *The Golden Bough* (New York: Macmillan, 1927), vol. 1, pp. 164ff. discuss the magic of precious stones among the ancient Greeks and non-Jewish societies in the nineteenth century.
41. The Georgian amulet was photographed by Beth Hatefutsoth, Tel Aviv, Israel, Doc. 2.219.8; and the Iraqi carnelian is in the collection of the Sir Isaac Wolfson Museum, Heikhal Shlomo, Jerusalem.
42. Aldabi, M., 1887, *op. cit.*, p. 112, recommended that a woman wear a belt of silk netting to protect against miscarriage. *Sefer ha-toledet*, British Library, London, Montefiore ms. 420, f. 28r. suggested a soft, comfortable binding. Luntz, E., 1720, *op. cit*, no. 44 recommended a canvas binding to protect pregnancy.
43. Ploss, H.H., and M. and P. Bartels, 1935, *op. cit.*, p. 438, mention the use of protective bindings by Jews in late pregnancy during the Ottoman Empire, noting that not only Jews but other locals also adhere to this custom. Molkho, M., "Leida ve-yaldut bein Yehudei Saloniki," *Edot* 2 (1947): 257. Personal communication from a Jewish woman from Tunisia, now living in Ness Ziona, Israel and another, who practiced as a midwife many years ago in Tunisia, now living in Ashdod, Israel. Patai, R., 1983, *op. cit.*, p. 363. Brauer, E., in *The Jews of Kurdistan*, edited by R. Patai (Detroit: Wayne State University Press, 1993), 150.
44. Allouch-Benayoun, J., and D. Bensimon, *Les Juifs d'Algerie* (Toulouse: Privat, 1989), 145. Brauer, E., 1993, *op. cit.*, p. 150. The Israel Museum has several examples of amuletic padlocks used by Jewish women to protect pregnancy. Personal communication about this custom in Georgia from Ms. Lily Magal.
45. Luntz, A.M., "Minhagei ahinu be-eretz ha-kodesh be-dat ve-hayyei ha-am," *Yeda Am* 14 (1968): 3–5. M. Reischer and A. Almaliah also wrote of the custom of using a thread measured around Rachel's tomb to protect against miscarriage.
46. This was practiced in Poland and Palestine in the late nineteenth century: Rozenberg, Y.Y., 1911, *op. cit.*, p. 61, *me'uberet*. O'Hana, R., *Mareh ha-yeladim* (Jerusalem: 1901), 105b. In this second reference, this advice is taken from "a Babylonian manuscript book." In a personal communication, Israeli gynecologist Dr. S. Daniel reported that she has observed this practice among her ultra-Orthodox patients in Rehovot and B'nei Brak, Israel.
47. Leibowitz, J.O., and S. Marcus, *Sefer ha-nisyonot: The Book of Medical Experiences Attributed to Abraham ibn Ezra* (Jerusalem: Magnes Press, 1984), 231; Binesh, B., *op. cit.*, p. 19a; and O'Hana, R., 1901, *op. cit.*, pp. 16b, 69a.
48. The Israel Museum has several examples in the Feuchtwanger collection, e.g., no. 776, and the Jewish Museum of Switzerland also has an example, JMS 513. Both no. 776 and JMS 513 are written out in the name of a particular woman; they were made for personal use, by request. A reddish stone, marble sized with a hole through the center, uninscribed, is in the collection of the Sir Isaac Wolfson Museum (see note 41). In Israel today it is not hard to find an amulet of this sort; for example,

Rabbi Barukh Abuhatzeira, the son of the Baba Sali, in Netivot, will write such an amulet. He is the best known of the miracle rabbis of Moroccan Jewry. The Ethiopian community in Israel has its own faith healers, as does the Yemenite community. A reddish preservation stone can be borrowed today in the Ungarin quarter in Jerusalem, and in B'nei Brak, Israel.

49. *B. Sanhedrin* 46b–47a.

50. Goitein, S.D., *A Mediterranean Society* (Berkeley: University of California, 1978), vol. 3, p. 230.

51. Dahan, H., *Otzar ha-pitgamim shel Yehudei Marocco* (Tel Aviv: Stavit, 1983), no. 168.

52. National Council of Jewish Women, New York Section, 9 East 69th Street, New York, NY 10021 (212) 535-5900. Yad Elisha, Jerusalem, 02-632213 or 02-6518439. See also, for example, Borg, S., and J. Lasker, *When Pregnancy Fails* (Boston: Beacon Press, 1989); Savage, J.A., *Mourning Unlived Lives* (Wilmette, IL: Chiron Books, 1989), for a psychoanalytic discussion; Kohn, I., and P.L. Moffitt, with I.A. Wilkins, *A Silent Sorrow: Pregnancy Loss Guidance and Support for You and Your Family* (New York: Delacorte Press, a division of Bantam Doubleday Dell, 1992). People might also find comfort in Kushner, H., *When Bad Things Happen to Good People* (New York: Avon Books, 1983).

53. Jewish Women's Research Center, New York, no. 1910, also no. 2359. See also Grossman, S., "Finding Comfort after Miscarriage," in *Daughters of the King*, edited by S. Grossman and R. Haut (Philadelphia: Jewish Publication Society, 1992), 284ff.

54. Adelman, P.V., "The Womb and the Word: A Fertility Ritual for Hannah," in *Four Centuries of Jewish Women's Spirituality*, edited by E.M. Umansky and D. Ashton. (Boston: Beacon Press, 1992), 247–257.

55. Feld, M., "Healing After a Miscarriage," *Response*, Spring, 1985. This poem has been published again more recently in Umansky, E.M., and D. Ashton, *op. cit.*, pp. 221–222.

7. Midwives

1. Genesis 35:17, 38:28; Exodus 1:15ff.; I Samuel 4:20. The Bible refers to a midwife as a *meyaledet*, or birth helper.

2. *Exodus Rabbah* 1:13, *Ecclesiastes Rabbah* 7:1. Legend tells that the mother of the Baal Shem Tov was a midwife; it is fitting that the mother of a holy man should be a righteous woman with both the character and profession of Jochebed. Ben-Amos, D., and J.R. Mintz, *In Praise of the Ba'al Shem Tov* (Bloomington: Indiana University Press, 1972), 7, 159.

3. *B. Sotah* 11b; and Rashi. *Exodus Rabbah* 1:13 and *Ecclesiastes Rabbah* 7:1 expand on other possible roots of the names of the midwives. The Hebrew words I refer to are *shafar* (to clean or swaddle), *she-paru* (they were fertile), *shafru* (their deeds were pleasing), and *po'ah* (to cry out); the rabbis chose others, too.

4. This was suggested in the thirteenth century by Meir B. Barukh of Rotenberg, Germany and in the early fourteenth century by Jacob ben Asher of Spain in their respective commentaries to Exodus 1:15, but not by Rashi. Thus, intubation as a means to resuscitate a newborn was a method used in the thirteenth century and not earlier: Weinberg, M., "Makor atik al haḥayyat ha-yelod," *Koroth* 10 (1994): 63–64.

5. Josephus: *Jewish Antiquities*, translated by H.St.J. Thackeray (Cambridge, MA, and London: Harvard University Press, and William Heinemann, 1926–1965), book 2, chap. 9:2, pp. 253–254. Preuss, J., *Biblical and Talmudic Medicine*, 2nd ed. (Brooklyn: Hebrew Publication Company, 1983), 37. *Encyclopedia Judaica* (Jerusalem: Keter, 1974), vol. 14, p. 1410.

6. *Rosh Hashanah* 2:5; *Shabbat* 18:3. The Talmud also uses the word *ḥayah*, or the Aramaic *ḥayeta*, for a midwife but also for a pregnant and parturient woman, and the Aramaic *molada*, meaning *meyaledet*, birth helper; *Hullin* 4:3, *B. Avodah Zarah* 26a.

7. *Sefer ha-toledet [Book on Generation]*, British Library, London, Montefiore ms. 420, f. 26r.

8. *The Book on Generation* guided the midwife through her postnatal duties, too. A similar handbook for midwives was written by a female obstetrician, Malka Berlant, who studied at the Vilna Academy: Berlant, M., *Die Glückliche Mutter* (Vilna: 1836). Zborowski, M., and E. Herzog, *Life Is with People* (New York: Schocken, 1962), 313, mentions the Eastern European midwife's postnatal duties, whereas Aslan, M., and R. Nissim, *Yehudei Iraq* (Tel Aviv: Ofer, 1982), 11, tell of the Jewish midwife's duties

in Iraq; and see Sternberg, G., *Stefanesti: Portrait of a Romanian Shtetl* (Oxford: Pergamon Press, 1984), 83, 126, for the duties of a midwife in a Romanian shtetl. The Old Yishuv Court Museum in Jerusalem, the Rishon Lezion History Museum in Rishon Lezion, and the Hameiri House in Safed all have midwives' artifacts and documents from the local Jewish midwives who practiced in these towns in the late nineteenth and early twentieth centuries.

9. Sternberg, G., 1984, *op. cit.*, p. 83. *Tosefta Shabbat* 7:11.

10. Malka E., *Essai d'ethnographie traditionelle des Mellah* (Rabat: 1946), 22–23.

11. Hacohen, Eliyahu ben Shlomo Avraham, *Shevet mussar* (Jerusalem: Y. Rubinstein, 1963), part 2, chap. 24.

12. Cardin, N.B., *Out of the Depths I Call to You* (Northvale, NJ: Jason Aronson, 1992), 124–127.

13. Ben Simhon, R., *Yahadut Marocco* (Lod: Orot Yahadut ha-magreb, 1994), 41–42; my translation.

14. *Genesis Rabbah* 60:3; *Shabbat* 18:3; *B. Shabbat* 128b; *Tosefta Baba Batra* 2:2.

15. Cambridge University Library, TS NS Box 320, f. 33.

16. *Pinkas Frankfurt am Main*, J.N.U.L. ms. 4–662, item 261 concerns the employment by the community of a midwife in 1656. Avron, D., ed., *Pinkas ha-casherim shel kehillat Pozna, 1621–1835* (Jerusalem: 1966), 219, reports that the Jewish community of Posen employed a midwife, Yentel, wife of Rabbi Henoch, in 1675, and notes her salary. Wachstein, B., *Urkunden un Akten zur Geschichte der Juden in Eisenstadt* (Vienna: 1926), 540–541, item 336 concerns the employment of a midwife from 1744 to 1748 and her emoluments, whereas item 337 concerns the employment of another midwife in the same community in 1823. Other examples can be found in Marcus, J.R., *Communal Sick-Care in the German Ghetto* (Cincinnati: Hebrew University College Press, 1947), 48–51, 137; and in Bloom, H.I., *The Economic Activities of the Jews of Amsterdam in the Seventeenth and Eighteenth Centuries* (Port Washington, NY: Kennikot Press, 1937; also 1967 reprint), 109 n. 126. The Rishon Lezion Museum in Israel has a copy of the contract between the local community and a midwife in 1902.

17. Marcus, J.R., 1947, *op. cit.*, p. 51.

18. Malka, E., 1946, *op. cit.*, p. 19. Mathieu, J., "Notes sur l'enfance Juive du Mellah de Casablanca," *Bulletin de l'Institut d'Hygiene du Maroc* 7 (1947): 26. Goulven, J., *Mellahs de Rabati-Salé* (Paris: 1927), 11. Ben Simhon, R., 1994, *op. cit.*, p. 41. Aslan, M., and R. Nissim, 1982, *op. cit.*, p. 11, and Mrs. Selime of Neveh Monosson in Israel, formerly a midwife in Baghdad, personal communication.

19. Melammed, R. Levine, "Medieval and Early Modern Sephardi Women," in *Jewish Women: in Historical Perspective*, edited by J.R. Baskin (Detroit: Wayne State University Press, 1991), 120.

20. Joel Cahen, personal communication.

21. Armistead, S.G., and J.H. Silverman, ed., "Judeo-Spanish Ballad Chapbooks of Y.A. Yona," in *Folk Literature of the Sephardic Jews* (Berkeley: University of California, 1971), vol. 1, p. 185ff. I have rewritten Armistead and Silverman's translation, which is a verse-by-verse translation of the ballad, to render the gist of the tale. These editors reproduce Yona's ballad in the original Judeo–Spanish, their English translation, an analysis of motifs, and a survey of all other known versions of this tale, comparing forms from the Spanish peninsula and other versions in Moroccan Judeo–Spanish and Eastern Judeo–Spanish (Greece, Turkey, and Palestine).

22. *Avodah Zarah* 2:1; *B. Avodah Zarah* 26a; *J. Avodah Zarah* 2:1:7.

23. Pansier, P., *Les Medecins juifs à Avignon aux treizième, quatorzième et quinzième siècles* (Janus: 1910), 428. The second instance is cited in Blumenfeld-Kozinski, R., *Not of Woman Born* (Ithaca, NY: Cornell University Press, 1990), 103. An example of anti-Semitism in connection with childbirth is found in a broadsheet printed in Strasbourg in 1574, reproduced in Raphael, F., and R. Weyl, *Les Juifs en Alsace* (Toulouse: Collection Franco-Judaica, 1977), 37. Shatzmiller, J., *Jews, Medicine and Medieval Society* (Berkeley: University of California Press, 1994), 14ff., tells of the licensing procedures imposed on the medical profession from the twelfth century onward in Christian Europe, which often discriminated against Jewish practitioners and fined those deemed inadequately qualified. *Ibid.*, p. 81 tells of cases where Jewish women were jailed for administering drugs—in one case a woman was accused of causing an abortion, and p. 83 quotes a warning in a late medieval Jewish moral treatise not to perform medical work for Christians because if anything goes wrong, the Jew will be accused of murdering Gentiles.

24. Institoris, *Malleus maleficarum*, translated and edited by M. Summers (London: Pushkin Press, 1948). Documentation of witch-midwives can be found in Forbes, T.R., *The Midwife and the Witch* (New Haven: Yale University Press, 1966), and in Witkowski, A., *Histoire des accouchements chez tous les peuples* (Paris: 1887), 160ff, and of the European witch craze in Russell, J.B., *A History of Witchcraft* (London: Thames and Hudson, 1980), 72ff.

25. Shulvass, M.A., *The Jews in the World of the Renaissance* (Leiden: E.J. Brill, 1973), 331.

26. Hsia, R. Po-Chia, *The Myth of Ritual Murder: Jews and Magic in Reformation Germany* (New Haven: Yale University Press, 1988), 205–207.

27. Katzenellenbogen, P., *Yesh manḥilin* (Jerusalem: 1986), sign. 23.

28. Noy, D., ed., *Folktales of Israel* (Chicago: University of Chicago Press, 1963), 24–27. Another version of this story was told by S. Ben-Omri, in his book *Ha-shed Tintal* (Hezlya: published by the author, 1987), 91–98, about a well-known midwife in Baghdad. A different version was told in Brauer, E., in *The Jews of Kurdistan* (Detroit: Wayne State University Press, 1993), edited by R. Patai, pp. 153–154.

29. Grunwald, M., "Tales, Songs, and Folkways of Sephardic Jews," *Folklore Research Center Studies* 6 (1982): 205, 225–227.

30. Sadeh, P., *Jewish Folktales* (New York: Doubleday, 1989), 169–172. Sadeh notices a similarity between the demons of this tale and the water demon, Deydushka Vodyani, of Russian folklore, and therefore assumes a Slavic influence in this Jewish tale. He has taken this tale from a mid-nineteenth-century book by Rabbi Tsvi Hirsh Kaidvar [sic]. It is probable that the origin of Sadeh's text are the tales of Posen, by Zvi Hirsch Kaidenover (d. 1712). However, there is an Iraqi version of this tale, according to D.S. Sassoon, told again by Ben-Omri, 1987, *op. cit.*, pp. 98ff.

31. Yehosha, Y., *Yaldut be-yerushalayim ha-yeshanah* (Jerusalem: R. Mass, 1966), 85–86.

32. *Encyclopedia Judaica* (Jerusalem: Keter, 1972), vol. 8, p. 1035, fig.2, and *Ibid.*, pp. 286, 1033.

33. Marcus, J.R., 1947, *op. cit.*, pp. 8, 13, 173 and n. 191, 186ff.

34. *Ibid.*, p. 188, taken from Hanauer, W., *Frankfurt am Krankenhaus*, 19.

35. For example, Cramer, A., *Vollstandige Gesetzsammlung für die Judenschaft in den königlichen Staaten* (Prague: 1790), vol. 1, pp. 251–252, item 132, quotes a directive to Jewish communities in Bohemia, dated 1787, to send some of their women to train as midwives. For another example, from England, see "The Training of Midwives," *Jewish Chronicle*, (November 11, 1904): 8–9.

36. Wolf, L., ed., *The Legal Sufferings of the Jews in Russia* (London: T. Fisher Unwin, 1912), 31, 87ff.

37. Silman, M., M. Siegel-Kellner, and T. Naaman, *A History of the Midwife* (Jerusalem: Gefen, 1991), 14–15. Malka, E., 1946, *op. cit.*, pp. 19–29; Mathieu, J., 1947, *op. cit.*, p. 25. Both these essays on Moroccan Jews report that only the very poorest patients and the most complicated cases were delivered in hospital. The same was true in Palestine in the early twentieth century: Mrs. Havah Karlan, personal communication.

38. Marks, L., "'Dear Old Mother Levy's': The Jewish Maternity Home and Sick Room Helps Society 1895–1939," History Workshop National Conference, 1988. Another Jewish charity, also concerned with the terrible situation in London's immigrant East End at the close of the nineteenth century, opened a home to help unmarried pregnant Jewish girls. The home offered birthing facilities and then placed the baby in a foster home; the girl could stay for up to one year, during which time charitable women educated her for domestic service and found her suitable employment.

39. Towler, J., and J. Bramall, *Midwives in History and Society* (London: Croom Helm, 1986).

40. Friedenwald, H., "Notes on the History of Jewish Hospitals," chap. 37 in *The Jews and Medicine*, vol. 2, (Baltimore: Johns Hopkins University Press, 1944).

41. Mrs. Karlan, personal communication, 1989.

8. Giving Birth

1. The Greek translation of the Septuagint, made some three centuries before the Christian era, translates the similar Hebrew word in both phrases as *lupe*, which refers to the emotion of suffering rather than physical pain: Wessel, H., "Childbirth in the Bible," *Koroth* 9 (1988): 270–280.

2. Genesis 4:1, 4:2, 4:25.

3. Genesis 35:16, regarding her hard labor; Genesis 31:32, regarding the curse for her having hidden the idols.

4. See also Isaiah 66:7–8; Jeremiah 4:31, 22:23, 49:24; Hosea 13:13; Micah 4:10; Psalm 48:7.

5. *Leviticus Rabbah* 14:4.

6. *B. Yoma* 20b; *B. Niddah* 31a; amazingly, the Talmud explained that the baby is born in the position assumed during sexual intercourse; while both lie face downward in the womb, only the female fetus turns to face upward before delivery, and this turning intensifies the pains. The talmudic rationale is surely based on the preference for baby boys because there is in fact no sex difference in fetal positions. Aldabi repeats this wisdom and adds that a boy is born face downward toward the dust from which the first male was created, whereas a girl is born facing up to the rib, from where the first female was created: Aldabi, M., *Sh'vilei emunah* (Warsaw: 1887), sign. 5, part 4, p. 113.

7. *B. Niddah* 31b.

8. *B. Sotah* 12b; *Exodus Rabbah* 1:20.

9. *Shabbat* 2:6, *B. Shabbat* 32b.

10. *B. Eruvin* 100b; *Genesis Rabbah* 20:6.

11. *Pirkei de Rabbi Eliezer*, edited and translated by G. Friedlander (New York: Hermon Press, 1981), chap. 14, p. 100. Saldarini, A.J., trans., *The Fathers According to Rabbi Nathan* (Leiden: E.J. Brill, 1975), 251–252.

12. Zohar II, 219b–220a. See English translation and explanations by I. Tishby, in *The Wisdom of the Zohar*, edited by F. Lachower and I. Tishby (Oxford: Oxford University Press, 1989), 738–740, 755.

13. For the snake's lust for Eve, see *B. Yevamot* 103b, *B. Avodah Zarah* 22b, and *B. Shabbat* 146a; *Pirkei de Rabbi Eliezer, op. cit.*, chap. 21, p. 150, and also Ginzberg, L., *Legends of the Jews* (Philadelphia: Jewish Publication Society, 1947), 105–106. Concerning the hind, see *B. Yoma* 29a. and *B. Baba Batra* 16b.

14. For fetal presentation and physique, see *Sefer ha-toledet* (fourteenth century), British Library, London, Montefiore ms. 420, ff. 39v–40r; Aldabi, M. (fourteenth century), 1887, *op. cit.*, sign. 5, part 4, p. 112–113; Cohn, Tobias, *Ma'aseh tuvya* (Venice: 1707), *Gan na'ul*, chap. 17. Regarding planetary influences, Saturn, for example, was responsible for immobility and illness, and if this planet dominated the heavens at the time of birth, the delivery would be prolonged and difficult: Barkai, R., "A Medieval Treatise on Obstetrics," *Medical History* 33 (1989): 101–102. For rabbinic references, see note 15 below.

15. Judah ben Samuel (the Pious), of Regensburg, *Sefer Hasidim*, edited by R. Margoliyot (Jerusalem: 1957), sign. 486. Paquda, Bahya ben Joseph ibn, *The Book of Direction to the Duties of the Heart* (London: Routledge and Kegan Paul, 1973), 151. Hacohen, Eliyahu ben Shlomo Avraham, *Shevet mussar* (Jerusalem: Y. Rubinstein, 1963), part 2, chap. 24. Cardin, N.B., *Out of the Depths I Call to You* (Northvale, NJ: Jason Aronson, 1992), 126, includes the transcript of a midwife's prayer asking God to silence those who speak against the birthing woman and to remember her meritorious deeds.

16. Weissler, C., "Mitzvot built into the body," in *Jews and Their Bodies*, edited by H.E. Schwartz (New York: State University of New York, 1992). Also see Weissler, C., "The traditional piety of Ashkenazic women," *Jewish Spirituality from the Sixteenth Century to the Present*, edited by A. Green (New York: Crossroad, 1987), 273 n. 49.

17. Yerushalmi, Moses ben Hanokh, *Brantspiegel* (Basel: 1602), chap. 34, p. 121a.

18. Katzenellenbogen, P., *Yesh manhilin* (Jerusalem: 1986), sign. 24. Pinhas Katzenellenbogen (1691–1761) quoted the Talmud as his source for this theory.

19. Ovadia, D., *Kehillot Zafro* (Jerusalem: 1975), vol. 3, p. 84.

20. Pain relief had not been offered in the previous births of most of the pregnant women that I interviewed in Israel, in 1984, and, in the absence of prenatal preparation, the pain of childbirth was often unexpected and shocking. One of the outcomes of prenatal classes is that women are now aware that they can ask for and receive some type of pain relief.

21. *Song of Songs Rabbah* 11.14.8; *Deuteronomy Rabbah* 2:11. *Sefer Hasidim, op. cit.*, 1957, sign. 487 instructs anyone in the house of a woman giving birth to pray for God's mercy and that the baby be

born under a lucky star. Azulai, H.Y.D., *Sefer avodat ha-kodesh* (Pressburg: 1818), 102, para. 4: this prayer is for a husband to recite for his wife when she goes into labor. It pleads "If she has had any sin, may You forgive and cleanse it through that which she is suffering, the pains of her labor. May the sound of her crying out ascend to Your Throne of Glory. Seal the mouth of her accusers . . . bestow goodness on the worthy and non-worthy alike."

22. *Shimmush tehillim* (Cracow: 1648), see under Psalm 20. This is not the same listing as reproduced in English by M. Grunwald in *The Jewish Encyclopedia* (London: 1901–1905), under "Bibliomancy" (vol. 3, p. 203). I do not know which edition he used. G. Scholem presumed that *Shimmush tehillim* dates from the gaonic period: Scholem, G., *Kabbalah* (New York: Meridian, 1978), 359.

23. Pollack, H., *Jewish Folkways in Germanic Lands (1648–1806)* (Cambridge, MA: Massachusetts Institute of Technology Press, 1971), 17. Tirshom, Joseph, *Shoshan yesod olam* (c. 1550), Sassoon ms. 290, item 1616.

24. Luntz, Eliahu ben Moshe, *Toldot Adam* (Zolkiew: 1720), no. 150. Binesh, Binyamin, *Sefer amta-ḥat Binyamin* (Wilmersdorf: 1716), 16b, recommended reciting the psalm twelve times, followed by meditations on the holy Names in it. Berekhiah ben Moses of Modena, *Ma'avar Yabok* (Vienna: 1857), 22 (first edition was 1626), recommended reciting it twelve times, referring the reader to Horowitz, I., *Shnei luḥot ha-brit*, first printed posthumously in Amsterdam in 1649. Cardin, N.B., 1992, *op. cit.*, pp. xi, 90–91, instructed the woman to recite Psalm 20 three times, and the copy of the psalm includes kabbalistic changes in the spelling of the divine Name. Here the psalm is recited in feminine ("May God answer you" where "you" is feminine). This change is recommended also in Rozenberg, Y.Y., *Rafael ha-malakh* (Piotrkow: 1911), *makshah le-yaled*, although Azulai, H.Y.D., 1818, *op. cit.*, p. 102, para. 4, specifically warned against converting the psalm to the feminine, and instructed that the psalm should be recited twelve times. *Kol t'khinah*, 1824, *op. cit.*, p. 10 instructed a pregnant woman to recite Psalm 20 every day from the start of the ninth month until she gave birth.

25. Epstein, Y.M., 1984, *op. cit.*, Binesh, B., 1716, *op. cit.*, Cardin, N.B., 1992, *op. cit.*

26. Itzḥaki, I., *Laḥash ve-kame'a* (Tel Aviv: Shakked, 1976), 133.

27. The Parma Library has a fifteenth-century Hebrew manuscript which includes a prayer for a woman sitting on the birthstool (Parma: 1706), ms. 1124, p. 68. Solomon, Jacob ben Abraham, *Ma'aneh lashon* (Frankfurt: 1726), sign. 31 and 32, p. 50–51: this prayer (first published in Prague in 1615) should be recited at the cemetery by anyone concerned for the well-being of a woman about to have a child or having difficulty in birthing. It invokes the merit of Sarah and the other matriarchs. Epstein, Yehiel Michl, *Seder tefillah derekh yesharah* (Frankfurt an der Oder: 1703), 27: this Yiddish prayer for a birthing woman invokes the merit of Sarah and Rachel and Hannah and all the barren women who eventually gave birth and requests that the pregnant woman be relieved from the decree on Eve. The same prayer is found in Aaron Berekhiah ben Moses of Modena, 1857, *op. cit.*, pp. 21–22, and in Binesh, B., 1716, *op. cit.*, pp. 17a–b, which also includes the prayer from *Ma'aneh lashon* and requests that God who heard the prayers of the matriarchs should hear this prayer, too. The first edition was published in Venice in 1626. "*Tkhine* for a woman who is about to have a child," in *Rokhl Weeps for Her Children* (Vilna: 1910), copied and translated in Klirs, T.G., comp., *The Merit of Our Mothers: A Bilingual Anthology of Jewish Women's Prayers* (Cincinnati: Hebrew Union College Press, 1993), 128–129: here in this Yiddish prayer, the merits of Sarah, Rebekah, Rachel, and Leah are called on, as well as the merit of the prophetesses, Miriam, Deborah, Hannah, and Huldah. Cardin, N.B., 1992, *op. cit.*, pp. 72–75 and 106–107: a prayer recited by an Italian Jewish woman in the late eighteenth century during the entire pregnancy begs that as God heard the prayers of Sarah, Rebekah, Leah, and Rachel, so may God hear this prayer and furthermore release this woman from the punishment of Eve. One of several childbirth prayers in Cardin's collection invokes the merit of Hannah. Another book of supplications used by another Italian Jewish woman in the early nineteenth century instructs on the giving of charity on the first day of the ninth month, with a prayer for easy birth, and invokes the merits of Sarah, Rebekah, Rachel, Leah, Hannah, and "all the pious, righteous, and worthy women"; *Kol t'khinah* (Trieste: 1824), 12, 14.

28. See note 16 above. See Nahmanides, Commentary to Leviticus 23:40. The *etrog* symbolizes the Shekhinah.

29. Hoffman-Krayer, E., *Handwörterbuch des deutschen Aberglaubens* (1927), vol. 4, p. 815, reports the use of the *etrog* at the birth of Frederick William IV. Schudt, J.J., *Jüdische Merkwurdigkeiten*, 1717, vol. 2, book 6, chap. 26, p. 8; and Bodenschatz, J., *Kirchliche Verfassung der heutige Juden* (Leipzig and Frankfurt: 1748–1749), reported its use by Jews in early eighteenth-century Germany. Its use in nineteenth-century Holland is reported in Beem, H., *Joden van Leeuwarden* (1974), 226, and in Bavaria, in Ploss, H.H., and M. and P. Bartels, *Woman*, edited by J. Dingwall (London: Heinemann, 1935), vol. 3, p. 19. Isaac Pallache, rabbi of Amsterdam, recorded the making of an *etrog* potion, Weisberg, Y.D., *Sefer otzar ha-brit* (Jerusalem; Makhon Torah ha-brit, 1986), vol. 1, p. 36, citing Pallache's *Yafe la-lev*, sign. 664:15. The Polish prayer book is Rozenberg, Y.Y., 1911, *op. cit., me'uberet.* Yemenite Jews used an *etrog* "nipple" as a charm for a safe pregnancy: personal communication from an elderly woman, Mrs. Hannah Aqua, who practiced midwifery in Yemen, now living in Kfar Gvirol, Israel.

30. *Seder tkhines u-vakoshes* (Fürth: 1762), no. 100. No. 89 repeats the *Tze'ena u-re'ena* prayer.

31. "*Tkhine* for a Pregnant Woman When She Is About to Give Birth," in *Rokhl Weeps for Her Children*, 1910, in *The Merit of Our Mothers . . .*, 1993, *op. cit.*, pp. 126–127.

32. Sore bas Toyvim, *Shloyshe she'orim* (Vilna: 1838), translated by C. Weissler, in Weissler, C., 1987, *op. cit.*, p. 259.

33. Neuda, F., *Duties of the Heart*, translated by R. Vulture (Vienna: Jos. Schlesinger, c. 1900), 112; my adaptation. The prayer book in which it is found, *Stunden der Andacht*, was first printed in Prague in 1857 and then went through over two dozen editions by the 1920s. A later revised version was made for the special conditions of Nazi Germany.

34. For example, Aaron Berekhiah of Modena, 1857, *op. cit.*, p. 21b, Epstein, Y.M., 1703, *op. cit.*, p. 27, Solomon, Jacob ben Abraham, 1726, *op. cit.*, sign. 32, p. 50b, and Azulai, H.D., 1818, *op. cit.*, p. 102, part 4.

35. Ginzberg, L., 1947, *op. cit.*, vol. 1, p. 106.

36. Luntz, E., 1720, *op. cit.*, no. 159. Nahman of Bratslav, *Likkutei etzot, Banim*, no. 11. For this practice in Iraq, see Aslan, M., and R. Nissim, *Yehudei Iraq* (Tel Aviv: Ofer, 1982), 12, and in North Africa, see Ovadia, D., 1975, *op. cit.*

37. Simner, Zechariah ben Yacov, *Sefer zekhirah* (Wilmersdorf: 1729), 27. This book of Jewish folk remedies was especially popular in Eastern Europe and was frequently reprinted in the eighteenth and nineteenth centuries. See also Grunwald, M., "Charms and Magic Recipes," *Edot* 1 (1945): 241–248, no. 48 (187). Pictorial depictions of this custom among Ashkenazi Jews, dating from the early eighteenth century, can be found in Kirchner, J.C., *Jüdische Ceremonial* (Nurnberg: 1726), and Bodenshatz, J., *Kirchliche Verfassung der Heutige Juden* (Leipzig: 1748–1749). This custom was also practiced by Sephardic Jews in North Africa and in the Balkans, see Ben Simhon, R., *Yahadut Marocco* (Lod: Orot Yahadut ha-magreb, 1994), 32–33, and Banbanashti, D., *Yehudei Saloniki* (Jerusalem: Kriyat Sefer, 1973), 62. Patai, R., *On Jewish Folklore* (Detroit: Wayne State University Press, 1983), 380.

38. Buber, M., *Tales of the Hasidim: Later Masters* (New York: Schocken, 1948), 91–92.

39. Howe, I., and E. Greenberg, ed., *A Treasury of Yiddish Poetry* (New York: Holt, Rinehart and Winston, 1969), 202.

40. Zlotnik, Y. (Elzet, J.L.), "*Me-minhagei Israel,*" *Reshumot* 1 (1918): 366, tells of the custom of visiting graves to supplicate. Frankfort, Simeon ben Israel Judah, *Sefer ha-hayyim* (Amsterdam: 1703), was bilingual, the first half in Hebrew, the second half in Yiddish, with prayers for reciting at the grave. Many later editions were printed. Thanks to Mrs. Y. Eizen for the explanation of the Yiddish words.

41. Molkho, M., "*Leidah ve-yaldut bein Yehudei Saloniki,*" *Edot* 2 (1947): 258.

42. B. *Baba Batra* 9a, 19b.

43. *Kol t'khinah*, 1824, *op. cit.*, p. 11b; Epstein, Y.M., *Kitzur shnei luhot ha-brit* (Jerusalem: 1984), 136.

44. Dubnow, S., ed., *Pinkas ha-medinah* (Berlin: 1925), *Takkanah* 1551b.

45. Molkho, M., 1947, *op. cit.*, p. 259; Mathieu, J., "Notes sur l'enfance juive du Mellah de Casablanca," *Bulletin de l'Institut d'Hygiène du Maroc* 7 (1947): 27; Patai, R., 1983, *op. cit.*, p. 381.

46. Brauer, E., in *The Jews of Kurdistan* (Detroit: Wayne State University Press, 1993), edited by R. Patai, p. 155.

47. B. *Shabbat* 128b.

48. Molkho, M., 1947, *op. cit.*, reports this custom. Also Ploss, H.H., and M. and P. Bartels, 1935, *op. cit.*, vol. 2, chap. 25, tell that in the villages in Russia, at the turn of the century, women gave birth in the bath house. A Jewish midwife who had worked in Baghdad in the first half of the twentieth century used a warmed stone. A hot-water bottle was later used instead, recommended by a woman of Yemenite origin who had given birth to sixteen healthy babies.

49. Barkai, R., *Les infortunes de Dinah: Le livre de la génération* (Paris: Editions du Cerf, 1991), 142–146, 185–191. This is a translation of *Sefer ha-toledet* (a fourteenth-century Hebrew medical manuscript). See also Barkai, R., 1989, *op. cit.*, pp. 115 ff., a translation of another fourteenth century Hebrew medical manuscript on easing delivery (Bibliothèque Nationale, Paris, ms. héb. 1120, ff. 66v–67r). Cohn, T., 1707, *op. cit.*, chap. 17 offers medicinal remedies for easing delivery.

50. Aldabi, M., 1887, *op. cit.*, sign. 4, part 5; my translation.

51. Bernstein, M., ed., *Two Remedy Books in Yiddish from 1474 and 1508* (Bloomington: Indiana University Press, 1960), p. 301; Simner, Z., 1709, *op. cit.*, p. 27a; Binesh, B., 1716, *op. cit.*, p. 19a; Yitzhaki, Y., 1976, *op. cit.*, p. 131–132.

52. Pollack, H. 1971, I., p. 17; Grunwald, M., "Tales, Songs, and Folkways of Sephardic Jews," *Folklore Research Center Studies* 6 (1982): 226; Patai, R., 1983, *op. cit.*, p. 374 and n. 313.

53. The quotation is from Judah ben Enoch, a German rabbi of Polish origin whose responsa were published together with his father's and his son's in *Hinukh beit Yehudah*, in 1708. See also Lampronti, I., ed., *Paḥad Itzhak* (Livorno: 1834), *yoledet*. Kirchner, J.C., 1726, *op. cit.*, p. 149, also refers to this custom, and similarly Bodenshatz, J., 1748–1749, *op. cit.*, vol. 4, pp. 56–57. See also Patai, R., 1983, *op. cit.*, p. 380, ref. n. 390. Hayyim Pallache, in his remedy book *Refu'ah ve-ḥayyim* (Izmir: 1873) chap. 9, p. 336 mentions this custom and rules against it.

54. Grunwald, M., 1982, *op. cit.*, p. 225. Nahum, Y.L., *Me-tzefonot yehudei Teiman* (Tel Aviv: 1961), 139. Patai, R., 1983, *op. cit.*, p. 379. Grunwald, M., "Bibliomancy," *The Jewish Encyclopedia* (1901–1906), vol. 3, pp. 202–203, reports the use of the Torah scroll in the birthing room to facilitate delivery. Kleeblatt, N., and Wertkin, ed., *The Jewish Heritage in American Folk Art* (New York), 81, and Beukers, M., and Waale, R., *Tracing An-sky* (Zwolle: Waanders, 1992), are catalogues of museum exhibitions displaying *pinkasim* used in this way.

55. Ben-Ami, I., *Ha'aratzat ha-k'doshim* (Jerusalem: Magnes Press, 1984), 59, 522. Ben Simhon, R., 1994, *op. cit.*, p. 34.

56. Zborowski, M., and E. Herzog, *Life Is with People* (New York: Schocken, 1962), 315. This documents the custom in Eastern Europe. Dr. Bracha Yaniv reported that this was practiced in her family, in Poland, in the early twentieth century (personal communication). Fraser, J.G, *The Golden Bough* (New York: Macmillan, 1927), vol. 3, pp. 294ff., examines the opening of knots to ease childbirth in many non-Jewish societies.

57. Exodus 22:17 and Deuteronomy 18:9–14 warn against magic and sorcery. *J. Shabbat* 6:8b warns against the use of biblical verses to calm a child, whereas *B. Shabbat* 66b–67a pronounces no objection to reciting such incantations in this way, especially against demons. *Song of Songs Rabbah* 2:16 mentions that Rabbi Hanina uttered an incantation over Rabbi Yohanan. The Jerusalem Talmud, *J. Sotah* 1:4:2 mentions women skilled in incantations. J. Preuss gives evidence that the recitation of incantations is a heathen custom that Jews learned, and although some efforts were made to reject such behavior, it nevertheless had a captive audience that chose to use it at times: Preuss, J., *Biblical and Talmudic Medicine*, 2nd ed., edited by F. Rosner (Brooklyn: Hebrew Publication Company, 1983), 144–146. In the face of this custom, some rabbis accepted it, as long it was remedial and not black magic.

58. Jakobovits, I., *Jewish Medical Ethics* (New York: Bloch, 1975), 22. Maimonides, M., *The Guide for the Perplexed*, translated by M. Friedlander (London: Trubner, 1885), vol. 3, chap. 37, p. 170, invokes against idolatrous practices, including incantations.

59. Naveh, J., and S. Shaked, *Magic Spells and Formulae* (Jerusalem: Magnes Press, 1993), 149, transcribing and translating T.S. K. 1.15 f.1 lines 6–10, from the Cairo *Geniza*.

60. Bernstein, M., 1973, *op. cit.*, p. 295. Manuscript H.B. XI/17, Wurtemberg National Library, Stuttgart, item 1001; *Sefer Razi'el ha-malakh* (Israel: Meirav, undated), 147, a modern printing of *Sefer Razi'el*, first published in Amsterdam in 1701; Binesh, B., 1716, *op. cit.*, p. 18b, and O'Hana R., *Mareh*

ha-yeladim (Jerusalem: 1901), 70b. Also all the prayer books mentioned in note 27 above, except for that edited by T. G. Klirs. A fifteenth-century Italian manuscript (Parma: 1706, ms. 1124, p. 74), includes an incantation for a woman on a birthstool, but unfortunately the microfilm printout was illegible. See also Cardin, N.B., 1992, *op. cit.*, pp. 96–97; and Sperling, A.I., *Ta'amei ha-minhagim ve-makor ha-dinim* (Jerusalem: Eshkol, 1961), 567–568.

61. Tirshom, Joseph, *Shoshan yesod olam*, c. 1550, Sassoon ms. 290, item 651. Zlotnick, Y., 1918, *op. cit.* Grunwald, M., 1945, *op. cit.*, no. 40 (185), from an Ashkenazi manuscript in the State Library of Hamburg. Hamoi, A., *Ha'ah nafshenu* (Izmir: 1870). *Refu'ah ve-hayyim me-yerushalayim* (Jerusalem: Bakall, 1974), 66a. Rozenberg, Y.Y., 1911, *op. cit., makshah leyaled.*

62. Cardin, N.B., 1992, *op. cit.*, pp. 100–103; *Kol t'khinah*, 1824, *op. cit.*, pp. 14a–b.

63. Leibowitz, J.O., and S. Marcus, *Sefer ha-nisyonot: The Book of Medical Experiences Attributed to Abraham ibn Ezra* (Jerusalem: Magnes Press, 1984), 239–245, with explanation on p. 70ff. Sheshet Benveniste offered some identical advice in his *Sefer ha-toladah* (Bodleian Library Neub. ms. 2142, f. 255b), and Naveh, J., and S. Shaked, 1993, *op. cit.*, p. 229, found another example in a *Geniza* fragment (T.-S. Arabic 49.54). See also the list of charms and remedy books in the Selected Bibliography; all these offer instructions for easy delivery.

64. *Sefer Razi'el ha-malakh, op. cit.*, p. 147.

65. Kaplan, A., *Meditation and the Bible* (York Beach, ME: Samuel Weiser, 1992), chap. 7 describes the secret society of practical kabbalists and the origins of *Toldot Adam*. Luntz, E., 1720, *op. cit.*, no. 158, is attributed to Nahmanides. Other formulas for amulets for easing delivery are offered in nos. 17, 29, and 92. Simner, Z., 1729, *op. cit.*, p. 27, quotes a powerful amulet, that must be removed after birthing, as "proven."

66. Ben-Yaakov, A., *Otzar Ha-segullot* (Jerusalem: 1991), chap. 10, part 6. Itzhaki, I., 1976, *op. cit.*, p. 135, includes a formula from *Sefer Razi'el ha-malakh* and another from *Sefer zekhirah*.

67. Lampronti, I., Pakad Itzhak (Livorno: 1834), vol. 5, *makshah le-yaled.*

68. Portaleone, Abraham, *Shiltei ha-gibborim* (Mantua: 1612), 66a.

69. Zlotnik, Y., 1918, *op. cit.*, p. 366.

70. Rozenberg, Y.Y., 1911, *op. cit., makshah le-yaled*, last entry.

71. Personal communication from a midwife in Jerusalem who works in the ultra-Orthodox community, 1995.

72. For a guide to Jewish meditation, see Kaplan, A., 1992, *op. cit.*

73. Rosenthal, D.S., *A Joyful Mother of Children* (Jerusalem: Feldheim, 1982); Cardin, N.B., 1992, *op. cit.*; and Klirs, T.G., 1992, *op. cit.*, all have different examples of such prayers, with English translations.

9. Death in Childbirth

1. Genesis 35:16–19.

2. Rachel had stolen her father's idols, unbeknown to Jacob. When her father accused Jacob of the theft, Jacob knew nothing of it and promised that whoever had stolen them would not be allowed to live: Genesis 31:32. The interpretation that Rachel died in childbirth because of this curse is found in *Genesis Rabbah* 74:9, and *Pirkei de Rabbi Eliezer*, edited and translated by G. Friedlander (New York: Hermon Press, 1981), chap. 36, pp. 274–275.

3. *Shabbat* 2:6, *B. Shabbat* 32b.

4. *B. Arakhin* 7a.

5. This law is believed to date from c. 715 B.C.E., proclaimed under King Numa Pompilius: Blumenfeld-Kozinski, R., *Not of Woman Born* (Ithaca, NY: Cornell University Press, 1990), 143ff.

6. Ilan, T., *Jewish Women in Greco-Roman Palestine* (Tübingen: J.C.B. Mohr [Paul Siebeck], 1995), 117–118.

7. Benveniste, S., *Ha-ma'amar be-toladah*, Oxford, Bodleian NeuB. 2142, f.255a suggested a strong binding to expel a dead fetus. Leibowitz, J.O., and S. Marcus, *Sefer ha-nisyonot: The Book of Medical Experiences Attributed to Abraham ibn Ezra* (Jerusalem: Magnes Press, 1984), chap. 5, p. 233, tells how to expel a dead fetus, giving the mother a drink or a fumigation. *Sefer ha-toledet*, British Library, London, Montefiore ms. 420, offered instructions on how to remove a dead fetus from a live mother.

Aldabi, M., *Sh'vilei emunah* (Warsaw: 1887), part 5, sign. 1, p. 113, on the extraction of a dead fetus with medicines and fumigations, according to the methods of the ancient Greeks. Zacuto Lusitanus, Abraham, *Medici et philosophi, praxis historiarum* (Lyon: 1644), book 3, chap. 17, p. 509, offered four recipes for expelling a dead fetus. Cohn, T., *Ma'asei Tuvya* (Venice: 1707), *Gan na'ul*, chap. 18 explained that a doctor was sometimes called on to cut out the baby when a pregnant mother had died. And the popular eighteenth-century remedy books offered advice for removing a dead fetus from a mother's womb, but often this involved giving the mother a drink or a fumigation; the former advice proves that this was for cases when the mother was still alive. Zimmels, H.J., *Magicians, Theologians and Doctors* (London: Edward Goldston & Sons, 1952), 69, reports that Hayyim Halberstam (1793–1876), a hasidic rabbi in Galicia, prohibited a doctor from using a knife on a woman who had just died to extract a baby thought to be still alive. The rabbi must have thought it impossible to save the infant's life. The case of the Russian Jewish woman is reported in Ploss, H.H., and M. and P. Bartels, *Woman*, edited by E.J. Dingwall (London: Heinemann, 1935), vol. 3, p. 412.

8. Zimmels, H.J., 1952, *op. cit.*, p. 69. Ploss, H.H., and M. and P. Bartels, 1935, *op. cit.*, vol. 3, p. 412, reported that Jewish women in Beirut took care that the baby was dead before burying a pregnant woman.

9. Ascher, B.H., *The Book of Life (Sefer ha-ḥayyim and kitzur ma'aneh lashon)* (London: Shapiro, Vallentine, 1922), 203–204. An earlier edition was printed in London in 1847. These ideas were taken directly from *Sefer ha-ḥayyim*, first published in Amsterdam in 1703. Ploss, H.H., and M. and P. Bartels, 1935, *op. cit.*, also cite this special burial practice among Jews of South Russia around 1900.

10. There is an engraving of the Jewish cemetery of Endingen and Lengnau, by J.C. Ulrich, *Sammlung Juedischer Geschichte* (Basle: 1768), showing a section for women who died in childbirth. This is reproduced in *Encyclopedia Judaica*, vol. 6, p. 738. My thanks to Prof. D. Sperber for bringing this to my attention. Joel Cahen researched Jewish customs in Dutch villages and discovered that this was common among Jews in Holland, too: Joel Cahen, personal communication. For the references and discussion of the ritual impurity and purification of a woman after childbirth, see Chapter 12.

11. Weisberg, J.D., *Sefer otzar ha-brit* (Jerusalem: Makhon Torat ha-brit, 1986), vol. 1, p. 235, citing Medini, Hayim Hezekiah, *Sedei ḥemed* (Warsaw: 1891–1912), *avelot*, sign. 141, p. 1412. Medini was born in Jerusalem, lived later in Constantinople, served as rabbi in the Crimea, and eventually became Chief Sephardic Rabbi in the Holy Land, living in Hebron until his death. In this encyclopedic work, he mentions that the ritual before burying a pregnant woman was the custom in some Jewish communities.

12. Goitein, S.D., "*Tzeva'ot me-mitzrayim me-tekufat ha-genizah*," *S'funot* 8 (1964): 119ff.

13. *Tosefta Makkot* 2:5.

14. *B. Sanhedrin* 72b.

15. *J. Shabbat* 14:4, *J. Sanhedrin* 8:9:3c,d.

16. Feldman, D.M., *Marital Relations, Birth Control and Abortion in Jewish Law* (New York: Schocken, 1978), 275ff.

17. *Niddah* 5:1. The postnatal purification laws are mentioned in Chapter 12.

18. Soranus, *Gynecology* (Baltimore: Johns Hopkins University Press, 1956), translated by O. Temkin, book 4. This translation is based on medieval Latin and Greek manuscripts, so it may be that Soranus did in fact write about this subject, but his words were excluded by later copyists because they were no longer relevant. We cannot know.

19. The Persian poet Firdousi described in couplets the successful birth of Rustam by caesarean section, with the mother under anesthesia. At about the same time, another Persian, the physician Avicenna (ibn Sina), explained in writing how to extract a dead baby surgically from a live mother. His predecessors, Rhazes and Abulcasis, described only embryotomy and the tools needed for this procedure.

20. The first Western description of a caesarean section performed on a live woman is found in François Rousset's publication in 1581, *Traitté nouveau de l'hystérotomotokie, ou enfantement caesarien*. He was fiercely criticized by his colleagues for his undertaking caesarean sections on live women.

21. Rashi to *B. Niddah* 40a; see Preuss, J., *Biblical and Talmudic Medicine*, 2nd ed. (Brooklyn: Hebrew Publication Company, 1983), 425.

22. *Tosafot* to *B. Hullin* 69b; *Sanhedrin* 47b; *Ketubbot* 4b; *Shabbat* 152b; *Yevamot* 102b.

23. Zimmels, H.J., 1952, *op. cit.*, p. 69, citing for example Moses Isserles.

24. Soranus' obstetric treatise was adapted to Hebrew: *Sefer ha-toledet*, British Library, London, Montefiore ms.420. Instructions for intervention in a difficult birth by embryotomy are given 42v–43v. ff. The eleventh-century Arabic philosopher, Avicenna (ibn Sina), also wrote extensively on obstetrics and gynecology. His work was translated into Hebrew in the thirteenth century and influenced both Jewish and Christian physicians: a summary of his writing on obstetrics is found in Meyerhof, M., and D. Joannides, *La gynecologue et l'obstetrique chez Avicenna (ibn Sina), et leurs rapports avec celles des Grecs* (Cairo: R. Schindler, 1938). He gave directions on how to extract a dead fetus and he leaned heavily on the ancient Greeks and Galen. Avicenna also advised that a woman who had great difficulty in birthing should not be seated on a birthstool or obstetric chair. Aldabi, in the fourteenth century, also limited his discussion of difficult births to the extraction of a dead fetus with medicines and fumigations, according to the methods of the ancient Greeks, and made no mention of caesarean section: Aldabi, M., 1887, *op. cit.*, part 5, sign. 1, p. 113. For another medieval Hebrew treatise on the difficulties of birth, see Barkai, R., "A Medieval Treatise on Obstetrics," *Medical History* 33 (1989): 115. This is a chapter entitled *Mekoshi ha-leidah*. The manuscript translated here is in the Bibliothèque Nationale, ms. Héb. 1120, and dates from the fourteenth century. Another medieval variant of this chapter is in British Library, London, ms. or. 10766.

25. Castro, Rodrigo de, *Universa muliebrum morborum* (Cologne: 1689), book 4, chap. 7, p. 202. This book was first published some 60 years earlier. Cardoso, Isaac, *Philosophia libera* (Venice: 1678), book 6, chap. 100, pp. 691–693.

26. Cohn, T., 1707, *op. cit.*, chap. 18; my translation.

27. Witkowski, A., *Histoire des accouchements chez tous les peuples* (Paris: 1887), 629. Also Ploss, H.H., and M. and P. Bartels, 1935, *op. cit.*, vol. 3, chap. 5.

28. Aridor, E., "Ha-tzeira ha-me'ushpezet be-matzav kasheh . . .," *Ha'aretz* Feb. 7, 1992: 1a.

29. Psalms 119:71; Job 1:15ff.

30. II Samuel 12:14; *Shabbat* 2:6; Gaon, Sa'adia, *The Book of Beliefs and Opinions* (New Haven: Yale University Press, 1948), 214, 295.

31. Zohar II, 96a–b, III, 113a.

32. Judah ben Samuel of Regensburg (Judah the Pious), *Sefer Hasidim*, edited by R. Margoliyot (Jerusalem: Mossad harav Kook, 1957), signs. 244, 246, 264, 460, 502, 509, refer to causes for infant death. The story of the rabbi is related in sign. 501.

33. Bin-Gorion, E., *Me-makor Israel* (Bloomington: Indiana University Press, 1976), 877, no. 298.

34. *B. Shabbat* 135b; *B. Mo'ed Katan* 24b.

35. Numbers 18:16, *B. Niddah* 44b.

36. *Tosafot* to Mo'ed Katan 24a–b. Maimonides, M., *The Guide for the Perplexed*, 2nd ed., translated by M. Friedlander (New York: Dover, 1956), 379.

37. Ecclesiastes 6:3–4; *B. Kiddushin* 80b; *Mo'ed Katan* 24a–b. Weisberg, J.D., *Sefer otzar ha-brit* (Jerusalem: Makhon Torat ha-brit, 1986), vol. 1, pp. 234–235; and Jakobovits, I., *Jewish Medical Ethics* (New York: Bloch, 1975), 199–200, citing, for example, Nahshon Gaon of Sura, Babylonia in the late ninth century; Abraham ben Isaac of Narbonne (twelfth century); Asheri (1250–1327) of Toledo; *Shulḥan arukh, Yoreh Deah*, 263:6; and Ezekiel ben Judah Landau (eighteenth century, Prague) for circumcision of a *nefel*. In contrast, Jacob and Gershom Ha-gozer, Germany, thirteenth century, and Isaac of Vienna, also thirteenth century, as well as Sephardic rabbi Hayim David Yosef Azulai, in the eighteenth century, opposed circumcision of a *nefel*. Ezekiel 32:24 tells that the uncircumcised will suffer Gehenna, whereas *Genesis Rabbah* 48:8 tells that Abraham sits at the gate of Gehenna to save the circumcised: Theodor, J., and C. Albeck, eds., *Genesis Rabbah* (Jerusalem: Wahrmann Books, 1964), 483.

38. Weisberg, J.D., 1986, *op. cit.*, cites Hayim Hezekiah Medini (1832–1904), rabbi in Crimea and later Chief Sephardic rabbi of Hebron, for the naming of a female *nefel*.

39. Thanks to Shelly Allon for the recording of Rabbi Howard Deitchee's lecture of May 1, 1987, "*Nefel* in Halakhah."

40. Borg, S., and J. Lasker, *When Pregnancy Fails* (London: Routledge and Kegan Paul, 1982). See also Kohn, I., and Moffitt, P.L., with Wilkins, I.A., *A Silent Sorrow: Pregnancy Loss Guidance and Support for You and Your Family* (New York: Delacorte Press, a division of Bantam Doubleday Dell, 1992). People may also find comfort in Kushner, H., *When Bad Things Happen to Good People* (New York: Avon Books, 1983). For the support group in Israel, Yad Elisha, and their explanatory brochure for bereaved parents and their friends, call 02-632213 or 02-6518439.

41. "Pregnancy Loss Support Program, Jewish Women's Resource Center," National Council of Jewish Women, 9 East 69 Street, New York, NY 10021, tel. (212) 535-5900. In Israel: Yad Elisha, Jerusalem, tel. 02-5632213 or 02-6518439.

42. Chagall, B., *First Encounter* (New York: Schocken, 1983), 275–276.

43. Roskies, D.G., ed., *The Literature of Destruction*, translated from Yiddish into English by C.K. Williams (Philadelphia: Jewish Publication Society, 1989), 494–495.

10. Lilith, The Demon Who Threatens Women in Childbirth

1. Albright, W.F., "An Aramean Magical Text in Hebrew from the Seventh Century B.C.," *BASOR* 76 (1939): 5–11.

2. Kerényi, C., *The Gods of the Greeks* (Harmondsworth: Penguin, 1958), 34–35.

3. Conybeare, F.C., "The Testament of Solomon," *Jewish Quarterly Review* 11 (1899): 29–30 (chaps. 57–59).

4. Lilith is mentioned in *B. Niddah* 24b, *B. Eruvin* 100b, and *B. Shabbat* 151b. A son of Lilith is mentioned in *B. Baba Batra* 73b. The Lilin are mentioned in *B. Eruvin* 18b and in *Genesis Rabbah* 20:11 and 24:6. *The Chronicles of Yerahmeel*, of unknown date (studied by M. Gaster), supposed that Adam had been visited by Lilith when he slept alone during the 130 years of his separation from Eve, and from these visits, the Lilin, demons and spirits, were created.

5. Morgan, M.A., ed., *Sefer ha-razim: The Book of Mysteries* (Chico, CA: Scholars Press for the Society of Biblical Literature, 1983), 54.

6. Naveh, J., and S. Shakked, *Magic Bowls and Amulets* (Jerusalem: Magnes Press, 1985). For description of the magic bowls see pp. 189–197, plates 28, 29.

7. *Ibid.*, pp. 104–110.

8. Gaster, M., "Two Thousand Years of a Charm Against a Child-Stealing Witch," in *Studies and Texts* (New York: Ktav, 1971), vol. 2, pp. 1005–1038.

9. See Naveh, J., and S. Shaked, 1985, *op. cit.*, pp. 111ff., appendix to amulet 15.

10. Yasif, E., *Sippurei Ben Sira be-yamei ha-beinayim* (Jerusalem: Magnes Press, 1984), 232.

11. Genesis 1:27.

12. Theodor, J., and C. Albeck, ed., *Genesis Rabbah* (Jerusalem: Mekitzei Nirdamim, 1964), 22:7, p. 213, and 17:7, p. 158.

13. See his story about virgin pregnancy in Chapter 4.

14. Dan, J., "Samael, Lilith, and the Concept of Evil in Early Kabbalah," *Association for Jewish Studies Review* 5 (1980): 19–25. For manuscript transcript, see Yasif, E., 1985, *op. cit.*, p. 232.

15. Zohar I, 19b, 55a, 148a–b; II, 96a; III, 77a.

16. Zohar III, 19a; I, 34b.

17. Zohar III, 76b-77a.

18. Zohar II, 96a–b.

19. Lachower, F., and I. Tishby, ed., *The Wisdom of the Zohar* (Oxford: Oxford University Press, 1989), vol. 2, p. 756.

20. Scholem, G., *Kabbalah* (New York: Meridian, 1978), 359, and Gaster, M., 1971, *op. cit*, e.g., p. 1027, where a fifteenth-century Syriac version is provided in English translation.

21. Abrahams, I., *Hebrew Ethical Wills* (Philadelphia: Jewish Publication Society, 1954), 48.

22. Patai, R., *The Hebrew Goddess* (Detroit: Wayne State University Press, 1990), 235, citing Naphtali ben Jacob Elhanan Bacharach, *Emek ha-melekh* (Amsterdam: 1648), chap. 11, 19c.

23. Scholem, G., 1978, *op. cit.*, pp. 358–359, quoting Hayyim Vital, *Sefer ha-likkutim* (1913), 6b.

24. Scholem, G., 1978, *op. cit.*, p. 359, quoting *Sefer ha-likkutim* (1913), 78c, and *Emek ha-melekh* (1648), 130b.

25. Simner, Zekhariah ben Yacov, *Sefer zekhirah* (Hamburg: 1709), 53b. Remedy books included this last warning, adding an incantation to send away the demon, with the recommendation that Psalm 91 should be recited three times. See also Zborowski, M., and E. Herzog, *Life Is with People* (New York: Schocken, 1972), 316, and Ben Simhon, R., *Yahadut Marocco* (Lod: Orot Yahadut ha-magreb, 1994), 124.

26. Lida, D., *Sod ha-shem* (Berlin: 1710), 20a; this reference is given by Scholem, G., 1978, *op. cit.*, p. 359, but I was not able to find this source and therefore do not know whether it is identical to or different from that of Azulai. Azulai, H.D., *Sefer avodat ha-kodesh* (Warsaw: 1864), *Yosef be-seder*, sign. 6. This section is not reprinted in all editions of *Sefer avodat ha-kodesh*.

27. Naveh, J., and S. Shaked, 1985, *op. cit.*, p. 119, includes a reproduction of an eighteenth-century amulet with our text on it (my translation). Gaster, M., 1971, *op. cit.*, pp. 1025ff has also translated this text. It also appears in translation in the exhibition catalogue *Magic and Superstition in the Jewish Tradition* (Chicago: Spertus College of Judaica Press, 1975), no. 190; the opening two lines are in Yiddish. This amulet, which is printed with a woodcut decoration, is in the Feuchtwanger collection of the Israel Museum. Similar copies of this popular amulet are in the Scholem Collection of the Jewish National University Library, Jerusalem, in the Jewish Theological Seminary Library, in the collections of Mr. I. Einhorn and of Mr. B. Gross of Tel Aviv, and no doubt in other collections, too. The story was sometimes copied out on to a simple card, without the illustrations: The Jewish Museum in Basel has a few examples of these. The same story was reproduced on North African amulets, often decorated with a *Magen David* star, and a hand against the Evil Eye, and examples of these are also in the Israel Museum (Aliks collection), in the Scholem Collection, in the collections of Einhorn and Gross, at the Judah L. Magnes Museum in Berkeley, California, and surely elsewhere.

28. Baharav, Z., *Shishim sippurei am* (Ya'ad: 1977), 212–213; my translation.

29. Itzhak Einhorn has an example of such a stone in his collection of amulets. Juhasz, E. ed., *Sephardi Jews in the Ottoman Empire* (Jerusalem: Israel Museum, 1990), 260, documents this custom. The Israel Museum has several examples of such head-dresses used by Jews during the Ottoman Empire. The Jewish Museum in Athens also has examples of these.

30. *B. Shabbat* 66b. In fact, amulets were not always dedicated maternally.

31. For example, Bill Gross Collection, 27.11.16, a printed copy of one of the *Sefer Razi'el* amulets, India(?), nineteenth century.

32. For example, the handwritten copies in *Sefer brit tamim*, the *pinkas* (notebook), of Isaac ben Abraham Ger, of Leeuwarden, Holland, who performed circumcisions in the early nineteenth century.

33. Eisenman, R.H., and M. Wise, *The Dead Sea Scrolls Uncovered* (Shaftesbury: Element, 1992), 266.

34. Schiffman, L.H., and M.D. Swartz, *Hebrew and Aramaic Incantation Texts from the Cairo Geniza* (Sheffield: Academic Press, 1992), 69ff. The childbirth amulet is in the Cambridge University Library, England, TS K1.18 and 30.

35. *Sefer Razi'el (The Book of Raziel)* (Amsterdam: 1701), 43b, reprinted in *Razi'el ha-malakh* (Israel: Meirav), 147b; my translation. This has been reprinted on amulets issued in Jerusalem in the early twentieth century and used by Jews in Georgia in Eastern Europe, and as far east as India. Many collectors have copies of such printed amulets, for example, Mr. I. Einhorn and Mr. B. Gross in Tel Aviv, the Scholem Collection in the Jewish National University Library, Jerusalem, and in the collection of the Old Yishuv Court Museum in Jerusalem and in the Rishon Lezion History Museum.

36. Trachtenberg, J., *Jewish Magic and Superstition* (New York: Atheneum, 1982), 90ff., provides an interesting review of the many magical names of God commonly used in Jewish magic.

37. For several examples, see *Encyclopedia Judaica*, vol. 2, p. 963.

38. See note 31. The adjuration appears together with these drawings in *Sefer Razi'el* and copied onto printed amulets.

39. Trachtenberg, J., 1982, *op. cit.*, p. 112. The talmudic source is *B. Shavuot* 15b. *J. Shabbat* 6:8b mentioned the use of biblical verses as incantations for a child's well-being.

40. *Razi'el ha-malakh, op. cit.*, p. 147a.

41. *Shimmush tehillim* (Cracow: 1648), see Psalm 126. Trachtenberg, J., 1982, *op. cit.*, p. 109. Scholem, G., 1978, *op. cit.*, p. 359.

42. Goitein, S.D., *A Mediterranean Society* (Berkeley: University of California, 1978), vol. 3, p. 226.

43. *Tosefta Shabbat* 6:4. Fraser, J.G., *The Golden Bough* (New York: Macmillan, 1927), vol. 1, pp. 159ff., documents the belief in the magic of iron in non-Jewish societies.

44. Cambridge University Library, TS K1.30, lines 27–30, translated by L.H. Schiffman and M.D. Swartz.

45. It was recognized by Eleazar of Worms, who reasoned that its effect on the demons could be due to its being manmade and the product of civilization, and the connection of this metal with the four biblical women was made by Israel Isserlein (1390–1460). See Trachtenberg, J., 1982, *op. cit.*, pp. 160, 313 n. 14.

46. Patai, R., *On Jewish Folklore* (Detroit: Wayne State University Press, 1983), 397.

47. Zafrani, M., *Mille ans de vie juive au Maroc* (Maisonneuve & Larose, 1983), 51–54. Ben Simhon, R., *Yahadut Marocco* (Lod: Orot Yahadut ha-magreb, 1994), 55ff. Mrs. Havivah Fenton, Lyons, France, 1988, personal communication.

48. Patai, R., 1983, *op. cit.*, pp. 242, 404.

49. Ben-Yaakov, A., *Otzar ha-segullot* (Jerusalem: 1991), 234ff. This image has been reprinted on amulets issued in Jerusalem in the early twentieth century and used by Jews in Eastern Europe, too. Many collectors have copies of such printed amulets, for example, Mr. I. Einhorn and Mr. B. Gross in Tel Aviv, the Scholem Collection in the Jewish National University Library in Jerusalem, and in the collection of the Old Yishuv Court Museum in Jerusalem and in the Rishon Lezion History Museum.

50. Musée Alsacien, Strasbourg; Jewish Museum, Basel.

51. Katzenellenbogen, P., *Yesh manḥilin* (Jerusalem:1986), sign. 24, 31, 32.

52. The controversy is summarized in *Encyclopedia Judaica*, vol. 6, pp. 722–723, 1076.

53. Koltuv, B.B., *The Book of Lilith* (York Beach, ME: Nicolas Hays, 1986).

54. Cantor, A., "The Lilith Question," in *On Being a Jewish Feminist*, edited by S. Heschel (New York: Schocken, 1983), 40–50. In addition, a Jewish feminist magazine is called *Lilith*, edited by S.W. Schneider (New York).

11. The First Week

1. Rappoport, A.S., *The Folklore of the Jews* (London: Soncino Press, 1937), 91.

2. Preuss, J., *Biblical and Talmudic Medicine*, 2nd ed. (Brooklyn: Hebrew Publication Company, 1983), 402ff. The usual practice of salting a newborn is referred to in Ezekiel 16:4. See also Patai, R., *On Jewish Folklore* (Detroit: Wayne State University Press, 1983), 88–90.

3. Ezekiel 16:4–5. *Tosefta Shabbat* 12:13e mentions a custom of bathing a newborn in wine. Customs in Yemen and Morocco: personal communication by elderly women and midwives in Israel. Ben Simhon, R., *Yahadut Marocco* (Lod: Orot Yahadut ha-magreb, 1994), 43 and n. 32. Rappoport, A.S., 1937, *op. cit.*, p. 93.

4. Zlotnik, Y. (Elzet, J.L.), "Me-minhagei Israel," *Reshumot* 1 (1918): 363, no. 61.

5. *B. Shabbat* 31b, 147b. Jews in the shtetl sometimes removed the hair on a baby boy's forehead to create a high brow, for a high brow was a sign of wisdom: Zborowski, M., and E. Herzog, *Life Is with People* (New York: Schocken, 1962), 315.

6. Dunn, J., *Distress and Comfort* (London: Fontana/Open Books, 1977), 28–29, 114. Controlled experiments in the 1960s showed that swaddling is in fact effective in calming babies, decreasing motor activity and crying as well as promoting sleep. For example, Lipton, E.L., A. Steinschneider, and J.B. Richmond, "Autonomic Function in the Neonate. II. Physiological Effects of Motor Restraint," *Psychosomatic Medicine* 22 (1960): 57–65. Dunn's book provides useful insight into why babies cry and how to calm them.

7. *B. Shabbat* 129b; *J. Shabbat* 18:16c.

8. Alper, R., *Anshei Peki'in* (Tel Aviv: Am Oved, 1960), 108.

9. A governess in talmudic times recommended rubbing the afterbirth on the chest of the infant if the baby was having trouble breathing, or on its lower half if the baby was too thin or too fat (*B. Hullin* 77a, *B. Shabbat* 134a). See also Patai, R., 1983, *op. cit.*, pp. 357, 393: In the early twentieth century, Moroccan Jews salted the placenta against evil spirits before burial when the baby was a boy, but the placenta of a girl was discarded. Polish and Russian Jews buried the afterbirth; Egyptian Jews preserved it in a hidden place. In Kurdistan, it was sometimes used for medicinal purposes.

10. *Ketubbot* 5:5; *J. Ketubbot* 5:6:2b.

11. *B. Baba Metzia* 87a; *B. Shabbat* 53b.

12. For talmudic advice, see *B. Ketubbot* 60b; for medieval advice see for example, Benveniste's treatise, *Ha-ma'amar be-toladah*, Bodleian Library Neub. no. 2142, *Sefer ha-toledet*, British Museum, Montefiore ms. 420, ff. 30a–32b; A late fifteenth-and early sixteenth-century Yiddish remedy book also has such recipes, see M. Bernstein, "Two Remedy Books in Yiddish," in *Studies in Jewish and Bibilical Folklore*, edited by R. Patai, F. Utley, and D. Noy (New York: Haskell House, 1973), HB XI/17, item 569. In addition to nutritional advice for nursing mothers, Simner, Zekhariah ben Yacov, 1729, *op. cit.*, 26b–27a warns women not to become angry while nursing, because anger could cause loss of milk and even a fever. Most printed remedy books dating from the eighteenth century and later include recommendations for encouraging and stopping milk flow, for example O'Hana, R., *Mareh ha-yeladim* (Jerusalem: 1901), recently reprinted in Mea She'arim, Jerusalem (1990), 108, and Rozenberg, Y.Y., *Rafael ha-malakh* (Piotrkow: 1911), 60. Interviewees reported the advice in their own ethnic communities; mothers and grandmothers continue to pass on this folk wisdom to women who breast-feed today. See also note 21 below.

13. *B. Gittin* 89a. Simner, Zekhariah ben Yacov, 1729, *op. cit.*, p. 26b; Shtal, A., *Mishpaḥah ve-giddul yeladim be-yahadut ha-mizraḥ* (Jerusalem: Academon, 1993), 395, no. 678 quotes Rabbi Yosef Hayyim of Baghdad. *Ibid.*, p. 384, para. 9, and pp. 394–395, notes other sources revealing that, in the nineteenth and early twentieth centuries, Ashkenazi, Sephardic, and Middle Eastern Jewish women nursed their babies in front of strangers, sometimes covering the breast with a scarf.

14. Judah ben Samuel of Regensburg (Judah the Pious), *Sefer Hasidim*, edited by R. Margoliyot (Jerusalem: Mossad ha-rav Kook, 1957), sign. 55 of testament, p. 29. Margoliyot traces the custom of nursing first with the left breast to tenth-century sources, and points out that the connection among the left breast, the heart, and wisdom is made in the Talmud (*B. Berakhot* 10a). The addition that this custom does not apply to girls came from a Moroccan rabbi in Jerusalem, Jacob Hagiz (1620–1674). Several references to this custom are offered by Weisberg, Y.D., *Sefer otzar ha-brit* (Jerusalem: Makhon Torat Ha-brit, 1986), vol. 1, p. 199 n. 1. A right-handed woman would nurse her infant from the left breast more comfortably than from the other, leaving the right hand free for use.

15. *Gittin* 7:6; *J. Sotah* 4.3:2; *Tosefta Niddah* 2:3b. For the custom to wean a son after one year, see Zborowski, M., and E. Herzog, 1962, *op. cit.*, p. 328, and among Sephardim, see note 21 below.

16. *B. Ketubbot* 37a, 60b; *B. Yevamot* 35a. For the belief among Sephardic and Middle Eastern Jews that a pregnant woman's milk is bad for her nursling, see Shtal, A., 1993, *op. cit.*, p. 395. The same was true among Eastern European Jews: Zborowski, M., and E. Herzog, 1962, *op. cit.*, p. 327.

17. *Ketubbot* 5:4; *B. Ketubbot* 60b; *J. Ketubbot* 5:6:2; *B. Yevamot* 42b; *Tosefta Niddah* 2:2–4. Also in the later Codes of Jewish law. Other reasons for delaying remarriage when a woman is nursing is that a new husband could distract her from her baby, and he might not have paid for a wet nurse for a child not his own, should one have been required.

18. Zimmels, H.J., *Magicians, Theologians and Doctors* (London: Edward Goldston & Sons, 1952), 75–76.

19. O'Hana, R., 1990, *op. cit.*, p. 159 citing rabbinic responsa and a case known to the author. (This book was originally published in 1901, and the author tells that he learned of the case when he was young.)

20. Eliyahu ben Shlomo Avraham Hacohen (1650–1729), rabbi of Izmir, instructed women regarding their prayers: *Shevet mussar* (Jerusalem: Y. Rubinstein, 1963), part 2, chap. 24. This prayer was copied out into the personal prayer books of Italian Jewish women in the late eighteenth and early

nineteenth centuries: see Cardin, N.B., *Out of the Depths I Call to You: A Book of Prayers for the Married Jewish Woman* (Northvale, NJ: Jason Aronson, 1992), 110–111, and *Kol t'khinah (The Voice of Supplication)* (Trieste: 1824), 20.

21. Papo, E., *Pele yo'etz* (Jerusalem: 1967), 249; my translation. Zohar IV, 19a.

22. For nursing on demand, see *Tosefta Sotah* 4:3d; Eastern Europe: Sternberg, G., *Stefanesti: Portrait of a Romanian Shtetl* (Oxford: Pergamon Press, 1984), 128; Zborowski, M., and E. Herzog, 1962, *op. cit.*, p. 325. Djerba: Hadad, B., *Sefer Djerba Yehudit* (Jerusalem: Beit ha-otzer ha-ivri, 1979), 24. Persia: Mizrahi, H., *Yehudei Paras* (Tel Aviv: Dvir, 1959), 75. Shtal, A., 1993, *op. cit.*, pp. 382–383, para. 5, quoting Mahel, M., *Sefer gidul banim lefi yesodot hokhmat harefu'ah* (Lemberg: 1821), 66, 126, and *Falksgesundt* 12 (1926): 198.

23. Shtal, A., 1993, *op. cit.*, p. 394, no. 674; my translation.

24. Genesis 24:59; II Kings 11:2; *Ketubbot* 5:4–5; *B. Ketubbot* 60b; *J. Ketubbot* 5:6:2b; *B. Shabbat* 53b.

25. *Sefer ha-toledet, op. cit.*, ms. 420, f. 31r; my translation. The advice stems from Greco-Roman times. Similar advice was offered in later handbooks, published as recently as 1920 in Vilna, cited by Shtal, A., 1993, *op. cit.*

26. Friedenwald, H., *The Jews and Medicine* (Baltimore: Johns Hopkins University Press, 1944), vol. 1, p. 359.

27. *Avodah Zarah* 2:1; *J. Avodah Zarah* 2:1:8a; *B. Ketubbot* 60b; *J. Ketubbot* 5:6:2ff. For attitudes toward the wet nurse in the early twentieth century, see Zborowski, M., and E. Herzog, 1962, *op. cit.*, p. 326–327, and Shtal, A., 1993, *op. cit.*, noting the use of wet-nurses in Sephardic Jewish communities and Jewish communities in Moslem lands as well as the reluctance to hire a Gentile midwife among the Jews of Yemen.

28. Goitein, S.D., *A Mediterranean Society* (Berkeley: University of California, 1978), vol. 1, p. 127 n. 7.

29. Pansier, P., *Les Medecins juifs à Avignon aux treizième, quatorzième et quinzième siècles* (Janus: 1910), 428.

30. Dubnow, S., ed., *Pinkas ha-medinah* (Berlin: 1925), 69, item 326.

31. Wetstein, P.H., ed., *Kadmoniyyot me-pinkasa'ot yeshanim* (Cracow: 1892), 42, no. 20.

32. *B. Eruvin* 41b. *Sefer ha-toledet* offered similar advice.

33. *B. Shabbat* 129b.

34. *B. Niddah* 9a.

35. Gamlieli, N.B., *Ahavat teiman: ha-shira ha-amamit ha-teimanit, shirat nashim* (Tel Aviv: Afikim, 1979), 203; my translation.

36. The text of *birkat ha-gomel* comes from *B. Berakhot* 54b. Eliyahu ben Shlomo Avraham Hacohen (1650–1729), rabbi of Izmir, instructed women to offer their prayers of thanksgiving at the synagogue when they were strong enough to attend, if necessary a few weeks after delivery, and to recite the prayer of deliverance from great danger; Hacohen, E., 1963, *op. cit.*, part 2, chap. 24. *The Authorised Daily Prayer Book*, 3rd ed., translated by S. Singer (London: 1892), 312–313. Neuda, F., *Hours of Devotion*, translated by R. Vulture (Vienna: Jos. Schlesinger, c. 1900), 112–113. Klirs, T.G., comp., *The Merit of Our Mothers: A Bilingual Anthology of Jewish Women's Prayers* (Cincinnati: Hebrew Union College Press, 1993), offers a Yiddish version of the prayer, taken from an early twentieth-century prayer book, but allegedly written by seventeenth-century Sore bas Toyvim, because it is written in her name. Cardin, N.B., 1992, *op. cit.*, pp. 108, 116. See Strassfeld, S., and M. Strassfeld, *The Second Jewish Catalogue* (Philadelphia: Jewish Publication Society, 1976), 37, for a modern version.

37. Yemenite Jews referred to a new mother as *hoyo* (reborn): Rabbanit Kappach, personal communication. The Arabic word *khlas* (deliverance) was used by North African Jews: Zafrani, H., *Mille ans de vie juive au Maroc* (Maisonneuve & Larose, 1983), 51. *Kimpetorn* (indulgence) was the Yiddish term for a postnatal mother: Zborowski, M., and E. Herzog, 1962, *op. cit.*, p. 315.

38. Muchawsky-Schnapper, E., "Symbolic Decorations for a Woman after Childbirth in San'a," *Israel Museum Journal* 7 (1988): 64–65.

39. Weisberg, Y.D., *Sefer otzar ha-brit* (Jerusalem: Machon Torat Ha-brit, 1986), vol. 1, 87–89. Weisberg provides the references to this custom by a fifteenth-century German rabbi, Israel Isserlein, and later by Yair Bacharach, another German rabbi, in the seventeenth century, and by Jacob Emden in the eighteenth century. The legend of the womb experience was told in Chapter 5.

40. Zunser, M.S., *Yesterday—A Memoir of a Russian Jewish Family* (New York: Harper & Row, 1978), 105–107.

41. Goldman, E., *Living My Life* (New York: Alfred A. Knopf, 1931), 185–186.

42. Shtal, A., *Mishpakhah ve-giddul yeladim be-yahadut ha-mizrah* (Jerusalem: Academon, 1993), 331ff.

43. Papo, E., 1967, *op. cit.*, p. 36.

44. Hayyim, Y., *Hukei nashim* (Jerusalem: 1979), 39; my translation. Hayyim Pallache, of Izmir, Turkey, noticed, too, in the midnineteenth century, that a woman could be in critical danger after the birth of a girl for this reason. For a woman's depression and a father's anger at the birth of a daughter, especially if it is not the first daughter, among Jews in Persia, see Mizrahi, H., *Yehudei Paras* (Tel Aviv: Dvir, 1959), 70.

45. Marcus, J.R., *Communal Sick-Care in the German Ghetto* (Cincinnati: Hebrew University College Press, 1947), 12, 206, for example. The Jewish Theological Seminary Library in New York holds the *pinkas* of a society that helped lying-in women in Reggio, Italy, in the seventeenth century (mss. 9728, 9729). The statutes of a women's society to support needy lying-in women is in the collection of Manfred Lehmann of Florida. These statutes were drawn up in Hamburg in 1829. A similar women's society that still functions today in Jerusalem, *Ezer Yoldot*, was founded in 1908. There is a modern lying-in home for ultra-Orthodox women in Telshe Stone, Israel.

46. Hogrefe, J., O'Keefe: *The Life of an American Legend* (Bantam Books, 1994), 138, reports that this was the fate of Kitty Steiglitz, daughter of photographer, Arthur Steiglitz.

47. *B. Yevamot* 42b. Bleich, J.D., "Abortion in Halakhic Literature," in *Jewish Bioethics*, edited by F. Rosner and J.D. Bleich. (New York: Sanhedrin Press, 1979), 157–158. Wolkind, S., and E. Zajicek, ed., *Pregnancy: A Psychological and Social Study* (London: Academic Press, 1981), chaps. 4 and 11, a study of psychiatric vulnerability in mothers.

48. Goitein, S.D., 1978, *op. cit.*, p. 226 (medieval times). For modern times (late nineteenth and early twentieth century), see Brauer, E., *Ethnologie der Jemenitischen Juden* (Heidelberg: 1934), 184. Brauer, E., *The Jews of Kurdistan* (Detroit: Wayne State University Press, 1993), 160–161. Goulven, J., *Mellahs de Rabati-Salé* (Paris: 1927), 11. Mathieu, J., "Notes sur l'enfance juive du Mellah de Casablanca," *Bulletin de l'Institut d'Hygiene du Maroc* 7 (1947): 28. Aslan, M., and R. Nissim, *Yehudei Iraq* (Tel Aviv: Ofer, 1982), 13–14.

49. Grunwald, M., "Tales, Songs and Folkways of Sephardic Jews," *Folklore Research Center Studies* 6 (1982): 205; my translation.

50. Ratzhabi, Y., "Shirat ha-ishah ha-yehudit be-teiman," *Yeda Am* 5 (1957): 87–88. Gamlieli, N.B., 1979, *op. cit.*, p. 203.

51. Leifer, D.I., and M. Leifer, "On the Birth of a Daughter," in *The Jewish Woman*, edited by E. Koltun (New York: Schocken, 1976), 21–30.

52. The Phonoteque of the Jewish National University Library, Jerusalem, has a collection of such recordings, as yet poorly catalogued and mostly of poor quality. Beth Hatefutsoth, The Museum of the Jewish Diaspora, Ramat Aviv, has also collected some recordings and sells tapes of traditional Jewish music, including some lullabies and welcoming songs.

53. For the week of the son, see *B. Sanhedrin* 32b; *B. Baba Kamma* 80a; *B. Baba Batra* 60b. For the week of a daughter, see Nahmanides, *Torat ha-adam* 35b, cited in the Soncino translation of *B. Baba Batra* 60b.

54. *B. Sanhedrin* 32b; Hurwitz, S., ed., *Mahzor Vitry* (Nurnberg: J. Bulka, 1923), *Hilkhot Milah*, sign. 505 (France, twelfth century); Anav, Zedakiah ben Avraham, *Shibbolei ha-leket*, edited by S. Mirsky (Jerusalem: Sura, 1966), *Hilkhot Milah*, sign. 7 (Italy, thirteenth century).

55. *B. Baba Batra* 60b; *B. Baba Kamma* 80a and *Tosafot*. Goitein, S.D., 1978, *op. cit.*, vol. 1, p. 232, refers to medieval North Africa; Mat, Moses B. Abraham, *Matteh Moshe* (London: 1958; 2nd ed., Jerusalem: Oftzar ha-poskim, 1978), 383, refers to the custom in Galicia in the sixteenth century to celebrate a *se'udat mitzvah*, a feast, on the Shabbat eve after a boy is born. Weisberg, Y.D., 1986, *op. cit.*, p. 85ff. reviews the rabbinic literature. Morocco: Ovadia, D., *Kehillot Zafro* (Jerusalem: Makhon le-heker toldot kehillot Yehudei Marocco, 1975), vol. 3, pp. 84ff. Libya: Slouschz, N., *Sefer ha-masa'ot, masa'ei be-eretz Luv* (Tel Aviv: 1943), vol. 2, p. 92. Persia: Mizrahi, H., 1959, *op. cit.*, pp. 72–73. Kurdistan: Brauer, E., in

The Jews of Kurdistan (Detroit: Wayne State University Press, 1993), 160–162. Yemen: Kappah, Y., *Halikhot teiman* (Jerusalem: Ben Zvi Institute, 1963), 160–178. Eastern Europe: Zborowski, M., and E. Herzog, *Life Is with People* (New York: Schocken, 1962), 318. Today, see Weisberg, Y.D., *ibid*, and Schauss, H., *The Lifetime of a Jew* (New York: Union of America Hebrew Congregations, 1950), 56.

56. Ovadia, D. 1975, *op. cit.*, vol. 3. p. 86 (Morocco); Slouschz, N., *Travels in North Africa* (Philadelphia: Jewish Publication Society, 1927), 434 (Morocco). Brauer, E., 1993, *op. cit.*, pp. 163–164 re: Night of *Shashah* (Kurdistan); Iraq: Aslan, M., and R. Nissim, *Yehudei Iraq* (Tel Aviv: Ofer, 1982), 15–17, Night of *Shashah* (Iraq). Mizrahi, H., 1959, *op. cit.*, p. 72 (Persia). Muchawsky-Schnapper, E., 1988, *op. cit.*, p. 64.

57. Dobrinsky, H., *A Treasury of Sephardic Laws and Customs* (New York: Yeshiva University Press, 1986), 28.

58. Sternberg, G., *Stefanesti: Portrait of a Romanian Shtetl* (Oxford: Pergamon Press, 1984), 127. Diamant, A., *The Jewish Baby Book* (New York: Summit Books, 1988), 206, refers to modern customs on this day.

59. Horowitz, E., "The Eve of Circumcision: A Chapter in the History of Jewish Nightlife," *Journal of Social History* 23 (1989): 48 and n. 18. This paper has been reprinted in Ruderman, D.B., ed., *Essential Papers on Jewish Culture in Renaissance and Baroque Italy* (New York: New York University Press, 1992), 554–588.

60. Moellin, Jacob b. Moses, *Sefer Maharil* (Sabionetta: 1556), *Hilkhot Milah*, para. 17, describes how the candle was made. Many editions were printed subsequently. Pollack, H., *Jewish Folkways in Germanic Lands (1648–1806)* (Cambridge, MA: Massachusetts Institute of Technology Press, 1971), 18, mentions the account of this custom in the *Minhagimbuch* of Furth (eighteenth century). Rabbi Juspa Shammes recounts in the *Sefer minhagim* of Worms, sign. 236–245, that a large candle (*ner tamid*), must burn for three days. When twins were born, twenty-four candles were lit.

61. Extrapolation from Weissler, C., "The traditional piety of Ashkenazic women," in *Jewish Spirituality from the Sixteenth Century to the Present*, edited by A. Green (New York: Crossroad, 1987), 253ff., for women's prayers while making candles for Yom Kippur.

62. *B. Berakhot* 5a; *Mahzor Vitry*, 1923, *op. cit.*, 70; Weisberg, Y.D., 1986, *op. cit.*, p. 112, quoting Asher Anschel of Przemysl (seventeenth century), *Zokher ha-brit*, sign. 16.

63. Sternberg, G., 1984, *op. cit.*, p. 126. Ben Simhon, R., 1994, *op. cit.*, p. 51, 67. Yehudit Vernick, personal communication.

64. Kehimkar, H.S., *The History of the Bene Israel of India* (Tel Aviv: Dayag Press, 1937), 117–118. Slapak, O., *Yehudei Hodu* (Jerusalem: Israel Museum, 1995), 155.

12. Ceremonies of Welcome: Rituals

1. Weisberg, J.D., *Sefer otzar ha-brit* (Jerusalem: Makhon Torat ha-brit, 1986), vol. 1, 239ff., probably cites all the reasons in the rabbinic literature.

2. Genesis 34:14. The word *arel* (having a foreskin) was frequently used as a term of contempt: Judges 14:3; 15:18; I Samuel 14:6, 17:26, 36; 31:4; and II Samuel 1:20.

3. Exodus 4:24–26; I Kings 19:10; Joshua 5:2–9; Ezekiel 32:21, 24; *The Book of Jubilees* 15:33–34, in Charles, R.H. ed., *The Apocrypha and Pseudepigraphia of the Old Testament* (Oxford: Clarendon Press, 1913), vol. 1.

4. For the forbidding of circumcision by the Hellenists, see I Maccabees 1: 48; II Maccabees 6:10, in Charles, R.H., *Ibid.*, vol. 2. Hadrian's prohibition stimulated the Bar Kokhba revolt (*Encyclopedia Judaica* [Jerusalem: Keter, 1972], vol. 9, pp. 246, 248). The Apostolic ruling against circumcision is reported in Acts 15. See also Signer, M., "To See Ourselves as Others See Us: Circumcision in Antiquity and the Middle Ages," in *Berit Mila in the Reform Context*, edited by L.M. Barth (Berit Mila Board of Reform Judaism, 1990), 119–122.

5. For example, Mishnah, *Shabbat* 19 and talmudic commentary on this chapter. *Nedarim* 3:11 gives a list of praises for why circumcision is a great mitzvah, see also *B. Nedarim* 31b–32a; *B. Shabbat* 137b; *Genesis Rabbah* 46:9.

6. In the fourth century, Ambrose of Milan, a fierce hater of Jews, attacked circumcision and pro-claimed it abolished since the death of Jesus. In Babylonia, *B. Sanhedrin* 32b; *B. Baba Batra* 60b; *B. Nedarim* 32a. In Palestine, *Genesis Rabbah* 46 argues for and against circumcision in the form of a dia-logue between God and Abraham. *Genesis Rabbah* 11:6.

7. Marcus, J.R., *The Jew in the Medieval World* (New York: Atheneum, 1981), 21.

8. Ezekiel 32:24 tells that the uncircumcised will suffer Gehenna, whereas *Genesis Rabbah* 48:8 tells that Abraham sits at the gate of Gehenna to save the circumcised: Theodor, J., and C. Albeck, ed., *Genesis Rabbah* (Jerusalem: Wahrmann Books, 1964), 483. For the rabbinic literature about the cir-cumcision of a dead infant, see Jakobovits, I., *Jewish Medical Ethics* (New York: Bloch, 1975), 199–200. *Pirkei de Rabbi Eliezer*, edited and translated by G. Friedlander (New York: Hermon Press, 1981), chap. 29, declares that circumcision is redemptive.

9. Circumcision appeared under the heading of the Laws of Shabbat in the thirteenth century *Sefer ha-roke'ah* of Eleazar of Worms (Jerusalem: 1967), pp. 59ff. It formed a topic in its own right in the twelfth-century *Mahzor Vitry*, Hurwitz, S., ed. (Numberg: J. Bulka, 1923), and in the thirteenth-century compendium of Jewish law by Anav, Zedakiah ben Abraham ha-rofeh, *Shibbolei ha-leket*, edit-ed by S. Mirsky (Jerusalem: Sura, 1966). Also in the thirteenth century, two German circumcisers, Jacob and Gershom Hagozer (father and son), composed the first book on the laws of circumcision and every aspect of the subject: Glassberg, J., *Zikhron brit ha-rishonim* (1892). The laws were also col-lated in the *Shulhan arukh*, see Ganzfried, S., *Code of Jewish Law, Kitzur Shulhan arukh*, translated by H.E. Goldin (New York: Hebrew Publishing Company, 1961), chap. 163.

10. Maimonides, M., *Guide for the Perplexed*, 2nd ed., translated by M. Friedlander (New York: Dover, 1956), 378. Signer, M., 1990, *op. cit.*, pp. 124–125, quotes *Sefer Nitzahon Vetus* and Isaac ben Yedi'ah in retort to the Christian accusation of sexual immorality.

11. Weisberg, J.D., 1986, *op. cit.*, vol. 1, pp. 242–243 quotes the Zohar, *Yalkut Shimoni*, and Rabbi Jacob Ha-gozer, all thirteenth-century sources, regarding circumcision as a sacrifice; *Ibid.*, p. 245 quotes the Zohar and *Menorat ha-ma'or* regarding the Shekhinah.

12. Yerushalmi, Y.H., *From Spanish Court to Italian Ghetto, Isaac Cardoso: A Study in Seventeenth Century Marranism and Jewish Apologetics* (New York: Columbia University Press, 1971), 367, 380, 387. In addition to Cardoso, Isaac Abrabanel (1437–1508), in his commentary to Genesis 17:9, states the importance of circumcision in his commentary on the Torah; he stresses that circumcision is a divine command-ment that differentiates God's people from other peoples, and the mark of this covenant is irremovable, reminding humankind constantly of the holy Covenant. He also notes that removal of the foreskin reduces the power of the genital organ and its animalistic behavior, and he points out that this enables conception to take place in holiness.

13. *Frankfurter Journal*, 15 July 1843; Trier, S.A., ed., *Rabbinische Gutachten über die Beschneidung* (Frankfurt: 1844). For the views about circumcision of Reform Jews today, see Barth, L.M., ed., *Berit Milah in the Reform Context* (Berit Mila Board of Reform Judaism, 1990). The Central Archives for Jewish History, Jerusalem, AHW/698; an exercise book with a record of sixteen boys not circumcised between the years 1844 and 1851, it was kept in the safe of the Hamburg Jewish community. The archives have a similar one from Frankfurt, from the same period.

14. Sider, F., *Seven Folktales from Boryslaw*, edited by O. Schnitzer (Haifa: Israel Folktales Archives, 1968), vol. 19, pp. 17ff; my translation.

15. Horowitz, E., "The Eve of Circumcision: A Chapter in the History of Jewish Nightlife," *Journal of Social History* 23 (1989): 45–69.

16. Zohar I, 93a–b.

17. Finkelstein, L., *Jewish Self-Government in the Middle Ages* (Philadelphia: Jewish Publication Society, 1924), 244.

18. Beinart, H., *The Jewish Life of the Conversos* (Jerusalem: Magnes Press, 1981), 279–280.

19. Carmi, T., ed. and trans., *The Penguin Book of Hebrew Verse* (London: Penguin, 1981), 451.

20. Mat, Moses B. Abraham, *Matteh Moshe* (London: 1958), 383a. Mat was a Galician rabbi who lived

in the second half of the sixteenth century. His book, a compendium of Jewish laws that includes also many customs regarding circumcision, was first published in Cracow in around 1590.

21. Horowitz, E., 1989, *op. cit.*, pp. 49, 63 nn 24, 26, 27.

22. Buxtorf, J., *Synagoga Judaica* (Basel: 1603), chap. 2.

23. Cohen, M.R., "Leon da Modena's *Riti*: A Seventeenth-Century Plea for Toleration of Jews," *Jewish Social Studies* 34 (1972): 287–289.

24. Pollack, H., *Jewish Folkways in Germanic Lands (1648–1806)* (Cambridge, MA: Massachusetts Institute of Technology Press, 1971), 19.

25. The accounts were by Giulio Morosini, who was baptized in 1649, and probably wrote about scenes in which he himself had participated, and by Rabbi Corcos of Rome, in the 1727 statutes of a confraternity founded in an attempt to promote religious content into the celebrations on the eve of a circumcision; see Horowitz, E., 1989, *op. cit.*, pp. 50, 55, 57–58.

26. The story has been told by Ben-Yehezkel, M., *Sefer ha-ma'asiyot*, 4th ed. (Tel Aviv: Dvir, 1977), vol. 4, pp. 9–12; in English, Sadeh, P., *Jewish Folktales* (New York: Doubleday, 1989), 348–350.

27. Fus, D., *Seven Bags of Gold*, edited by O. Schnitzler (Haifa: Israel Folk Archives, 1969, no. 25), 23–26; my translation.

28. It was once known in Ashkenaz as *Weizennacht* (wheat night) because wheat pretzels were served: the association between wheat and circumcision was taken from the Bible. Ripe wheat has to be prepared to make bread; so also a baby boy needs to be prepared (circumcision) before he becomes accepted into the community. More commonly it was known as *Wachnacht*, or *Vakhnakht*, from the German *wachen* (to stay awake) and *nacht* (night) among Ashkenazi Jews, and *La Veglia* (the [night of] vigilance) among Italian-speaking Jews, because members of the household stayed awake through the night in the room of mother and baby: see Horowitz, E., 1989, *op. cit.*, p. 49. Among the Sephardic Jews in the Ottoman Empire, this night was known as *La Viola, Velen,* or *Bilada,* meaning "watchfulness" and "without misfortune." *Belo-da* in the local vernacular means "without harm or tragedy." However, the name may have emerged instead from the joyous exclamation of *ben yaldah* (she delivered a son): Tsarfati, S., *El cadra* (Israel: published by author, 1987), 93. Slouschz, N., *Travels in Africa* (Philadelphia: Jewish Publication Society, 1927), 435, reported that this night was called *Talamon* in northern Morocco. Jews in the Holy Land in the nineteenth century referred to *Lel Tara*, the night when the Tara lamp, a traditional seven-branched lamp, was brought from the synagogue and kept burning in the lying-in room. The Old Yishuv Court Museum in Jerusalem and the Land of Israel Museum in Tel Aviv have such lamps in their collections. In Yemen, this night was referred to as *Lilat Elzaba* (night of vigilance): Zadok, M., *Yehudei teiman: toldoteihem ve-orkhot hayyeihem* (Tel Aviv: Am Oved, 1967), 213. In other communities, the night is named after the preparations for the next day. Thus, in Iraq and India it was called *Lel Ikd Elias,* when Elijah's chair was prepared for the next day. *Elias,* in Arbic, means "myrtle" as well as "Elijah." Myrtle has been used in burial, wedding, and birth ceremonies since talmudic times to protect against evil powers: Brauer, E., in *The Jews of Kurdistan*, edited by R. Patai (Detroit: Wayne State University Press, 1993), 164–166. Persian Jews named this night *Leil Brit Itzhak*: Mizrahi, H., *Yehudei paras* (Tel Aviv: Dvir, 1959), 72–73.

29. Horowitz, E., 1989, *op. cit.*, pp. 52ff., and Weisberg, Y.D., 1986, *op. cit.*, p. 112, have reviewed this literature from different angles, drawing, for example, on Aaron Berekhiah ben Moses of Modena, *Ma'avar Yabok* (Vienna: 1857; the first edition was Venice in 1626).

30. Halpern, I., ed., *Takkanot medinat Mehrin* (1952), 9.

31. Horowitz, E., 1989, *op. cit.*, p. 53. Also *Ibid.*, p. 58, for late eighteenth-century rulings limiting the drinking of coffee to those who studied all night, at *La Veglia* in Ancona and Mantua.

32. Schudt, J.J., *Jüdische Merkwürdigkeiten* (Frankfurt and Leipzig: 1717), part 4, book 3, pp. 74, 90.

33. Horowitz, E., 1989, *op. cit.*, p. 54 nn. 53–55, provides publication details. For a modern reproduction of these texts, see Weisberg, Y.D., 1986, *op. cit.*, pp. 255ff.

34. Wassertil, A., ed., *Yalkut minhagim* (Israel Ministry of Education and Culture, 1977), on Tunisian Jews. A similar story, not from Tunisia, was told by Hayyim Yosef David Azulai (Weisberg, Y.D., 1986, *op. cit.*, p. 113, n. 16).

35. Attias, M., *Romancot ve-shirei am be-yahadut sepharadit* (Jerusalem: Ben Zvi Institute, 1961), 46–47. Molkho, M., "Leidah ve-yaldut bein Yehudei Saloniki," *Edot* 2 (1947): 262.

36. Weisberg, Y.D., 1986, *op. cit.*, p. 112–3. Zborowski, M., and E. Herzog, *Life Is with People* (New York: Schocken, 1962), 318.

37. Sassoon, S., *A History of the Jews of Baghdad* (Letchworth: 1949), 182–183. Also Isaac, I.A., *A Short Account of the Calcutta Jews* (Calcutta: 1917), 9; Brauer, E., *Ethnologie der Jemenitischen Juden* (Heidelberg: 1934), 193; Brauer, E., 1993, *op. cit.*, pp. 164–166; Dobrinsky, H., *A Treasury of Sephardic Laws and Customs* (New York: Yeshiva University Press, 1986), 5 (Syria). Malka, E., *Essai d'ethnographie traditionelle des Mellah* (Rabat: 1946), 32.

38. Nahum, Y.L., *Me-tzefonot yehudei teiman* (Tel Aviv: 1961), 145: in Yemen, a sign was made on the house where a circumcision was to be performed. A special herb was inserted in a crack near the front door, and Jews who passed by noticed it and entered the house to take a part in the ceremony. Yemenite Jews tell that this custom originated from an earlier period when a king had forbidden the Jews to practice circumcision. Like the *Marranos*, they continued to observe the ritual in secret, but made a sign that enabled other Jews to join them. Regarding the haircut, see Ben Simhon, R., *Yahadut Marocco* (Lod: Orot Yahadut ha-magreb, 1994), 78. Fraser, J.G., *The Golden Bough* (New York: Macmillan, 1927), vol. 3, pp. 258ff., explains the significance of ceremonial hair cutting in some non-Jewish societies.

39. Zouarch, P., *Yahadut Luv* (Tel Aviv: Va'ad ha-kehillot Luv be-Israel, 1982), 386–390. Hadad, B., *Sefer Djerba yehudit* (Jerusalem: Beit ha-otzer ha-ivri, 1979), 114. Today in Djerba: Keren T. Friedman, personal communication.

40. *B. Shabbat* 137b. Schauss, H., *The Lifetime of a Jew* (New York: Union of America Hebrew Congregations, 1950), chaps. 1–4, for accounts of how the circumcision has been performed in specific communities from ancient to modern times. Matzner-Bekerman, S., *The Jewish Child: Halakhic Perspectives* (New York: Ktav, 1984), chap. 4, provides guidelines for parents to perform the postnatal rituals according to Jewish law. Or see Strassfeld, S., and M. Strassfeld, eds., *The Second Jewish Catalogue* (Philadelphia: Jewish Publication Society, 1976), 23–30.

41. Sometimes the father performs the job of *sandek*, but more often it is a grandparent or a rabbi or some other person who will serve as a role model for the boy. The word *sandek* derives from the Greek *syndikos*, which is the same word in late Latin and means a delegate, someone entrusted with a special affair. This name, which was not mentioned in the Talmud, implies that this role was formalized in Byzantine times. *Yalkut Shimoni* (Jerusalem: 1960), vol. 2, Psalm 35 discussed the origins of this word.

Judeo-Arabic speakers have said the word comes from the Arabic word *sandouk*, meaning a box, because it was once the custom for the *mohel* to bring all his equipment in a long narrow box. After emptying the box in the room of the circumcision, he placed it below the mezuzzah, and the *sandek* sat on this during the rite. The *sandek* was thus he who sat on the *sandouk*. Another explanation is that *sandek* is derived from the Hebrew *shen dak*, literally a "thin tooth," which refers to the thin tooth of flint used by Zipporah to circumcise her son (Exodus 4:25): Ben Simhon, R., 1994, *op. cit.*, p. 92.

A kabbalistic interpretation proposed that the four Hebrew letters of the word form the initials of four Hebrew words—*sod, nahash, dam, kodesh*, which depict mystical aspects of the rite, in kabbalistic imagery: Pritzker, A., "Brito shel Avraham avinu," *Yeda Am* 1 (1954): 22.

In medieval Germany, the circumcision was held in the synagogue. It was necessary for a woman to bring the baby from his mother to the door of the synagogue where, for reasons of modesty, she passed him to her husband. Originally, the wife of the *sandek* performed this role, but in the nineteenth century, Ashkenazi Jews created an extra role of honor by having a couple carry the baby in turn, and another man act as *sandek*. Nineteenth-century rabbis theorized about the root of the words *kvatter* and *kvatterin*: they may have come from *kapitorin*, a word for bindings, from the Hebrew word for incense, *ketoret*, or from a medieval German word for godfather. Orthodox Jews consider it a mitzvah to ask a childless couple to take the roles of *kvatter* and *kvatterin*.

42. *B. Sanhedrin* 32b; *Deuteronomy Rabbah* 9:1.

43. Goitein, S.D., *A Mediterranean Society* (Berkeley: University of California, 1978), vol. 1, p. 232 attests to the large numbers who attended circumcisions in medieval North Africa. For an example of a ruling limiting these numbers, in 1418, representatives of Jewish communities throughout Italy published a ruling permitting only ten Jewish men and five Jewish women to be invited to a circumcision feast, in addition to relatives, and second cousins were not to be counted as relatives: Finkelstein, L., 1924, *op. cit.*, p. 243 n. 17, p. 294 n. 4. See also Marcus, J.R., 1981, *op. cit.*, p. 195, quoting from the National Jewish Council of Lithuania, 1637.

44. Marcus, J.R., *Communal Sick-Care in the German Ghetto* (Cincinnati: Hebrew University College Press, 1947), 9, 187–189. Community records document these societies, often called *Ba'alei Brit Avraham* in past centuries.

45. *B. Hullin* 9a; *B. Sanhedrin* 17b. I thank Prof. Daniel Sperber for bringing to my attention the fact that there were women *mohalot* in Renaissance Italy. Nineteenth- and early twentieth-century *mohel* diplomas (attesting that the man is qualified to practice this ritual) have been preserved in some Judaica collections, such as the London Museum of Jewish Life, the Sir Isaac and Lady Wolfson Museum in Heichal Schlomo, Jerusalem, and the Museum of Jewish Art at Kiryat Banot, Jerusalem. Specially minted coins that a *mohel* in Amsterdam gave in 1851 as a gift to a boy he circumcised have also been preserved in these Judaica collections.

46. *Pirkei de Rabbi Eliezer*, 1981, *op. cit.*, chap. 29; the custom is first mentioned in this eighth- or ninth-century source. It was also mentioned by R. Jacob Nissim of Kairwan, c. 970 C.E. and again in later medieval sources, such as *Maḥzor Vitry, op. cit., Hilkhot milah*, sign. 505; Judah ben Samuel of Regensburg, *Sefer Hasidim*, 2nd ed., edited by J.H. Wistinetzki (Frankfurt: 1924), sign. 1044; *Yalkut Shimoni*, 1960, *op. cit.*, vol. 1, p. 38, on Genesis 13:17, and the Zohar I, 93a, by which time the custom seems to have become well established. Weisberg, Y.D., 1986, *op. cit.*, p. 126, quotes Joshua Falk (d. 1614), who viewed Elijah's presence as a reward; the Zohar and later kabbalists viewed this as a punishment.

47. I Kings 17:17–24.

48. Bin-Gorion, E., *Memakor Israel* (Bloomington: Indiana University Press, 1976), 852–853.

49. Malachi 3:1, 23.

50. Schauss, H., 1950, *op. cit.*, pp. 35–36. Jacoby, R., "The Small Elijah Chair," *Journal of Jewish Art* 18 (1992): 73 and n. 49.

51. Weisberg, Y.D., 1986, *op. cit.*, p. 128 nn. 2 and 3; some Ashkenazim prepare two chairs, one each for the Prophet and *sandek*, the custom recorded in the *Maḥzor Vitry* (twelfth-century France), by Aharon Hacohen of Lunel in southern France, Jacob and Gershom Ha-gozer in thirteenth-century Germany, and Jacob Moellin, the Maharil, in fifteenth-century Germany. Others prepare one chair only, on which the *sandek* sits, the custom reported in Galicia by Moses ben Abraham Mat in the sixteenth century and by Yehiel Michl Epstein in the seventeenth century. Ovadia, D., *Kehillat Sefrou* (Jerusalem: Makhon le-heker toldot kehillot Yehudei Marocco, 1975), vol. 3, p. 86; in Sefrou, the *sandek* sat on the special chair, while another chair was put on a shelf on the wall for Elijah. In Italy, too, the *sandek* sits on the Chair of Elijah.

52. For pictures of Chairs of Elijah, see *Encyclopedia Judaica*, vol. 5, p. 306 (for a double chair, Germany, eighteenth century), vol. 9, p. 1140 (for an ornate Italian chair, seventeenth or eighteenth century). For the small Provençal chairs, see Jacoby, R., 1992, *op. cit.*, pp. 70–77.

53. Ben Simḥon, R., 1994, *op. cit.*, p. 78.

54. Kurt, Z., "Matehu shel eliahu ha-navi," *Yeda Am* 25 (1962): 64. Also, Hanegbi, Z., and B. Yaniv, *Afghanistan: Beit ha-knesset ve-ha-bayit ha-yehudi* (Hebrew University and Center for Jewish Studies, 1991), 81–82.

55. Exodus 13:2; Deuteronomy 21:17.

56. *The Jewish Encyclopedia*, 1901–1903, Child:27. The reference comes from Eleazar of Worms' *Ḥukkei ha-Torah*, which dates from 1309.

57. Exodus 11:5; Numbers 8:17.

58. Exodus 32:4, 26, 28; Numbers 3:41.

59. Numbers 18:15–16.

60. *Bekhorot* 8:1; *Kitzur Shulḥan Arukh*, 1961, *op. cit.*, vol. 4, chap. 164; *B. Kiddushin* 29a; *B. Pesaḥim* 121b for blessings; see *Siddur of Sa'adia Gaon* (Jerusalem: Mekitzei Nirdamim, 1941), 99–100. Sa'adia Gaon lived in the early tenth century. The ritual was first recorded in the *Siddur* of Rav Amram Gaon, half a century earlier.

61. *B. Niddah* 23a; *Bekhorot* 2:9. See Matzner-Bekerman, S., 1984, *op. cit.*, for guidelines on conduct-ing this ritual according to Jewish law.

62. Moellin, Jacob b. Moses, *Sefer Maharil* (Sabionetta: 1556), sign. 5.

63. *Shulḥan arukh*, edited by Z.H. Preisler and S. Havlin (Jerusalem: Ketuvim, 1993), *Yoreh De'ah*, 305:15.

64. This is in the collection of the Israel Museum.

65. *Sefer ha-roke'aḥ*, 1967, *op. cit., Hilkhot pidyon ha-ben ha-bekhor*, p. 246; *Sefer Maharil, op. cit., Hilkhot pidyon ha-ben*, sign. 1, 6.

66. This particular tray is in the collection of the Jewish Museum of New York. Other trays can be found in this and other Judaica collections. For an etching showing such a tray in use during a redemption ceremony, see Bodenschatz, J., *Kirchliche Verfassung der Heutige Juden* (Leipzig, 1748). Trays engraved with biblical scenes can be found on display in many Jewish museums.

67. Lawrence Salzmann, photograph, 1988; Gabbay, M., *Roots* (Beer Sheba: 1988), 20.

68. Goulven, J., *Mellahs de Rabati-Salé* (Paris: 1927), 16–17.

69. Dobrinsky, H., 1986, *op. cit.*, p. 8. Dina Yerushalmi, personal communication, 1994.

70. Molkho, M., 1947, *op. cit.*, p. 265.

71. Morad, E., *Nofei yaldut me-beit abba* (Stavit: 1985), 198; Aslan, M., and R. Nissim, *Yehudei Iraq* (Tel Aviv: Ofer, 1982), 23. Brauer, E., 1993, *op. cit.*, who documented Kurdistani Jewry, and Sassoon, D., 1949, *op. cit.*, who documented Iraqi Jewry, omitted mention of the redemption ritual in their obser-vations in the early twentieth century, probably because there was no *cohen* to do it.

72. Kehimkar, H.S., *The History of the Bene Israel of India* (Tel Aviv: Dayag, 1937), 124ff. Brauer, E., 1934, *op. cit.*, made no mention of this ritual, nor did Zadok, M., 1967, *op. cit.*, or Nahum, Y.L., 1961, *op. cit.*

73. Landau, J.M., *Jews in Nineteenth Century Egypt* (New York: New York University, 1969), 109.

74. Matzner-Bekerman, S., 1984, *op. cit.*, p. 55.

75. Leifer, D.I., and M. Leifer, "On the Birth of a Daughter," in *The Jewish Woman: New Perspectives*, edited by E. Koltun (New York: Schocken, 1976), 25. See also Diamant, A., 1988, *op. cit.*, pp. 199ff.

76. Beinart, H., 1981, *op. cit.*, pp. 279–280.

77. Slouschz, N., 1927, *op. cit.*, p. 435. Grunwald, M., "Tales, Songs, and Folkways of Sephardic Jews," *Folklore Research Center Studies* 6 (1982): 226–227. Molkho, M., 1947, *op. cit.*, pp. 264–265.

78. My translation. Idelsohn, A.Z., *Jewish Liturgy and its Development* (New York: Schocken, 1967), 168; Also Dobrinsky, H., 1986, *op. cit.*, p. 11.

79. Song of Songs 2:14 and, especially if the daughter was first-born, 6:9.

80. *Maḥzor Vitry, op. cit.*, p. 628. Jews in early thirteenth-century southern Germany may also have per-formed a cradle ceremony when they placed the Book of Leviticus next to the baby's head and gave the child a name (presumably a Yiddish or secular name for a boy, because he received his Jewish name at his circumcision): Patai, R., *On Jewish Folklore* (Detroit: Wayne State University Press, 1983), 410, quoting *Sefer Hasidim*; I was not able to find this in the editions I consulted.

81. This custom was reported in the seventeenth century by Joseph Hahn of Kleinsteinach, Bavaria, and in the eighteenth century by Joseph Steinhardt of Fürth. J.J. Schudt, J.C. Kirchner, and J. Bodenschatz all reported this custom in the first half of the eighteenth century in their books on Jewish life. Raphael, F., and R. Weyl, *Les Juifs en Alsace* (Toulouse: 1977), 88–89 reported the practice in Alsace, Alis Guggenheim painted this custom in Switzerland in around 1950 (the painting is now in the collection of the Israel Museum), and Joel Cahen found reports of this custom in southern Holland (Joel Cahen, personal communication, 1995).

82. Trachtenberg, J., *Jewish Magic and Superstition* (New York: Atheneum, 1982), 42 and notes. Also, Pollack, H., 1971, *op. cit.*, pp. 27–28, 217 n. 71; Raphael, F., and R. Weyl, 1977, *op. cit.*, pp. 89–90, pro-vide the sources and discussion on this topic; Schauss, H., 1950, *op. cit.*, pp. 44–47.

83. Jacob ben Isaac of Yanov, *Tsena u-rena* (Jerusalem: Makhon ha-ma'or, 1975), p. 40 on Genesis 3:16 and p. 258 n. 159.

84. Yemen: Brauer, E., 1934, *op. cit.* Syria: Dobrinsky, H., 1986, *op. cit.*, p. 3. Bukhara: Asherov, S., *Mesamarkand ad Petaḥ tikva* (Tel Aviv: Brit Yotzei Bovda, 1977), 67. Afghanistan: Laniado, E.I., *Yehudei mosul me-galut shomrom ad mivtzah ezra ve-neḥemiah* (Tirat Carmel: Institute for Research of Mosul Jews, 1981), 241. Iraq: Brauer, E., 1993, *op. cit.*, p. 164. Iran: Mizrahi, H., *Yehudei Paras* (Tel Aviv: Dvir, 1959), 72–73. For India, see note 86 below.

85. Genesis 30:20. Cohen, A., *Zeved ha-bat* (Jerusalem: Caneh, 1990), 9ff.

86. Kehimkar, H.S., 1937, *op. cit.*; Isaac, I.A., 1917, *op. cit.*, p. 9. Slapak, O., *Yehudei Hodu* (Jerusalem: Israel Museum, 1995), 142, 155. Concerning the custom now in Israel, Dr. Shalva Weil and Mrs. Flora Samuel, personal communications.

87. Tree planting as a girl-welcoming ceremony was pioneered in the United States by Rich and Treasure Cohen in 1981. See Diamant, A., 1988, *op. cit.*, pp. 193, 196, 209, regarding planting a tree in Israel on the occasion of a birth.

88. *B. Gittin* 57a.

89. Leifer, D.I., and M. Leifer, 1976, *op. cit.*, pp. 21–30. Schneider, S.W., *Jewish and Female* (New York: Touchstone [Simon and Schuster], 1985), 121–130. Strassfeld, S., and M. Strassfeld, 1976, *op. cit.*, pp. 30–37.

90. Reifman, T. Fishbein, ed., *Blessing the Birth of a Daughter: Jewish Naming Ceremonies for Girls* (Englewood, NJ: Ezrat Nashim, 1978).

91. Leviticus 11–17 discusses the sources of uncleanness and the purification requirements. Leviticus 18:19 forbids sexual relations when a woman is unclean. See *Encyclopedia Judaica*, vol. 13, pp. 1405ff., for discussion of Jewish attitudes to ritual purity and states of impurity. In fact, after the destruction of the Temple, the ritual purification following contact with the dead, the leprous, and male issues lapsed—only the laws regarding women's issues remained.

92. The ancient Babylonians and Hittites practiced postnatal purification rituals with incantations to drive out evil spirits, but there are no magical connotations in the Jewish ritual. Fraser, J.G., 1927, *op. cit.*, III:145–157. For the connection among cleanliness, purity, and holiness, see *B. Avodah Zarah* 20b.

93. Leviticus 12:2–8; *Niddah* 3, 4, 10:4–5 and talmudic commentaries; *Kitzur Shulḥan Arukh*, *op. cit.*, vol. 4, chap. 158.

94. See *Encyclopedia Judaica*, vol. 12, pp. 1146–1147, for rabbinic views on sexual relations after birth. See Patai, R., 1983, *op. cit.*, p. 411 for some local customs.

95. See Lamm, N., *A Hedge of Roses* (New York: Feldheim, 1977), chap. 5. Greenberg, B., *On Women and Judaism* (Philadelphia: Jewish Publication Society, 1981), 105ff. See Adler, R. "Tumah and Taharah; Ends and Beginnings" in *The Jewish Woman: New Perspectives*, edited by E. Koltun (New York: Schocken, 1976), 63–71, for a modern feminist view of these laws. For purification as healing and renewal, see Levitt, L., and S.A. Wasserman, "*Mikvah* Ceremony for Laura," in *Four Centuries of Jewish Women's Spirituality*, edited by E.M. Umansky and D. Ashton (Boston: Beacon Press, 1992), 321ff.

96. *The Book of Jubilees* 3:8–9; *B. Niddah* 30b; *Zohar V*, 43b–44a.

97. Schneider, S.W., 1985, *op. cit.*, p. 207. I am grateful to Deena Garber for a discussion on this topic.

98. Leslau, W., *Falasha Anthology* (New Haven: Yale University Press, 1951), xiv–xv.

99. Brauer, E., 1993, *op. cit.*, 158.

100. Kehimkar, H.S., 1937, *op. cit.*, pp. 111–127.

101. Brauer, E., 1934, *op. cit.*, p. 190; also Rabbanit Kappach, personal communication.

102. Personal communication from a Tunisian Jewish woman in Ness Tziona, Israel, 1987.

103. Leviticus 12:6–7.

104. *B. Niddah* 31b. See also note 83 above.

105. *Genesis Rabbah* 17:13. Weissler, C., "Mitzvot built into the body," in *Jews and Their Bodies*, edited by H.E. Schwartz. (New York: State University of New York, 1992).

106. Dr. Y. Latti, personal communication.

107. Genesis 21:8; I Samuel 1:24ff.

108. Dr. Y. Latti, personal communication.

109. Schauss, H., 1950, *op. cit.*, p. 81. Sephardic, North African, and Asian Jews did not celebrate this event, which was often helped by anointing the breast with an unpleasant-tasting substance that the infant would be sure to reject.

110. Strassfeld, S., and M. Strassfeld, 1976, *op. cit.*, pp. 43–45. See also Diamant, A., *op. cit.*, pp. 242–246; Schneider, S.W., *op. cit.*, p. 130.

13. Blessings and Hopes

1. *B. Shabbat* 137b.

2. For example, Sarah and Abraham laughed when they were told that a child, Isaac (Itzhak, "he will laugh"), would be born to them in their old age: Genesis 17:17–19. Rebekah's twin sons were called Esau and Jacob, derived from Hebrew words meaning "thick-haired" (Esau's appearance at birth), and "one that takes by the heel" (as Jacob was born with his hand on his brother's heel): Genesis 25:25–26. Leah named her children herself, as did Rachel, although Jacob altered the name of her younger son: Genesis 35:18.

3. *B. Shabbat* 137b.

4. *B. Yoma* 38b. A thorough review of naming customs throughout Jewish history can be found in Lauterbach, J.Z., "The naming of children in Jewish folklore, ritual and practice," in *Studies in Jewish Law, Custom and Folklore* (New York: Ktav, 1970).

5. See Lauterbach, J.Z., 1970, *op. cit.*, pp. 20ff. The naming customs of the Hasidei Ashkenaz are amply documented in Judah ben Samuel of Regensburg, *Sefer Hasidim*, edited by R. Margoliyot (Jerusalem: Mossad ha-rav Kook, 1957), sign. 51 in the testament, also sign. 244 and others. Trachtenberg, J., *Jewish Magic and Superstition* (New York: Atheneum, 1982), 287. Gluckel of Hameln (c. 1700) reported, in her memoirs, that her newborn baby was named after a close relative who had died.

6. Asheri, M., *Living Jewish* (Everest House, 1978), 49. Grunwald, M., "Tales, Songs, and Folkways of Sephardic Jews," *Folklore Research Center Studies* 6 (1982): 226. Ben Simhon, R., *Yahadut Marocco* (Lod: Orot Yahadut ha-magreb, 1994), 121, 123. Rozenberg, Y.Y., *Rafael ha-malakh* (Piotrkow: 1911), 18, under *banim*, quoting these and yet other customs from earlier sources. Information from Yemen is taken from a traveler to Yemen in 1857–1859, Jacob Saphir, see Lauterbach, 1970, *op. cit.*, p. 21.

7. *Birth Ceremonies* (Jewish Women's Resource Center: 1985); see, for example the ceremony for Rachel Sylvia Baran, 1981.

8. *Kiddushin* 4:1.

9. Throughout the ages, Jews who could trace their lineage back to King David were particularly esteemed. Johanan ha-sandlar, Hai Gaon, Rashi and his famous grandsons, Rabbenu Tam and Samuel ben Meir, were said to have had such lineage. More recently, the Hasidim were concerned to maintain genealogical records to prove their descent from a particular *tzaddik*. Moroccan families kept genealogical records that they sometimes included on a *ketubbah*. Italian Jewish families also kept family record books. Some Ashkenazi families have published their family record books.

10. Trachtenberg, J., 1982, *op. cit.*, p. 311 n. 1.

11. *B. Shabbat* 156a–b; *B. Nedarim* 32a. The Jews exiled in Babylon learned astrology from the Chaldeans of Southern Babylonia and possibly also from the Zoroastrians, but many talmudic scholars must have been familiar also with the astrology of the ancient Greeks and even the influential writings of Ptolemy of Alexandria in the second century.

12. Levy, R., and F. Cantera, ed., *Abraham ibn Ezra: The Beginning of Wisdom* (Baltimore: Johns Hopkins University Press, 1939), vol. 14, chap. 2, pp. 156ff. He leaned heavily on Ptolemy's *Almagest*.

13. Fenton, P.B., "Les manuscrits astrologiques de la Gueniza du Caire," in *Le monde Juif et l'astrologie*, edited by J. Halbronn (Milan: Arché, 1985), appendix. Isaacs, H., *Medical and Paramedical Manuscripts in the Cambridge Geniza Collection* (Cambridge: Cambridge University Press, 1994), citing TS. Ar.39.396. Goitein, S.D., *A Mediterranean Society* (Berkeley: University of California, 1978), vol. 3, p. 233.

14. Ms. Parma (2637), 336 f. 73.

15. Abraham bar Hiyya (Spain, early twelfth century), and Eleazar of Worms (Germany, c. 1200), rationalized that the stars affect people's behavior and are themselves controlled by God's will. The Hebrew poet was Immanuel of Rome (c. 1261–c. 1332); see his poem in Carmi, T., ed. and trans., *The Penguin Book of Hebrew Verse* (London: Penguin, 1981), 422–423. Barzilay, I., *Yosef Schlomo Delmedigo* (Leiden: E.J. Brill, 1974), 28. Delmedigo and his friend, Rabbi Leon da Modena (1571–1648), believed that the constellation at birth influenced one's personality; see also Cohen, M.R., ed., *The Autobiography of a Seventeenth Century Venetian Rabbi* (Princeton: Princeton University Press, 1988), 110. *Razi'el ha-malakh* (Israel: Meirav, undated), 68.

16. Graves, R., and R. Patai, *Hebrew Myths* (New York: Doubleday, 1964), 134ff. The story is from an early ninth-century midrash, *Pirkei de Rabbi Eliezer*, chap. 26. The Ladino ballad is thought to come from a twelfth-century rendering of the legend: Attias, M., *Romancot ve-shirei am be-yahadut sepharadit* (Jerusalem: Ben Zvi Institute, 1961), 236–238. Weich-Shahak, S., "Shirim sephardiim yehudiim le-brit milah," *Dohan* 12 (1989): 168–170. More recently, it has become popular in a modern Hebrew version, too, written and sung by Israeli Naomi Shemer.

17. British Library, London, Montefiore ms. 322, no. 2, second and last fly-leaf.

18. Lisbon National Library ms. II.72. My thanks to Mr. and Mrs. Mendel Metzger for information concerning medieval birth records.

19. Jewish National University Library, Jerusalem, ms. 4281, f. 398, and British Library, London, Montefiore ms. 220, II, f. 193.

20. Jewish National University Library, Jerusalem, mss. Yahudah, Hebr. nos. 2, 5, 32 and ms. Heb. octo. 580.

21. Jewish National University Library, Jerusalem, ms. 1240.

22. For example, British Library, London, Montefiore ms. 205 and 208 are German liturgical manuscripts containing inscriptions of births from the late fifteenth and early sixteenth centuries. The Israel Museum has a beautifully illuminated south German liturgical manuscript, redacted c. 1460, with birth inscriptions dating from the late seventeenth century.

23. A Dutch prayer book, printed in 1794, carries Hebrew inscriptions of children born to the owner: two boys in 1799 and 1800, followed by two girls, in 1803 and 1805. All four births are recorded with the hope that the child was born with *mazal tov* and would grow up to a life of Torah, the marriage canopy, and to perform good deeds. This item (ref. 25.1.7), is in the Gross Family Collection, Tel Aviv, which has several other examples of this custom in the rare books collection. In another example, a Jew from Germany traveled to Palestine in the late nineteenth century, to help found a Jewish village on the barren sand. Here his son was born, with *mazal tov*, in 1895. He noted this in Hebrew and in German on the endpaper of a book he had brought with him, a volume about Jewish principles, Joseph Albo, *Sefer ha-ikkarim* (Warsaw: 1877). (This fifteenth-century treatise was especially popular in the late nineteenth century, when it was seen to be an apologia for Judaism.) He would have registered the birth at the offices of the local Ottoman authorities some time later. A photograph of the endpaper inscription is displayed in the municipal museum of Rishon Lezion, Israel.

24. Family record, Pittsburgh, Pennsylvania, 1888, now owned by Mrs. Evelyn Glick Bloom, granddaughter of the artist. This and other examples were exhibited in an exhibition at the Museum of American Folk Art in New York: Kleeblatt, N.L., and Wertkin, G.C., eds. *The Jewish Heritage in American Folk Art* (New York: Universe Books, 1985).

25. Calimani, R., *The Ghetto of Venice* (New York: M. Evans and Co., 1987), 218–221, from a document in the records of the Cattaveri and preserved in the Venetian State Archives in the collection of the Magistracy of Inquisitors over the University of the Jews.

26. Moellin, Jacob b. Moses, *Sefer Maharil* (Sabionetta: 1556), *Hilkhot Milah*, sign. 24.

27. The Musée Alsacien in Strasbourg and The Jewish Museum of New York have some examples.

28. Schudt, J.J., *Jüdische Merkwürdigkeiten* (Frankfurt and Leipzig: 1717), part 4, book 3.

29. Eis, R., *Torah Binders of the Judah L. Magnes Museum* (Berkeley: Judah L. Magnes Museum, 1979), 15.

30. Raphael, F., and R. Weyl, *Les Juifs en Alsace* (Toulouse: 1977), 183–185.

31. Grossman, C., "Womanly Arts: A Study of Italian Torah Binders," *Journal of Jewish Art* 7 (1980): 35–43.

32. Juhasz, E., ed., *Sephardi Jews in the Ottoman Empire* (Jerusalem: Israel Museum, 1990), 256.

33. For instructions for making a *wimpl*, see Strassfeld, S., and M. Strassfeld, eds. *The Second Jewish Catalogue* (Philadelphia: Jewish Publication Society, 1976), 42–43.

34. Goitein, S.D., 1978, *op. cit.*, p. 226 n. 19.

35. Zeitlin, W., "Bibliotheca epistolographica," *Zeitschrift für Hebraische Bibliographie* 4 (1919): 32–33. The Jewish National University Library, Jerusalem, has at least thirty of these letter-writing manuals, *igronim*, including Johann Buxtorf's *Institutio epistolaris hebraica* (Basel: 1610), and many from all corners of Eastern Europe. For example, Frishman, D., *Igron shalem* (Warsaw: P. Kantrowitz, 1911), contains exemplars of letters of congratulations and blessings on the occasion of the birth of a son, an invitation to a circumcision feast, and the formula for replying, in Hebrew, Russian, Polish, and German.

36. For example, *Keryas-sh'ma bei a kimpetorn*, "reading *Shema* prayer" for the lying-in woman, depicted on a New Year card, Eastern Europe, c. 1900, Jewish Theological Seminary Library, New York; circumcision scenes in Tunisia and Algeria are depicted on a color postcard, reproduced in Silvain, G., *Images et traditions Juives* (Paris: Editions Astrid, 1980), 254–255, 400; circumcision was depicted by Hermann Junkers, and a redemption of the first-born scene by Hugo Elkan, Germany, 1898.

37. Attias, M., 1961, *op. cit.*, pp. 231ff (Judeo-Spanish); Lasseri, Y., *Ha-shirah ha-yehudit-amamit be-Morocco* (Tel Aviv: Ha-kibbutz ha-me'uhad, 1986), 37–41 (Morocco); See also the Yemenite song including the theme of deliverance of the mother after birth and the Balkan welcoming song quoted in Chapter 11, pp. 165 and 169. Danon, A., "Receuil de romances Judéo-Espagnoles," *Revue des Etudes Juives* 2 (1896): 138–139. Toledano, E., *Brit milah ve-minhage'ia* (Kiryat Yam: 1977), on the customs of Jews in Morocco.

38. Lasseri, Y., 1986, *op. cit.*, pp. 36–37; Ben Simhon, R., 1994, *op. cit.*, pp. 84–89.

39. Zafrani, H., *Mille ans de vie juive au Maroc* (Maisonneuve & Larose, 1983), 54.

40. Lasseri, Y., 1986, *op. cit.*, pp. 40–41; Maoz, B., *op. cit.*, pp. 65–66.

41. Ausubel, N., ed., *A Treasury of Jewish Folklore* (New York: Crown, 1948), 678, 681–682.

42. The lyric was written by Mordechai Gebirtig (1877–1942), in Yiddish. A translation and transcript can be found in the sleeve of the compact disc or tape of Jewish lullabies, *Sleep My Child* (Blue Hill Recordings, 1994).

43. Ausubel, N., 1948, *op. cit.*, pp. 680–681.

44. Mlotek, E.G., and J. Mlotek, comp., *Pearls of Yiddish Song* (New York: Education Department of Workman's Circle, 1988), 2–3. The lullaby is by Mikhl Gordon (1823–1890).

45. Ausubel, N., 1948, *op. cit.*, p. 679, has a transcript and translation of the male version of the lullaby. For the female version, see Sternberg, G., *Stefanesti: Portrait of a Romanian Shtetl* (Oxford: Pergamon Press, 1984), 176.

46. Sabar, Y., *The Folk Literature of the Kurdistani Jews* (New Haven: Yale University Press, 1982), 196. *Sleep My Child*, 1994, *op. cit.*, includes a Judeo-Spanish lullaby for a daughter, as well as a Yiddish lullaby for a daughter, nos. 4 and 14, with transcripts and English translations.

47. Ausubel, N., 1948, *op. cit.*, pp. 678, 684, 682; Mlotek, E.G., and J. Mlotek, 1988, *op. cit.*, pp. 4–5; the lullaby is by Moyshe Oysher (1906–1958); the Bessarabian song is cited in Sternberg, G., 1984, *op. cit.*, pp. 177–178.

48. A recording of it was made from a Jerusalem woman.

49. Kehimkar, H.S., *The History of the Bnei Israel of India* (Tel Aviv: Dayag, 1937), 120–122.

50. Weich-Shahak, S., 1989, *op. cit.*, p. 172.

51. Avishur, Y., ed., *Women's Folk Songs in Judaeo-Arabic from Jews in Iraq* (Tel Aviv: Iraqi Jews Traditional Culture Center Publication, 1987), 59ff, for an example of a lullaby expressing the tensions of living with one's in-laws; pp. 35ff. document the fantasy of the woman on the roof.

52. Diamant, A., *The Jewish Baby Book* (New York: Summit Books, 1988), 175, 194–195, 211ff., and for a directory of calligraphers in the United States, pp. 247–248. In Israel, contact artist Jeffrey Allon, 02-5632213.

53. The Phonoteque of the Jewish National University Library, Jerusalem, has collected many recordings of lullabies and newborn welcoming songs from many different Jewish communities. The music department of Beth Hatefutsoth, The Museum of the Jewish Diaspora, Tel Aviv, also has some recordings of such songs. YIVO, in New York, has recordings of Yiddish lullabies. There are some commercial recordings: Beth Hatefutsoth's compact disc, *Oasis* (Tel Aviv: 1996), features Jewish-Yemenite women's songs, translated from Arabic, edited by Shalom Seri, and sung by Lea Avraham. *Sleep My Child*, 1994, *op. cit.* (compact disc and cassette), has Yiddish and Judeo-Spanish lullabies. For cassettes, see *Yiddish Lullabies* (Israel: Jewish Music, 1991); *Ladino Folk Songs* (Boynton Beach, FL: Leisure Time Music, 1993); *Hakki Obadia, Iraqi Jewish and Iraqi Music* (New York: Global Village Music, 1993).

14. Final Reflections

1. Umansky, E.M., and D. Ashton, eds., *Four Hundred Years of Jewish Women's Spirituality* (Boston: Beacon Press, 1992).
2. For inspiring honor and fear, see Exodus 20:12 and Leviticus 19:3; for his educational duty, see Deuteronomy 6:7 and 11:19; for both these parental duties, see *B. Kiddushin* 29a–30b; for compassion, see Psalm 103:13; for discipline, Proverbs 19:18, 29:15; *B. Sotah* 47a; *Genesis Rabbah* 54:3. Psychologists now accept that infants, given the opportunity, are able to form emotional attachments to their fathers as well as to their mothers. Evidence remains inconclusive that the absence of a father in childhood and adolescence may affect the development of gender identity or, especially in the case of boys, the emergence of antisocial behavior. Perhaps in Jewish society, in the past few centuries, absence of a father may not have involved absence of a father figure for boys, because they spent most of their waking hours in male company, taught by a rabbi or other male teacher. A girl in a fatherless home had little opportunity to interact with men and thereby widen her experience, however, unless her family lived with her grandparents (which was common), or other relatives who provided her with a father figure. Perhaps the absence of a father figure is more serious now than in the past, for children who grow up isolated from the extended family, whose teachers are likely to be female, and who live in a society where the role of a father is no longer clearly defined. On the other hand, as sex roles have become eroded, it may be possible for one parent (father or mother) to raise children alone, to teach them how to love and feel secure, to master the environment, and to find a place in society. The increasing phenomenon of one-parent families may test this theory. Because Jewish society is still heavily biased by traditional parental roles, however, the lack of acceptance of this new parenting style, rather than the shortcomings of the single parent, may possibly create long-term effects on the growing child.
3. Genesis 37:3, 44:30. Maimonides, M., *Guide for the Perplexed*, 2nd ed., translated by M. Friedlander (New York: Dover, 1956), part 3, chap. 49. Zohar I, 233a. Mann, M.N., "Mothers and Fathers: A Conceptualization of Parental Roles," *Tradition* 21 (1983): 52–65.
4. A Jewish man, who maintained the traditional role differences between parents, usually felt obliged to find another wife if he were widowed or divorced, to avoid having his children placed in foster care. Research in Israel revealed that only a minority of men whose wives were pregnant for the first time intended to help with parenting in various ways: feeding, getting up at night, disciplining, seeking medical care, and taking the baby out for walks. After the birth, fathers in fact helped more at night than they had themselves predicted, but otherwise, they fulfilled their expectations: *The Jerusalem Post*, 20 Jan. 1985. In many ultra-Orthodox homes, the question of the man's helping in these ways is not even considered. A rabbi's 32-year-old wife, pregnant with her ninth child, said: "I look after the home—we have no such concept [of the husband helping in this], it just does not arise, I never think of such a thing."
5. *Kinnim* 3:3.
6. Schneider, S. W., *Jewish and Female* (New York: Touchstone [Simon and Schuster], 1985), 522ff. (childcare services), 543ff. (Jewish family services).
7. "Stars of David," 24 Lisa Lane, Reading, MA 01867. "Pregnancy Loss Support Program, Jewish

Women's Resource Center," National Council of Jewish Women, 9 East 69 Street, New York, NY 10021, tel. (212) 535-5900. See also Borg, S., and J. Lasker, *When Pregnancy Fails* (Boston: Beacon Press, 1989), appendix A and B. Yad Elisha in Jerusalem, 02-5632213 or 02-6518439.

8. The National Tay-Sachs and Allied Diseases Association, 385 Elliot Street, Newton MA 02164, tel. (617) 964-5508. For other specialist organizations, contact local Jewish family service or local health services.

9. Gold, M., "An Agenda for the Jewish Community," chap. 9 in *And Hannah Wept* (Philadelphia: Jewish Publication Society, 1988).

10. For the Orthodox view on these controversial issues, see Rosner, F., ed., *Medicine and Jewish Law* (Northvale, NJ: Jason Aronson, 1993), vol. 1, pp. 19–30, on secular and Jewish approaches to medical ethics, and pp. 105–122 on contraception and abortion; also Steinberg, A., "Gynecology and Infertility," pt. 4 of *Jewish Medical Law, Compiled and Edited from Tzitz Eliezer*, translated by D.B. Simons (New York: Bet Shammai, 1989). For a liberal view, see, for example, Borowitz, E.B., *Liberal Judaism* (New York: Union of American Hebrew Congregations, 1984), 392–395.

11. The literature on Jewish medical ethics includes Jakobovits, I., *Jewish Medical Ethics* (New York: Bloch, 1975); Rosner, F., and J.D. Bleich, eds., *Jewish Bioethics* (New York: Sanhedrin Press, 1979); and Grazi, R.V., *Be Fruitful and Multiply* (Jerusalem: Genesis, Feldheim, 1994), 177–208.

12. Lamm, M., *The Jewish Way in Love and Marriage* (San Francisco: Harper & Row, 1979), 132.

13. Epstein, H., *Children of the Holocaust* (New York: G.P. Putnam's Sons, 1979), 23–24. Borowitz, E., 1984, *op. cit.*, p. 451.

14. Frank, S., "The Population Panic," *Lilith* 1 (1977), 12–17. Schneider, S.W., 1985, *op. cit.*, p. 371ff. Israel's Central Bureau of Statistics has warned that the world Jewish population is shrinking because of its low birth rate and assimilation; Cullen, R.B., and M.J. Kubic, "A Numerical Nightmare," *Newsweek*, May 26, 1986, p. 13.

GLOSSARY

All italized words are Hebrew, unless specified otherwise.

Aggadah: Literally, "narrative." Rabbinic teaching containing narrative not concerned with religious laws. It includes homiletic expositions of the Bible, stories, legends, folklore, or maxims, sometimes seeking reasons for religious duties.

Akarah: A barren woman.

Amidah: Literally, "standing"; certain benedictions that are recited silently, standing, at each of the daily services (morning, afternoon, and evening).

Aramaic: An ancient northwestern Semitic language, spoken earlier than 700 b.c.e. Aramaic became the official language of Persia and the Near East from 700 to 300 b.c.e. and is found in biblical passages from that period. Later, the Bible was translated into this language, and the Dead Sea Scrolls, the Babylonian Talmud, and eventually also the Zohar were written in Aramaic.

Aravah: Willow, one of the four plants used during the celebration of Sukkot.

Ariri: Sterile, a childless man.

Ashkenaz, Ashkenazi, (pl. **Ashkenazim**): In the eleventh century, Ashkenaz referred to the area in the Rhine valley, near Mainz and Worms, where there were significant Jewish communities. Ashkenaz came to refer to the larger area of Germany in northwest Europe, and eventually the adjective, Ashkenazi, was used to describe all the descendants of these Jews, including those of the many who emigrated to Eastern Europe in the fifteenth and sixteenth centuries. Yiddish, a Judeo-German language, was spoken by and characterized Ashkenazi Jews. The customs of Ashkenazim often differed from those of the Sephardim.

Baal Shem: "Master of the Divine Name." Title, dating from the Middle Ages, given to a Jew, usually a kabbalist and a Hasid, who knew how to use the secret names of God. While the earlier masters were scholars, in the seventeenth and eighteenth centuries this title was applied to wonderworking Jews well-versed in practical Kabbalah. The name Baal Shem Tov applies to Israel ben Eliezer (c. 1720–1760).

Bar Mitzvah: Literally, "son of commandment"; a boy who, on reaching his thirteenth birthday, accepts the responsibility of fulfilling religious law. Also, the celebration of this event.

Barzel: Iron.

Bat Mitzvah: Literally, "daughter of commandment"; the festive initiation of a Jewish girl into adulthood at the age of twelve.

Be-etzev, Be-itzavon: In suffering, sorrow, pain, labor, toil.

Bekhorot: First-borns. The name of a tractate of Mishnah and Talmud on first-borns.

Ben (pl. *banim*): Son, boy.

Bilada: "Watchfulness"; "without misfortune." The name for the watchnight before the circumcision in some parts of North Africa. The name may have emerged from *Belo-da*, "without harm or tragedy" in Judeo-Arabic, or from the joyous exclamation of *ben yaldah*, "she delivered a son."

Bodgelt (Yiddish): Coins that the newborn's father and guests threw into the baby's bath and that the midwife kept for herself.

B'rakhah (pl. *berakhot*): "Blessing" or "benediction." Usually a fixed formula of blessing or thanksgiving recited in public services or privately. *Berakhot* is the name of the first tractate of the Talmud, which is about benedictions.

Brit: A covenant, pact. *Brit milah:* The covenant of circumcision. *Brit Itzhak:* Literally, the covenant of Isaac; the name of a book with special prayers for the first Friday night after a birth of a boy, or for the night before his circumcision; in some communities, the night before the circumcision is called *Brit Itzhak*.

Bubbeh (Yiddish): Granny, midwife.

Cohen: A priest or a person of a priestly family. In ancient times, the priests served in the Temple. Today, a *cohen* has certain rights, privileges, and prohibitions in Jewish ritual.

Conversos (Spanish): Converts to Christianity in Spain or Portugal at the time of the Inquisition on the Iberian peninsula. Many fled Spain and Portugal and returned to Judaism in their new homes when it was safe to do so.

Dead Sea Scrolls: Scrolls preserved in caves above the Dead Sea in the Judean desert that apparently belonged to a community of Jews, who were zealous and messianic, in the first century c.e. They include many biblical manuscripts, apocrypha, and pseudepigrapha, as well as community documents.

Duda (pl. *duda'im*): Usually translated as mandragora, or mandrake; the plant used by Rachel (Genesis 30:14–16) to help her relations with Jacob bear fruit.

Etrog: A citrus fruit, used together with a palm branch, myrtle, and willow in the Sukkot benediction.

Evil Eye: Malevolent effect caused by another person's glance. The Evil Eye was an accepted source of harm in the early Jewish literature, in mishnaic and talmudic times. Fear of the Evil Eye has never been a particularly Jewish phenomenon; it existed in the cultures of ancient Greece, Rome, Islam, and, further east, in the Buddhist and Hindu cultures. In each culture, measures were taken to avert the Evil Eye. Jews worldwide have taken many measures to avert the Evil Eye, especially in the form of amulets, incantations, herbs, and foods.

Fados (Judeo-Spanish): The festive naming celebration for a newborn girl among Sephardic Jews.

Gaon (pl. **geonim**), **gaonic:** Literally, "eminence"; the title of the heads of rabbinic academies, especially in Babylonia. The gaonic period was from the sixth to the eleventh centuries.

Gehenna (Gehinnom): A name derived from the valley of the sons of Hinnom, south of Jerusalem, where (according to the Bible) children were once burned by a cult. This name is used by Jews to refer to a place of torment reserved for the wicked after death.

Gemara (Aramaic): A popular term for the Talmud as a whole, although it is also used more specifically to refer to most of the discussions of the Mishnah within the Talmud.

Gematria: A method of interpreting words from their numeric configuration, used in ancient times by Babylonians and Greeks and by Jews since the second century, although perhaps earlier. Each letter of the alphabet is assigned a number according to specific rules. Different words adding up to the same number reached through *gematria* were interpreted to be equivalent. The rules for such calculations were developed especially by the Hasidei Ashkenaz in the twelfth and thirteenth centuries, and this method of interpretation was used extensively by Jews practicing mystical meditation and Kabbalah. By the sixteenth century, many different systems of *gematria* were documented and used in the centuries that followed by Jews all over the world.

Geniza: Literally, "store"; a depository for used and damaged Hebrew manuscripts and books. The best-known is the Cairo *Geniza*, from Fostat (Old Cairo), which was in use from the tenth to the nineteenth centuries. The oldest item is actually from the eighth century. This *Geniza* is an important source of material from the gaonic period and sheds light on Jewish life in the Mediterranean area in the Middle Ages.

Golem: Literally, "embryo," "shapeless matter," something unformed and imperfect. (This term came to be applied to manmade creatures.)

Hadas, Hatas (Judeo-Spanish): The celebration on the night before the circumcision in medieval Spain; the festive naming celebration for a newborn girl among Sephardic Jews.

Hadlakat nerot: The lighting of candles. It is the duty of the woman of the household to light the Sabbath candles.

Halakhah (pl. **halakhot**): A particular law or legal decision, or the generic term for the whole legal system of Judaism. The sections of rabbinic literature concerned with religious, ethical, civil, and criminal law are termed halakhah, as opposed to the nonlegal material, the aggadah. The main sources of halakhah are in the Written Law, believed to have been revealed at Sinai; the Oral Law, also believed to have been transmitted to Moses at Sinai, written down only later, in the Mishnah; and the sayings of the scribes, through the authority of the sages. Halakhah was codified only later, in the early Middle Ages, and updated codifications followed soon after, the most influential being the ninth-century *Halakhot g'dolot;* Maimonides's *Mishneh Torah* in the twelfth century; Jacob ben Asher's Tur Code (*Arba'ah turim*) in the early fourteenth century; and Joseph Caro's *Shulḥan arukh*, in the sixteenth century.

Halitzah: The ceremony, dictated in the Bible (Deuteronomy 25:7–10), that liberates a woman from levirate marriage.

Ḥallah: Literally, "the priest's share of the dough"; a religious ceremony performed over the finished dough; also the popular name for the Sabbath or holiday bread, a plaited loaf.

Hanukkah: Literally, "dedication"; the name of an eight-day festival to celebrate the dedication of the Hasmonean Temple by Judah Maccabee after its destruction by Antiochus IV Epiphanes, as related in the Books of Maccabees. Legend tells that a miracle happened: one small jar of undesecrated oil lasted eight days, long enough to prepare more.

Ha-shem: The (holy) Name; God.

Hasid (pl. **Hasidim**), **hasidic:** Literally, a "pietist"; this term refers to a person belonging to a mystical, religious movement, Hasidism, which emerged in the second half of the eighteenth century in southeastern Poland and spread, under the influence of pietists who were charismatic leaders, to win a massive following, especially among poor Jews. They taught that serving God must be joyful, to make God joyful, and encouraged dance and song in divine worship. They developed their own characteristic method of praying, which involved ecstatically attaching oneself to God by immersing oneself in contemplative prayer. They taught that human behavior should be governed by both love and fear of God, and many tales were told to reinforce this basic idea. Not everyone could do this, but there were especially holy men, *tzaddikim*, who could help others to reach up to God. The Hasidim are also characterized by their social organization, in which wealth is shared and the leader has his followers.

Hasidei Ashkenaz: Jewish pietists in medieval Germany characterized by their particular theology, symbolism, ethical views, and social doctrine. They shared a common spirituality, deriving strength from their devout service to God and the Jewish people. They were stricter than their contemporaries in obeying commandments, they led ascetic lives, and they preached the moral values of Judaism, for example, in *Sefer Hasidim*, attributed to Judah the Pious (d. 1217). The Hasidei Ashkenaz also passed on to future generations many mystical, esoteric texts about the unity and incorporeality of God.

Hekdesh (pl. **hekdeshim**): A term used since the Middle Ages to refer to funds used for communal needs, for the poor, or for fulfilling a duty such as ransoming a Jewish captive. It came to refer to property set aside for charitable functions, and eventually it signified a communal shelter for the poor and sick, as well as for itinerant Jews.

Heyalakh: Literally, "a little *heh*"; a medallion inscribed with the Hebrew letter *heh*, which is numerically equivalent to five and represents the five-shekel redemption fee.

Holah: This biblical word literally means a woman who writhes (in pain) and therefore is used to depict a travailing woman. The root of this verb is *ḥil*, from the Assyrian *ḥilu*, to writhe in fear, and not *ḥalah*, from the Assyrian *ḥalu*, meaning sickness or grief.

Hollekreisch: A cradle ceremony practiced by Jews in Bavaria in the fifteenth century that became a naming ceremony for Jewish girls in rural areas of the Rhineland and in Alsace, Switzerland, and southern Holland.

Ḥutz: "Out"; often used on childbirth amulets to keep Lilith away.

Kabbalah: Literally, something handed down by tradition. An esoteric form of mysticism that involves both communion with God and a particular understanding of the concept of God and creation. Kabbalists seek the hidden mysteries of God and the relationship between these, human life, and the creation of the universe. Since the beginning of the fourteenth century, the speculative elements of Kabbalah have been differentiated from the magical applications, or "practical" Kabbalah. Kabbalah was given a new direction in the late sixteenth century by the mystical theories and practices of Isaac Luria (Lurianic Kabbalah) and his small circle of mystics in Safed, Israel. The Lurianic theory of the drama of creation explained the forces of evil and the transmigration of souls.

Kaddish: Literally, "holy"; an ancient doxology, mostly in Aramaic, recited since the sixth century at the end of sections of the synagogue prayer service, and since the thirteenth century also by mourners remembering the dead.

Kiddush: "Sanctification"; also the name of the benediction pronounced upon the wine at the commencement of the Sabbath, on holidays, and during Jewish rituals.

Koilich Tanz (Yiddish): Literally, the dance [with the] plaited loaf (*Koilich*). Eastern European Jews have performed this dance at weddings to wish the bride and bridegroom abundance, especially of fertility.

Kosher: Ritually correct and faultless, applied to food prepared according to Jewish dietary laws, to parchment correctly treated for the writing of holy words on it, and to mezuzzot that are fashioned according to Jewish law.

Kvatter, Kvatterin (Yiddish): Godfather and godmother, a couple given a role of honor at the circumcision ceremony.

K'vorim reissen (Yiddish): Literally, "to tear [at] the graves." Jews went to the grave of a holy person and measured it with a piece of string, which they then tore up to use as candle wicks. They burned the candles in the synagogue.

La Veglia, La Viola, *Lilat Elzaba:* The name given to the night of vigilance before the circumcision among Italian Jews, Sephardic Jews, and Yemenite Jews, respectively.

Levirate marriage: The marriage between a widow whose husband died without offspring and the dead man's brother, as prescribed in Deuteronomy 25:5–6.

Levite: Descendent of Levi, son of Jacob and Leah. After the incident of the Golden Calf, the Levites were chosen to attend to the Ark and the sanctuary in place of the first-borns of the Israelites.

Mamzer: Usually translated "bastard." This label is given to a person conceived from a sexual relationship forbidden by Torah and punishable by divine punishment or death, that is, an incestuous or adulterous relationship. A *mamzer* is forbidden to marry a legitimate Jew, and any child born to a *mamzer* is also considered a *mamzer.*

Mappah (Hebrew), *Mape* (Yiddish): A Torah binder.

Marrano: A Christian of Spanish or Portuguese Jewish origin who maintained Jewish practices in secret. A *Marrano,* or his or her parents or ancestors, had been forced to convert from Judaism during persecutions and inquisitions between the late fourteenth and the late fifteenth centuries. Many fled Spain and Portugal.

Mazal: A star; luck.

Mazel tov: A good luck greeting.

Mezuzzah (pl. **mezuzzot**): Literally, "doorpost." The word now refers to the kosher parchment inscribed with the verses of Deuteronomy 6:4–9 and 11:13–21, which Jews affix, by biblical ruling, to the doorpost of rooms in the Jewish home. The parchment is rolled up and put into a small case, which is nailed to the right hand side of the doorpost. Jews have put mezuzzot on their doorposts since the period of the Second Temple. They have believed the mezuzzah has a protective effect on the home, but harm may occur if it is imperfect.

Midrash (pl. *midrashim*): "Exposition, interpretation." Homiletic exegesis of the Bible, rich in legends, parables, similes, and sayings. The early midrashim date from the fifth and sixth centuries; many midrashim date from the seventh to the end of the tenth centuries, and the late period refers to those written in the eleventh and twelfth centuries.

Mikveh: Ritual bath; a pool of clean water in which a Jew immerses for ritual purification.

Minhag (pl. *minhagim*): A custom.

Mi-shebeirakh: "May the One who blessed [the matriarchs or patriarchs, bless . . .]"; a blessing.

Mishnah: Literally, "repetition, teaching." The earliest codification of Jewish Oral Law, edited by Judah ha-Nasi (d. 225 c.e.), from earlier and contemporary rabbinic authorities. It is divided into six "orders," entitled Seeds, Festivals, Women, Damages, Holy Things, and Purities.

Mitzvah (pl. **mitzvot**): Commandment, precept, a religious duty. A good deed. There are traditionally 613 commandments: 248 positive mandates and 365 prohibitions. A benediction is usually recited before performing a mitzvah. Fulfilling mitzvot should be a joy; reward for performance of these duties is expected in the World to Come.

Mohel (pl. *mohalim*): Circumciser.

Mokh: A contraceptive tampon used in talmudic times.

Nefesh: The human soul, or the part of the soul that first enters the baby, before or at birth, and gives it vitality.

Nekevah: Female.

Neshamah: Spirit, the highest level of the human soul, responsible for rational and intellectual thought.

Nezek: Harm, indemnity.

Niddah: "A menstruating woman." According to biblical law (Leviticus 15:19ff.; 20:18), a woman is forbidden to have sexual relations with her husband during menstruation and for the seven days afterward, when she is considered impure; both partners may be punished by death for this sin. The Jewish laws pertaining to menstruating women and to women after childbirth (who also bleed for some days) were spelled out at great length in the Mishnaic Order, Purities, and in the Talmud in a whole tractate of ten chapters, entitled *Niddah*.

Onah: A husband's duty to respect his wife's sexual rights, to provide her with her conjugal dues.

Parokhet: The curtain covering the Ark of the Law.

Piadamento (Judeo-Spanish): "Day of the gifts"; a naming celebration for newborn girls.

Pinkas: A minute book kept by the community or a circumciser.

Piyyut (pl. **piyyutim**): Hebrew liturgical poem that embellishes private or public prayer. Some *piyyutim*, written in the land of Israel, date from talmudic times; others were composed all over the Diaspora until the early eighteenth century and were incorporated into the liturgy. Collections of *piyyutim* often included some local compositions. When the liturgy was printed, local differences were stabilized.

P'nim: Literally, "inside"; when used on childbirth amulets, the term refers to the inclusion of Adam and Eve in the invocation.

Pok (Aramaic): "Get out"; used in childbirth incantations and on amulets.

Rimon (pl. **rimonim**): Torah finials that crown the staves of the scroll.

Rosh Hodesh: Literally, "head of the month," the beginning of the month, that is, the new moon, celebrated in biblical times (Numbers 10:10). In talmudic times, it became a day when women could desist from hard work. Also since talmudic times, a special prayer has been recited on this night.

Rozhinkes mit Mandlen (Yiddish): Literally, "Raisins with Almonds," a well-known Yiddish lullaby.

Ru'ah: Anima, part of the human soul.

Sandek: The man who holds the baby boy during the circumcision ritual.

Sefer (pl. **sefarim; sifrei**): Book.

Sephardic Jew: A descendant of Jews who lived in Spain or Portugal before the expulsion in 1492. These Jews have spoken Judeo-Spanish. Their customs are slightly different from Ashkenazi Jews, but they maintain the same basic tenets of Judaism.

Shabbat: The Sabbath, the day of rest, starting at sundown on Friday evening and ending at sundown on Saturday evening. The special laws relating to the observance of the Sabbath are found in the first tractate of the Mishnah, Shabbat, and in subsequent commentaries.

Shabbat avi ha-ben: Literally, "the Shabbat of the father of the [newborn] son." The first Shabbat after the birth of a son, which Jews from North African and Asian communities have celebrated. The father is honored at the synagogue, and relatives and friends feast with him after the service.

Shaddai: A Name of God in the Bible; God appeared to the three patriarchs as *El Shaddai*, and in other biblical passages the word *Shaddai* appears on its own. Talmudic sages explained it to mean "the all-powerful," by breaking it up into *sha-* ("who") and *dai* ("enough"). Through the ages, this name has been used in particular for protective purposes. The letters of this name were interpreted to represent *shomer delatot Israel*, "guardian of the habitations of Israel," when it became customary to inscribe it on the back of the mezuzzah. Other meanings have been derived using *gematria*.

Shalom zakhar: Literally, "peace to the male child"; the name of the home celebration on the first Friday evening after the birth of a son, when friends and relatives visit and recite the *Shema* prayer, psalms, and other prayers, followed by festive foods, traditionally fruits and drinks, and sometimes also lentils and chickpeas.

Shashah: A Moslem version of Lilith. The Night of *Shashah* was clearly adapted from a local protective ritual, and was celebrated by Iraqi and Kurdistani Jews, on the sixth or seventh night after a birth. The neighborhood children gathered at the baby's home. An earthenware vessel was shattered, and the children gathered the shards to dip into saffron water. The shape of a hand was painted with this colored water on the wall behind the mother's bed for protection, and the children were given handfuls of popcorn amid shouts of "*Shashah, Shashah*." A baby girl was named at this ceremony.

Shekhinah: Divine Presence. Rabbinic sages used this term to mean the presence of God, whereas medieval Jewish philosophers used it to refer to the glory of God, an intermediary between God and humankind. Kabbalists have used this term to refer to the feminine principle in the divine world, the last principle in the divine hierarchy. Being the closest to the earthly world, she is the battleground between the divine powers of good and evil. The Shekhinah waxes and wanes with every good deed and every sin of each individual Jew and the Jewish people as a whole. Lurianic kabbalists imagined her exiled from the rest of the divine whole and taught that Jews should fulfill commandments to reunite her with the Holy One. The mystic tries to reach up to the Shekhinah when in communion with God.

Shema: Declaration of God's unity, consisting of Deuteronomy 6:4–9 and 11:13–21 and Numbers 15:37–41, recited by Jews twice daily, morning and evening.

Shir ha-ma'alot: A song of ascents; a Psalm, usually Psalm 121 or 126, when it appears in connection with childbirth.

Shir ha-malos-tsetl (Yiddish): A charm with a song of ascents (usually Psalm 121) written on it; used among Yiddish speakers to protect a woman in childbirth.

Shofar: An animal's horn used to produce trumpet sounds on special occasions. A musical instrument in ancient times, the shofar was also used to inspire awe. Since talmudic times, Jews have blown the shofar on the Jewish New Year, and eventually also on the Day of Atonement. In an extension of its use to inspire awe, it has also been used to frighten demons.

Shulḥan Arukh: Literally, "the prepared table"; Joseph Caro's code of Jewish law first published in Venice in 1565, which eventually became the authoritative code for world Jewry.

Siman tov: Literally, "a good sign"; often said together with *mazel tov*, as a blessing that the occasion bodes well for the future, or on its own among North African Jews, when a son is born.

Sukkot: The Feast of the Tabernacles, commemorating the booths in which the Children of Israel lived when in the wilderness, after their exodus from Egypt (Leviticus 23:39–43). The festival lasts seven days; the seventh day is known as Hoshanah Rabbah, after the words used in the prayers on that day, and the eighth day is the festival of Shemini Atzeret. In the Diaspora, the festivities are celebrated for an extra day. Four species of plants are used in this celebration—*etrog* (citron), myrtle, palm, and willow.

Talmud: A compilation of rabbinic commentaries on the Mishnah. A compilation was done both in Babylonia and in the land of Israel between the first half of the third century and the end of the fifth century. Discussion in the Talmud attempts to apply Mishnaic teaching to the daily life of the people and also addresses many questions that are purely theoretical. The Babylonian Talmud is more massive than that of the Land of Israel (six orders in the former, four in the latter) and has considerably more aggadah—in the land of Israel, aggadic material was generally collected separately into Midrashim. Both Talmuds rule on Jewish law, but the Babylonian Talmud is usually authoritative.

Tazri'a: A word appearing in Leviticus 12:2, *ishah ki tazri'a ve-yaldah*, "when a woman seminates and gives birth," or "when a woman conceives and gives birth." *Tazri'a* has been translated also as "she gives forth seed," because the word is derived from the Hebrew word for seed, *zera*.

T'khinah (pl. *t'khinot*) (Hebrew); *tkhines* (Yiddish): Private devotion. Such devotional prayers were popular from the sixteenth century to the early twentieth century and were formulated in Hebrew or in the local vernacular.

Torah: This word usually refers to the Pentateuch, although it can also refer to everything that Moses received from Sinai.

Tosafot: Literally, "additions"; commentaries on the Talmud, eventually the Bible and other texts, too, made in France and Germany between the twelfth and fourteenth centuries. New deductions regarding the source material were made in these commentaries. The most prominent tosafist was Jacob Tam. Printed editions of the Talmud today include the Tosafot commentary in the margin.

Tzaddik (pl. *tzaddikim*): A "righteous man," a person who has special relations with God and lives by his faith. In Hasidism, the *tzaddik* has mystical powers that enable him to draw close to God and to serve as an intermediary between God and other Jews.

Tzarah (pl. *tzarot*): Trouble, misfortune, anguish, distress; the distress of a woman in labor; also, a rival wife in a polygamous marriage.

Tzir (pl. *tzirim*): Literally, a (door) hinge; a woman's twists and turns during contractions; the contractions of labor.

Wachnacht (Yiddish): The name given by Ashkenazi Jews to the night of vigilance before a baby's circumcision.

Wimpl (Yiddish): A Torah binder, made from the swaddling cloth used at a boy's circumcision.

Yeshivah: An academy for the study of rabbinic literature.

Yeshu'a ha-ben: Literally, "salvation of the son"; also the feast on the first Shabbat after a son's birth.

Yetzer ha-ra: The evil inclination; an untamed natural impulse or instinct that can lead one to act in an evil manner, contrary to God's will. Traditionally, the antidote to this is the study of Torah and to follow the guidelines set by the Torah. This idea has been personified in the form of Satan, or the serpent, who tempts men and women to do evil deeds. In moderation, the evil inclination is a driving force that leads men to marry, to beget children, to build a house, and to work. When uncontrolled and allowed to dominate human behavior, however, it causes harm.

Yidschkerz, Yidish-kerts (Yiddish): Literally, "Jewish candle"; the candles made for burning during the circumcision. In the fifteenth century and until the nineteenth century, Jewish women in the Rhine valley made these candles ceremoniously on the fifth day after a boy's birth.

Yom Kippur: Day of Atonement; the holiest day in the Jewish year when Jews fast and atone for their sins.

Yotze dophen: Literally, "coming out of the wall [side]." This mishnaic term describes a special manner of delivery that is not through the normal birth canal, usually understood to refer to caesarean section.

Zakhar: Male.

Zera: Seed.

Zeved, Zeved ha-bat: Literally, "the gift," "the gift of a [newborn] daughter"; the ceremony or celebration for naming and welcoming a newborn daughter.

Zion: This term is used in the Bible to refer to Jerusalem, because it is the name of the hill and the city where King David built his capital. The association of Zion with the Temple, with a place where God dwells, and with the scene of messianic salvation, gave the word religious and emotional significance. Eventually, Zion came to mean the Jewish homeland, and hence Zionism has referred to the movement to establish a Jewish national home in Palestine.

Zohar: Literally, "splendor"; *Sefer ha-zohar, The Book of Splendor*, an important text of Jewish mysticism, written in Aramaic in the late thirteenth century. The main part is arranged according to the weekly portions of the Torah. The Zohar includes several discourses attributed to Simeon bar Yohai, a mystic who lived in Palestine in the middle of the second century. It also includes discourses about the celestial palaces in the Garden of Eden and the mysteries of divine emanations. The book was written by

Moses ben Shem Tov de Leon (c. 1240–1305) some time between 1270 and 1300, although one report dating from the early fourteenth century tells that Moses de Leon had copied the book from an ancient manuscript. Scholarly analysis today confirms the authorship of Moses de Leon. The work was first published in Italy in the sixteenth century. Parts of it were translated into Hebrew in the fourteenth century, with more translated in later centuries. Similarly, some parts of it were translated into Latin by Christian mystics in the sixteenth century or earlier. French translations followed and eventually (in the twentieth century), English too.

Z'mirot: Literally, "hymns, psalms"; this term also refers to "table songs" sung during meals.

HISTORICAL PERSONALITIES

Aaron: A Levite. Son of Amram and Jochebed, brother of Moses and Miriam. He married Elisheva. During Moses' absence on the mount, he fashioned a golden calf that became a cause of apostasy. However, he became high priest and founder of the priesthood in Israel. He wore a holy breastplate. (Exodus 28–32).

Abel: Second son of Adam and Eve, murdered by Cain, his older brother (Genesis 4:1–9).

Abitu, Abizu, Amzarfo, Hakash, Odem, Ikpodu, Iylu, Tatrota, Avinukta, Satruna, Kalicatiya, Tulatuy, Piratsha: Alternative names for Lilith.

Aboab, Isaac (end of fourteenth century): Spanish Jew who wrote an ethical treatise, *Menorat ha-me'or*. The third part is on observance of mitzvot, including the founding of a family.

Abraham: First patriarch. His marriage to Sarah was childless for many years, but she gave him her handmaid, Hagar, with whom he fathered Ishmael. Sarah eventually conceived in old age and bore Isaac (Genesis 11–25).

Abraham ben David of Posquières (Ravad) (c. 1125–1198): Talmudic authority and halakhist of Provence, southern France. He was the author of an influential code, *Ba'alei ha-nefesh* (first publ. Venice, 1602) and many other treatises.

Abraham ibn Ezra: See Ibn Ezra, Abraham.

Adam: First man, created by God in God's image (Genesis 1:27, 2:7) from whose rib God fashioned Eve (Genesis 2:22). Eve bore Adam three sons—Cain, Abel, and Seth. He died at age 930 after begetting more children (Genesis 5:4–5). Jewish legend tells that Lilith was the first wife that God created for Adam, but Adam did not like her. God therefore created Eve. Legend also tells that Adam begot children from spirits during his long separation from Eve.

Afarof: Raphael in *gematria*, an angel of God who, according to *The Testament of Solomon*, prevented the child-killing demon from harming a newborn.

Aldabi, Meir ben Isaac (c. 1310–c. 1360): Philosopher with rabbinic training, author of *Sh'vilei emunah*. The third part of this text is on family life, taken from Nahmanides's *Iggeret ha-kodesh*; the fourth part concerns embryology.

Alexander the Great (356–323 B.C.E.): King of Macedonia, who conquered most of the Near East and Asia and who granted privileges to the Jews.

Almoli, Solomon (before 1485–after 1542): Physician, philosopher, grammarian, and kabbalist. He was born in Spain, but he left as a child for Salonika, eventually settling in Constantinople, where he was physician to the sultan. His most popular work was his *Interpretation of Dreams*, first published as *Mefasher halomin* (Salonika, c. 1515) and later as *Pitron halomot*. This was translated into Yiddish (Amsterdam, 1694), and both versions were frequently reprinted until the early twentieth century.

Amatus Lusitanus (1511–1568): Born a Portuguese *Marrano*, he studied medicine in Spain, lectured on this subject in Italy, and served as physician to the Pope. He practiced Judaism openly after moving to Salonika in 1558 and published seven books of case studies (*Centuria*) as well as other texts.

Amram: Father of Aaron, Moses, and Miriam. (Exodus 6:18–20).

Amram ben Diwwan: Eighteenth-century Moroccan rabbi, whose burial site is a favorite pilgrimage.

Antiochus IV Epiphanes (c. 215–164 B.C.E.): Seleucid ruler of Syria who enforced hellenization on the peoples under his rule, including Judea. He stormed the city of Jerusalem, killed thousands of Jews, sold thousands more into slavery, and planted a Greek community in the citadel. He compelled the Jews under his rule to abandon the laws of Torah.

Aristotle (384–322 B.C.E.): Greek philosopher concerned with science and the phenomena of the world, whose many writings have been studied by philosophers through the ages.

Asaph Judaeus (Middle East, seventh century): Jewish physician whose medical writings quoted Hippocrates, Dioscorides, and Galen. He was religious and believed that some diseases were retribution for sins. He understood pathology in terms of the imbalances among the four humors (earth, air, fire, and water). He also had a social conscience and insisted that doctors treat poor patients without charge. He was concerned to safeguard the high ethical standards that he believed were necessary in his profession and composed an oath for qualifying physicians.

Ashkenazi, Jacob ben Isaac of Yanov: See Jacob ben Isaac Ashkenazi of Yanov.

Asmodeus, Ashmedai: King of the demons, but a friend in talmudic folklore. He first appeared in the apocryphal book of *Tobit*, and then again in the first-century C.E. *Testament of Solomon*. The Talmud depicts him as having foreknowledge and being a help to Solomon. His friendship with Solomon is a popular theme in Jewish folklore, and he was frequently invoked in kabbalistic incantations as a help to humankind.

Ayash, Judah (d. 1760): Rabbi of Algiers.

Azulai, Hayyim Yosef David (1724–1806): Born in Jerusalem, he became a leading scholar in the Ottoman Empire, a halakhist, a kabbalist, and an emissary for the Hebron yeshivah, traveling all over Europe and raising considerable sums of money for the yeshivah. He retired in Italy. In addition to his halakhic and travel writings, he wrote prayers and collected folktales.

Baal Shem Tov: See Israel ben Eliezer.

Bacharach, Naphtali ben Jacob Elhanan (first half of seventeenth century): A German-born Kabbalist who lived in Poland and wrote *Emek ha-melekh*, an important text of Lurianic Kabbalah based largely on earlier sources.

Bacharach, Yair Hayyim (1638–1702): German talmudic scholar with extensive knowledge in general sciences.

Baer, Yisakhar, of Radoshitz (d. 1843): Eastern European hasidic miracle worker, especially gifted in curing people possessed by demons.

Bahya ben Asher (thirteenth century): Spanish exegete and kabbalist, whose popular commentary on the Pentateuch drew on many different sources.

Bahya ibn Paquda (c. 1050–c. 1100): Spanish Jew, author of *Duties of the Heart*, an influential pietist work.

Basnage, Jacques C. (1653–1725): French Protestant historian who was the first to write a history of the Jews in the Christian era.

Ben Azzai, Shimon (early second century): Palestinian Jewish scholar who never had children.

Benjamin: Youngest son of Jacob by Rachel. She died after his delivery (Genesis 35:16–18).

Ben Sira: It is important to distinguish between Simeon ben Jesus ben Sira, who lived in the second century B.C.E. and who wrote *The Wisdom of Ben Sira*, known as Ecclesiasticus, which is included in the Apocrypha, and Ben Sira, son of Jeremiah, who is the subject of *The Alpha Beta of Ben Sira*, a satirical work of the gaonic period, of eastern origin.

Benveniste, Sheshet (c. 1131–1209): Spanish Jew, poet, diplomat, and physician to the kings of Aragon. He was the author of medical works.

Berekhiah ha-nakdan (c. 1200): A Jewish grammarian and translator who lived in Normandy and England and whose most famous work was a Hebrew collection of fables from many lands.

Bilhah: Servant girl of Rachel. While still childless, Rachel gave her to Jacob as a concubine so Rachel would have children through her. Bilhah bore two sons (Genesis 30:3ff.).

Binesh, Binyamin (late seventeenth century–early eighteenth century): Kabbalist author of *Sefer amtahat Binyamin*, a book of charms and remedies that includes prayers, too.

Bluwstein, Rahel (1890–1931): Russian Jewish woman who emigrated to the land of Israel and became a Hebrew poet. She died unmarried after a long tubercular illness that contributed to the sadness of her later work.

Brusha, Brosha, Broxa: Unwholesome night bird in medieval Spain and Provence, eventually thought of as a witch who harmed women in childbirth.

Caesar, (Gaius) Julius (100–40 B.C.E.): Roman general and statesman, conqueror of Gaul and dictator of the Roman people. He was born in the month that was later named July in his honor, but we do not know for certain about the nature of his birth. Pliny the Elder (23–79 C.E.) mentioned a surgical operation done on a mother who had died in childbirth to deliver her live baby, as in the case of "the first of the Caesars." The identity of the child is not clear from this text. Besides, Suetonius (69–140 C.E.) wrote that Julius Caesar's mother died during his conquest of Gaul. However, the legend that Julius Caesar was born through a cut in his dead mother's abdomen was well known in the Middle Ages and was widely accepted in the medical world of sixteenth-century Europe. Thus, François Rousset had this legend in mind when he coined the term "caesarean childbirth" in 1581, in his treatise on how to perform this operation on live women. For the fascinating etymology of the name of this operation, see the appendix of Blumenfeld-Kosinski, R., *Not of Woman Born* (Ithaca, NY: Cornell University Press, 1990) 143–154.

Cain: Son of Adam and Eve. He killed his brother Abel (Genesis 4:1–25).

Cardoso, Isaac (1604–1681): *Marrano* physician and philosopher. Born in Portugal, he became physician at the royal court of Madrid. Persecuted by the Inquisition, he fled to Italy where he openly embraced Judaism.

Castro, Rodrigo de (c. 1550–1627): *Marrano* physician from Lisbon, who settled in Hamburg, where he openly embraced Judaism and attended the King of Denmark. His treatise on gynecology was of scientific importance.

Chagall, Marc (1887–1985): Born in Vitebsk, he settled in France and became a prolific artist whose work often contained Jewish themes.

Cleopatra: The name of seven Egyptian queens in the second and first centuries B.C.E.. The last and most famous (69–30 B.C.E.) was mistress of Julius Caesar and later of Mark Antony and was the enemy of Herod. It is not clear whether the Cleopatra referred to in the Talmud is this last one.

Cohn, Tobias (1652–1729): Born in Eastern France, he received a traditional Jewish education. He studied medicine in Germany and Italy and then worked as a court physician in Turkey. He retired from his profession at the age of sixty-two and went to Jerusalem to end his days in Torah study. His encyclopedia *Ma'aseh Tuvya* showed that he was fully aware of the latest discoveries in medicine and astronomy, although he rejected some of these on religious grounds. He also rejected many superstitions and the miracles of kabbalists.

David: Achieved fame in his youth for his courage against Goliath. He became the second king of Israel. He was known for his musical and poetic talents. He fathered Solomon from Bathsheba.

Dinah: Daughter of Jacob and Leah (Genesis 30:21) and raped by Shechem, the Hivite (Genesis 34). Legend tells that she was destined to be male but Leah, while pregnant, prayed that she would give birth to a daughter. Another legend tells that when Dinah was raped, she conceived a daughter who later married Joseph.

Dioscorides (c. 40–c. 90): Greek physician and pharmacist, whose pharmacologic treatise, containing a thousand different drugs and descriptions of some six hundred plants used medicinally, was used by physicians until the end of the fifteenth century. It was translated into seven languages.

Duran, Simon ben Tzemah (1361–1444): Spanish rabbi, philosopher, and physician, well-versed also in mathematics and astronomy, who eventually became chief rabbi of Algiers. He was the author of a scientific encyclopedia, *Magen avot*.

Duran, Solomon ben Simon (c. 1400–1467): A rabbi of Algiers, son of Simon ben Tzemaḥ, and well-read in medicine and philosophy.

Eleazar the Great: Author of an ethical will, dated Venice, 1544, mentioning the dangers posed by Lilith.

Eleazar ben Judah of Worms (1176–1238): Last major scholar of Hasidei Ashkenaz. He lived mainly in Worms, where he witnessed anti-Semitic massacres in which he was wounded and his wife and two children were killed. A prolific writer, among his writings were a halakhic, ethical treatise, *Sefer ha-roke'ah*, and a mystical, theological text on creation. He was interested also in the exegesis of Holy Names.

Eli: A priest in the sanctuary of the Lord at Shiloh who noticed Hannah praying for a child. She conceived and bore a child (Samuel) soon after this, and when the child had been weaned, Hannah brought him to Eli to serve the Lord (I [see II kings under *Elijah*] Samuel 1).

Eliezer ben Hyrcanus (end of first century–early second century): One of the important scholars at the time of the destruction of the second Temple, who promoted the traditional, established halakhot and avoided contact with non-Jews. Many mishnaic laws are attributed to him.

Elijah (ninth century B.C.E.): Israelite prophet who triumphed over the pagans in Israel. It is told that he did not die but went to heaven in a chariot of fire (II Kings 1:8). He became a legendary figure, one who attends all circumcisions and whose task it is to herald the redemption of Israel. In Jewish mysticism, he is depicted as an angel who spent a short period on earth in human form. He becomes visible to chosen people, giving them divine insights. Folktales about Elijah abound, in which he is usually disguised as a poor man, healing, rewarding the poor, and protecting newborns.

Elijah Pinhas ben Meir (c. 1742–1821): Kabbalist and scholar in secular studies, who wrote an encyclopedia (*Sefer ha-brit*) that contributed to the enlightenment of Galician and German Jews, although he maintained a kabbalist conception of the universe.

Elisha: A prophet, annointed by Elijah to succeed him. He enabled the birth of the son of the Shunammite woman (II Kings 4:8ff.).

Elisheva: Wife of Aaron (Exodus 6:23).

Emden, Jacob (1697–1776): Ashkenazi halakhic authority, who was well-read in sciences and in Latin, German, and Dutch. He was a kabbalist and strongly anti-Shabbatean—he exposed hidden Shabbatean meanings and allusions. He published an edition of the prayer book with his commentaries (*Siddur Beit Ya'akov*), and a commentary on the Mishnah, and halakhic works.

Ephraim: Son of Joseph, who favored him over his older brother when blessing the two of them (Genesis 48:13–20).

Er: Eldest son of Judah. He married Tamar but died childless in punishment for wickedness (Genesis 38:6–7).

Esther: Beautiful heroine of the Book of Esther, made queen by King Ahasuerus, who did not know that she was a Jew. When she learned of a plan to exterminate all the Jews in the empire, Esther risked her life to save her people. The king complied with her request.

Eve: Wife of Adam and mother of all humankind, who was encouraged by the serpent to taste the forbidden fruit of the tree of knowledge in the Garden of Eden.

She, in turn, gave Adam to taste it, too, and for this she was punished with the pain of childbirth and submission to her husband. Legend tells that Samael (Satan) lusted after her and also that God fashioned Lilith from the dust before Eve.

Eybeschutz, Jonathan (1690/95–1764): Talmudist and kabbalist of Eastern European origin, who lived in Prague and eventually became the head of three communities in Germany. There he was accused of making use of Shabbatean formulas in the amulets he wrote. He denied the accusation, but the dispute raged for many years.

Falaquera, Shem Tov (c. 1225–1295): Spanish Jewish philosopher and translator. A prolific writer.

Frederick William IV (1795–1861): A king of Prussia.

Gabriel: An angel.

Galen (129–c. 200): Greek physician who studied in Greece as well as in Alexandria, and then achieved fame practicing medicine and lecturing in Rome. He studied anatomy from dissections and believed that human health depended on equilibrium among the four humors—phlegm, black bile, yellow bile, and blood. His many written treatises were studied by physicians and dominated the practice of medicine in the Western world until the sixteenth century. These works were translated into Latin, Arabic, and Syriac in the Middle Ages.

Gershom ben Judah of Mainz (c. 960–1028/40): Head of the rabbinic academy in Mainz, where he proposed enactments that had far-reaching consequences among Ashkenazi Jews, including his prohibition of polygamy and his disallowance of a husband's right to divorce without his wife's consent.

Gluckel of Hameln (1645–1724): German Jewish woman of an aristocratic family, who married at fourteen and raised twelve children (a thirteenth died). She was pious and well-read, and she managed her husband's business after he died. She wrote her memoirs in Yiddish, providing a touching view of Jewish life in Europe at the time.

Goldfaden, Abraham (1840–1908): Yiddish poet, dramatist, and composer of tunes for the plays he wrote for Yiddish theater. Born in the Ukraine, he lived in various parts of Eastern Europe and eventually in Paris, London, and Lemberg (near Lvov), and he died in New York. Some of the tunes he adapted from existing songs, and others became folksongs through their popularity. Best known of his tunes is *Rozhinkes mit Mandlen* from his operetta, *Shulamis.*

Goldman, Emma (1869–1940): Born in Lithuania, she emigrated to the United States when still a teenager. She qualified as a midwife in Vienna and worked as a midwife in the United States at the end of the nineteenth century. She soon became involved in anarchist activities and especially with teaching people about birth control, which generated animosity against her. She is best known for her anarchist activities and writings, which led to her deportation from the United States.

Graaf, Regnier de (1641–1673): Dutch physician who discovered the follicles of the ovary, known as graafian follicles.

Hadrian, Publius Aelius (76–138 C.E.): Roman Emperor at the time of the Bar Kokhba revolt (132–135) when the Jews were defeated by the Romans after a bitter struggle. Hadrian appeared to have been friendly to the Jews in the early years of his rule, but at the time of the Jewish revolt and especially after it, he issued vicious anti-Jewish decrees, including that against circumcision.

Hamoi (or Hammawi), Avraham (nineteenth century): Kabbalist and prolific writer who collected practical kabbalah in books he published in Izmir, *Ha'ah nafshenu* (1870), and *Devek me'ah* (1874). He also published anthologies of kabbalistically inspired, highly emotional prayers, *Beit din* (1858).

Hannah: Wife of Elkanah and mother of the prophet Samuel. She was childless for many years and taunted by her husband's other wife, Peninnah. She prayed for a son at the temple in Shiloh and was helped by the temple priest. She vowed to dedicate any son born to her to God (I Samuel 1). After weaning Samuel, she left him with the temple priest so he could be raised to serve God. She eventually had five more children.

Hannover, Nathan Nata (d. 1683): Eastern European kabbalist who followed the Lurianic school. Among the books he wrote was *Sha'arei tziyyon*, (1662), one of the most influential and widely circulated kabbalistic books. It is a collection of prayers that aroused the reader's imagination and emotions.

Hayyim, Yosef (c. 1835–1909): Rabbi of Baghdad, who wrote a book about Jewish laws regarding women.

Hera: Sister-wife of Zeus, queen of Olympian gods, and goddess of women, in Greek mythology. She was believed to protect women in childbirth.

Herod (73–4 B.C.E.): Appointed king of Judea by the Romans, he built massive fortresses and palaces and many other fine buildings and raised the level of prosperity in the land, but he caused political and family intrigues. He was a Jew (his mother was the daughter of a proselyte), but he was hated by the Hasmoneans, the ruling faction of Jews in the land at the time, because he murdered many of them and undermined their power and the authority of Torah. He loved Greek culture and was faithful to Rome, which gave him his power. Nevertheless, he wanted favor from the Jews and rebuilt the Temple and helped Jews in the Diaspora.

Hezekiah (eighth century B.C.E.): Ruler of Jerusalem (II Kings 18:9–10). A king of legendary piety, he strove to unite those of Davidic descent with the people of Judah before he was defeated by the Assyrians.

Hippocrates (c. 460–c. 377 B.C.): Greek physician, the first to study medicine scientifically and rationally, from clinical observations. His oath set the standards for medical ethics.

Hisda (c. 217–309): Babylonian sage of priestly family, frequently quoted in the Talmud. He married at sixteen, fathered seven sons and at least two daughters, and died at the age of ninety-two.

Hiyya (end of second century): Born in Babylonia, he moved to the land of Israel where he headed his own academy and was frequently consulted by the writer of the Mishnah. He was quoted in both Talmuds. His wife, Judith, suffered greatly in childbirth and swallowed a "cup of roots" to keep from conceiving again.

Hosea (eighth century B.C.E.): A prophet and the name of a book in the Bible.

Ibn Ezra, Abraham (1089–1164): Poet, grammarian, biblical commentator as well as physician, mathematician, astronomer, and philosopher. Born in Spain, he wandered through North Africa and spent years in Italy, too. He studied the stars and believed in astrology. He also believed that divine providence has its limitations and attempted to reconcile these beliefs with the existence of free will.

Ibn Gabirol, Solomon (1021–c. 1057): A major medieval Spanish Jewish poet, he also wrote philosophical and ethical treatises. Many of his religious poems have been included in the liturgy.

Ibn Ghayyat, Isaac ben Judah (1038–1089): Spanish Jew, an authority in halakhah, commentator and poet, and author of hundreds of *piyyutim*.

Isaac: Son of Abraham and Sarah, who was born in his mother's old age, fulfilling a divine promise (Genesis 12:4). God ordered Abraham to sacrifice him, and Abraham set out to do so; at the last moment, God provided a sheep instead for the burnt offering. Isaac married Rebekah and remained monogamous even though they remained childless for twenty years. Eventually, she bore twins, Esau and Jacob.

Isaac ben Solomon Luria: See Luria, Isaac ben Solomon.

Isaiah (eighth century B.C.E.): A prophet and the name of one of the books of Prophets in the Bible. He preached that God would punish Israel for their sins, for the corruption in his country, and prophesied that a remnant would survive and find justice and peace in Zion with the coming of a messianic king at the end of days. He believed that God would see to the destiny of Israel and preached faith in God's holiness. Legend tells that Isaiah warned King Hezekiah that he would die because he was childless and offered the king the opportunity to marry the prophet's daughter in the hope of a worthy son. However, the son born was wicked, as the king had feared.

Ishbili, Yom Tov ben Abraham (1250–1330): Spanish talmudist and spiritual leader.

Israel ben Eliezer, Baal Shem Tov (c. 1700–1760): Eastern European founder and first leader of Hasidism. Born of humble and aged parents, he lived a simple life until he was thirty-six years old, when he revealed his unusual mystical qualities. He then became a spiritual leader and miracle worker. He approached God through his ecstatic prayers and studied Torah, but showed no signs of talmudic scholarship. He was a *tzaddik*, who mixed with simple people, helping them to reach out to God and to repent for their sins. Legends were told of his supernatural gifts and of the miracles he performed.

Israel ben Shabbetai Hapstein: See Maggid of Koznitz.

Issachar: Ninth son of Jacob, and fifth of Leah, born after a long intermission from childbearing (Genesis 30:18).

Issachar Dov Roke'ah of Belz (1854–1927): Galician Hasid.

Jacob: Younger twin son of Isaac and Rebekah, destined to become the founder of a great nation. He had two wives, Leah and Rachel, daughters of Laban, and fathered children also from their two handmaids, Zilpah and Bilhah. He had twelve sons, who founded the twelve tribes of Israel, and one daughter, Dinah (Genesis 25–49).

Jacob ben Isaac Ashkenazi of Yanov (1550–1625): Polish rabbi who wrote an immensely popular book for women, *Tze'enah u-re'enah*, in Yiddish, to familiarize them with the Bible. This book included biblical passages and commentaries, the weekly readings, parables, allegories, legends, and admonitions about ethical conduct. It included tender descriptions of the matriarchs and the birth of Moses, and it depicted the rewards awaiting the righteous in the next world, as well as vivid scenes awaiting the wicked that encouraged repentance and charity.

Jacobs, Aletta (1854–1929): The first woman to study medicine at a Dutch university, she opened a clinic for working-class women and championed women's emancipation and pacifism.

Jeremiah (early seventh century–late sixth century B.C.E.): A prophet and the name of one of the books of the Prophets in the Bible, which records the oracles of the prophet, as well as details about his life, and recounts the destruction of Jerusalem and subsequent events in Judah and Egypt. Dismayed by the corruption of the people and impending doom, he never married, but urged the people of Israel to worship God and repent. His personal poems and confessions reveal his relationship with God. Jeremiah had an unusual personality, and therefore it is not surprising that several legends attest to unusual circumstances related to his birth; one tells that he was born circumcised, another tells that he was born with the ability to speak.

Job: The Book of Job is one of the Hagiographa in the Bible. Job was wealthy and pious but suffered numerous calamities intended to test his faith in God. God spoke to him, telling him that he should not question divine justice.

Jochebed: Wife of Amram, mother of Aaron, Moses, and Miriam (Exodus 2:1).

Joel Baal Shem Tov of Zamosz (d.1703): Head of a secret society of kabbalists and a wonderworker.

Joseph: Son of Jacob and Rachel, born after her long period of barrenness (Genesis 30:23–4). Jacob especially favored him, to his brothers' annoyance and jealousy. After being thrown in a pit and sold to passing travelers, Joseph reached Egypt, where he won the ruler's respect and achieved a position of honor and power. He was eventually reconciled with his brothers. Legend tells that he married his niece, daughter of Dinah.

Josephus Flavius (c. 38–after 100 C.E.): Born in Jerusalem, he took part in the Jewish war against the Romans, was captured, and then found favor with them and became a Roman citizen. He wrote *Jewish Antiquities*, about Jewish life and history, as well as *The Jewish War*.

Joshua ben Hananyah (late first–second century C.E.): Religious leader in Israel, responsible for some Jewish laws.

Judah: Fourth son of Jacob and Leah, father of three sons (Onan, Er, and Shelah) by his wife and father of twins from an unintentional relationship with Tamar, the widow of both Onan and Er (Genesis 38).

Judah ben Samuel, the Pious (ha-hasid) of Regensburg (c. 1150–1217): Leader and teacher of the Hasidei Ashkenaz, whose piety and humility set an example to others. In addition to the other works he wrote on theology, prayers, and even magic, he was the principal author of the ethical treatise, *Sefer Hasidim*. Legends about his life were spread posthumously, especially in the sixteenth and seventeenth centuries.

Katzenellenbogen, Pinhas, of Mehrin (1691–1765): Born to an established Polish family, he lived in Moravia and southeastern Germany and wrote detailed memoirs that reveal the daily life of a pious Ashkenazi Jew at that time.

Laban: Brother of Rebekah, father of Leah and Rachel (Genesis 29–31).

Lamashtu: Female demon in Babylonian mythology, who slew children, drank the blood of men, and caused nightmares.

Lamia: Child-eating female demon in Greek mythology, who also seduced sleeping men.

Lamech: Descendant of Seth. He had two wives, Adah and Tzillah (Genesis 4:19).

Lampronti, Isaac (1679–1756): Italian rabbi and physician, author of the encyclopedic *Pahad Itzhak*, in which he included views of other Italian rabbis.

Leah: Elder daughter of Laban and wife of Jacob. She gave birth to six sons and one daughter (Genesis 29–30).

Leeuwenhoek, Antonie van (1632–1723): Dutch microscopist and biologist, who ground especially accurate lenses for his microscope, which enabled him to discover spermatozoa, microbes, protozoa, and blood corpuscles.

Leone da Modena (1571–1648): Italian rabbi and an articulate writer. He was a child prodigy and had an unusual personality; although he delivered fine sermons, wrote verse and critiques of kabbalistic texts, he was addicted to gambling, frequented bad company, wrote amulets, enjoyed music, and acted in amateur theatrical performances. He wrote a frank and intimate autobiography, a treatise against gambling, and (in Italian) a book about Jewish customs, as well as many other books.

Levi ben Gershom (1288–1344): Mathematician, astronomer, philosopher, and biblical commentator who lived in southern France.

Lida, David (c. 1700): Kabbalist rabbi of Amsterdam.

Lili, Lilitu, and Ardat Lili: Demons in Babylonian mythology.

Lilith (pl. Lilin, Lilitin): Female demon in Jewish folklore, harlot, and mother of demon offspring, strangler of newborn babies, reputedly also the first wife of Adam, and the wife of Samael.

Lillake: Sumerian female demon.

Luntz, Eliahu ben Moshe: Baal Shem, author of *Toldot Adam* (1720), a book of mystical remedies. This may be Eliahu of Chelm (1537–1653), who founded a secret society of kabbalists. He is said to have been a wonder child who was unknown until he turned forty, and then emerged as a miracle worker and founded an academy, allegedly dying at the age of 116. His successor, Joel of Zamosc, also a Baal Shem, was thought to be a coauthor of *Toldot Adam*.

Luria, Isaac ben Solomon, "The Ari" (1534–1572): Kabbalist of Ashkenazi parentage who settled in Safed, Israel, where he expounded his mystical doctrines to disciples. Believed to be possessed by a holy spirit and to receive revelations from Elijah, he became a legendary figure. He developed an original theory about the cosmos, including how each Jew has a role in bringing about cosmic restitution. See the description of Lurianic Kabbalah under "Kabbalah" in the Glossary.

Lusitanus, Amatus: See Amatus Lusitanus.

Lusitanus, Abraham Zacuto: See Zacuto Lusitanus, Abraham.

Maggid of Koznitz, Israel ben Shabbetai Hapstein (1733–1814): Hasidic rabbi in Poland, ascetic disciple of Dov Baer, Maggid of Mezhirech. Israel ben Shabbetai was an eloquent preacher, known for his ecstatic mode of prayer. He was well-versed in Kabbalah, and he distributed remedies and amulets.

Maharil: See Moellin, Jacob Segal.

Maimonides, Moses ben Maimon, "Rambam" (1135–1204): Rabbinic authority, codifier of Jewish law, philosopher, and physician. He had an outstanding intellect and was a supreme rationalist. Born in Spain, he moved to Fez and eventually settled in Egypt, where he was physician to the local ruler of Egypt and where he headed the Jewish community. He wrote a commentary on the Mishnah, codified Jewish law in his *Mishneh Torah*, enumerated the commandments in his *Sefer ha-mitzvot*, and wrote his influential philosophical treatise, *The Guide for the Perplexed*, in which he expounded his views on God, creation, prophecy, the nature of evil, divine providence, and the basic principles of Judaism. He wrote many medical treatises as well, including a commentary on Hippocrates' aphorisms, and a collection of his own, based on Hippocrates, Galen, and Arab physicians. He wrote a dissertation on cohabitation, another on asthma, and another on poisons and their antidotes, as well as a pharmacopoeia.

Manasseh: Elder son of Joseph. Manasseh and his brother, Ephraim, were blessed together by their grandfather, Jacob (Genesis 48:20).

Manger, Itzik (1901–1969): Yiddish poet, dramatist, and novelist.

Manoah: Father of Samson (Judges 13:1–25).

Messiah: Descendant of David whom Jews, since the period of the Second Temple, have believed that God will raise up to reign over a restored kingdom of Israel.

Michael: An angel, often given the special designation of archangel and divine messenger, who attends the throne of God and defends the Jewish people.

Miriam: Sister of Moses and Aaron (Exodus 15:20, Numbers 26:59). Legend tells that she was one of the midwives of the Israelite women and that she encouraged her parents to have a child in spite of Pharaoh's decree.

Moellin, Jacob Segal, "Maharil" (c. 1360–1427): Most important and influential talmudist of his generation; head of the Jewish communities of Germany, Austria, and Bohemia. He formed his decisions on the basis of a thorough appraisal of the situation. He emphasized the importance of giving charity yet ensured that the poor retain their dignity. He enjoyed the traditional tunes of the liturgy and believed they should not be changed. His statements regarding Jewish law and custom were recorded by a pupil of his and eventually published as *Sefer Maharil*.

Mordecai: A Jew in the royal court of King Ahasuerus, advisor to Esther. His story is told in the Book of Esther.

Moses: Son of Amram and Jochebed, younger brother of Aaron and Miriam. National leader, prophet, and lawgiver, his life is documented in Exodus, Leviticus, Numbers, and Deuteronomy.

Moses ben Shem Tov de Leon (c. 1240–1305): Spanish kabbalist. He wrote many mystical texts and commentaries and, scholars believe, most of the Zohar, too.

Moshe Leib of Sasov (1745–1807): Eastern European hasidic rabbi, Torah scholar, and learned in Kabbalah. He composed hasidic melodies and dances.

Nahman of Bratslav (1772–1811): Hasid, *tzaddik*, the great-grandson of the Baal Shem Tov. He lived in Podolia and the Ukraine. He believed he was the *tzaddik* destined to be the Messiah. He taught the importance of faith and self-criticism and sought direct communion with God through prayer and meditation. He urged others to be joyful, to dance and enjoy melody, and to communicate with the *tzaddik*.

Nahmanides, Moses ben Nahman (1194–1270): Spanish rabbi, halakhist, philosopher, kabbalist, biblical commentator, poet, and physician.

Nebuchadnezzar (sixth century): Ruler of Babylon (605–562 B.C.E.) who conquered Palestine and destroyed the Temple in 586 B.C.E., sending most of the Jews into captivity and exile in Babylon.

Neuda, Fanny (1819–1894): Wife of a Moravian rabbi. After his death, she published a prayer book in German for women that became very popular in Central Europe.

Nimrod: Mentioned in the Bible as a great-grandson of Noah, he became a legendary figure in the Talmud and later rabbinic lore, for his rebellion against God, and idolatry. King of the world, he built the Tower of Babel for idol worship. Legend tells that on the night of Abraham's birth, Nimrod's astrologers predicted the infant's impressive future and that all kings would be dethroned; Nimrod issued a death warrant for all newborn babies, but the infant, of course, survived.

Noah: Son of Lamech, a righteous man, whom God decided to save from the Flood and who was blessed and commanded by God to "be fertile and increase" (Genesis 8:17, 9:1, 9:7).

Nuriel: An angel.

Obizuth: A female demon who strangled newborns, according to *The Testament of Solomon*.

Onan: Second son of Judah, who was given in levirate marriage as a husband to Tamar, his childless sister-in-law. Because her child would not be his, he spilled his seed to prevent her from conceiving, and God took his life for this sin (Genesis 38:7–10).

Onkinerah, David (sixteenth century): Possibly a native of Istanbul, he became the youngest and most gifted member of the Salonika Academy of poets.

Ouziel, Benzion (1880–1953): Sephardic Chief Rabbi of Israel from 1939 until his death.

Papo, Eliezer ben Itzhak (d. 1824): Sephardic rabbi of Silistria, Bulgaria, who compiled several prayer books and ethical treatises.

Peninnah: Second wife of Elkanah (I Samuel 1:1–2), mother of his children, less favored than his first wife, Hannah, whom she taunted on account of her childlessness.

Perilman, Yehudah L. (c. 1900): A rabbi of Minsk, who set a precedent when he ruled that a woman may destroy seed sown by rape.

Pharaoh: King of ancient Egypt.

Philo Judaeus (c. 20 B.C.E.–50 C.E.): Jewish Stoic philosopher of Alexandria.

Phinehas: Younger of Eli's sons, killed in battle by the Philistines when they captured the Ark, causing his wife's premature delivery (I Samuel 4:19).

Pliny the Elder (23–79 C.E.): Roman intellectual and author of encyclopedic *Natural History*, about cosmology and astronomy (book 2), human biology including pregnancy, birth, and caesarean birth (book 7), and medicine and drugs (books 20–32). It was not wholly accurate and included fabricated stories and fables, as well as magic and superstition, but it was a classic sourcebook in Europe until refuted in the late fifteenth century.

Potiphar: The Egyptian in Pharaoh's court who bought Joseph and whose wife desired to seduce Joseph (Genesis 39:1).

Puah: A Hebrew midwife in Egypt, ordered by Pharaoh to kill the Israelite newborn male infants (Exodus 1:15ff.).

Rachel: Dearly beloved wife of Jacob the patriarch, and daughter of Laban. She suffered greatly from barrenness but eventually bore Joseph and died while giving birth to Benjamin (Genesis 30).

Raphael: One of the archangels and an angel of healing. This angel is mentioned in the Talmud as having visited Abraham after his circumcision and is frequently invoked in magical texts.

Rashi, Solomon ben Isaac (1040–1105): The name "Rashi" comes from the initial letters of Rabbi Shlomo ben Itzhak, and this is how the leading commentator on the Bible and Talmud is referred to. He was an unusually brilliant man, whose father, legend has it, heard a heavenly voice foretell the birth of a son who would enlighten the world with his wisdom. When pregnant, his mother miraculously escaped harm. Rashi lived mostly in France, where he founded a great rabbinic school. Rashi's commentary to the Talmud was printed alongside the Talmud in its first printed edition and in most editions ever since.

Rebekah: Wife of Isaac. Barren for many years, she eventually gave birth to twins, Esau and Jacob (Genesis 25:21ff.).

Remak, Robert (1815–1865): German Jewish physician who carried out unpaid neurological and embryological research, because as a Jew he was denied a teaching position. He eventually became the first Jew to teach in Berlin, in recognition of his brilliant work.

Reuben: First-born son of Jacob and Leah, who found the mandrakes that helped Rachel to conceive (Genesis 30:14).

Rhazes (c. 865–923/932): Physician, philosopher, and alchemist, who lived in Persia and in Baghdad and who was familiar with Greek, Syrian, Arab, and Indian medicine. His influential medical treatises surveyed existing knowledge and included his own commentary from his own medical experience. They were translated into Latin and Greek and eventually into other languages, too.

Rousset, François (late sixteenth century): Rousset coined the term "caesarean childbirth" for the operation that he performed on live women who could not give birth otherwise, and claimed that he did this without endangering the lives of these women or their babies. He was the first physician in Europe to make this claim and to operate in this way on live women—this work had been done previously by barber-surgeons, and Rousset generated much criticism from his medical colleagues.

Rustam: Legendary hero in Iranian mythology, who was delivered from his mother's side (by caesarean section) while she was anesthetized with wine. She was sewn up and felt no pain, because she slept a whole day and night. Her wound was healed with remedies. This description, in rhyming couplets, was written in the *Shah namah* (The Book of Kings) of Persian poet Firdousi in 1010, which went on to tell of the amazing feats of the hero whose life began in such an unusual manner.

Ruth: The Moabite daughter-in-law of Naomi. Both were widowed in Moab and returned together to Bethlehem, where Ruth married her late husband's kinsman. This levirate marriage restored the continuity of the dead man's name, and the son born was the grandfather of King David. Her story is told in the Book of Ruth.

Sa'adia Gaon (882–942): Born in Egypt, he became a leader of Babylonian Jewry and a great scholar, the head of the rabbinic academy at Sura. He wrote many monographs on Jewish law and a major book on philosophy, he translated the Bible into Arabic, with commentaries, and he arranged the liturgy into a book of prayers for the whole year, in Arabic, which was used in medieval times by Jews in Egypt and other countries where Arabic was the vernacular. He wrote many *piyyutim* and supplications. He was also a linguist and Hebrew grammarian and was well-read in the sciences.

Saladin (1138–1193): Vizier of Egypt and founder of the dynasty of Ayyubid sultans. He dethroned the last Fatimid sultan of Egypt, seized control of Syria after the death of its ruler, and shortly after conquered Jerusalem and most of Israel, although he eventually signed a peace treaty with England over the crusader occupation of the coastal region. Saladin was tolerant to Jews; he greatly honored Maimonides, who was his court physician.

Samael: A common name for Satan, chief of the devils in *The Testament of Solomon*; guardian angel of Esau in early rabbinic tradition; chief of the devils and angel of death in later aggadah; partner of Lilith as leaders of the impure Other Side (world of evil) in medieval Kabbalah.

Samson: Son of Manoah, born after a long period of childlessness, following an announcement from an angel of the Lord, who predicted the boy would be a nazirite from birth and would deliver Israel from the Philistines. The angel told Manoah's wife not to drink intoxicating liquid when pregnant or eat anything unclean because her son was consecrated to God (Judges 13). He grew into a man with superhuman strength that came from his uncut hair, but women were his downfall.

Samuel: Israelite judge and prophet at the time of the founding of the monarchy in the eleventh century B.C.E. He was born after his mother's long period of childlessness. When praying for a son, his mother, Hannah, vowed the son who would be born to her to a nazirite life in the sanctuary at Shiloh (I Samuel 1).

Saoshyans: Son of Zoroaster (sixth century B.C.E.) and savior of the world in the Zoroastrian religion. He was miraculously conceived by a young woman who swam in a lake where Zoroaster's seed was preserved. Zoroastrianism was the influential religion of Persia until the rise of Islam.

Sarah: Wife of Abraham, who was barren for many years. She eventually offered Abraham her handmaid, Hagar, so that she could bear him a child for her. This caused much tension between the two women. Sarah eventually bore a son, as God had promised, at the age of ninety and thus became the first of the four matriarchs (Genesis 21:2).

Satan: Originally used in the Bible to refer to an antagonistic adversary, Satan first appeared as an angel in the Prophets, as prosecutor in the celestial court, a subordinate to God. In the Apocrypha he represents the forces of evil. In early talmudic times, Satan referred to an impersonal force of evil, but he soon became identified with Samael, the angel of death, and the evil inclination. Although sometimes a tempter, Satan is more often the accuser, and Jews today still fear giving Satan a cause for accusing them. Satan was deemed responsible for all the sins in the Bible. Kabbalists introduced the reciting of six biblical verses before blowing the shofar (the sound is believed to confuse Satan); the initial letters of these form *kera satan*, "tear Satan," a term invoked on many protective amulets.

Shabbetai Zvi (1626–1676): Born in Izmir (Smyrna in his day), he was well educated in the traditional Jewish sources and in Kabbalah. He soon showed signs of manic-depressive psychosis. When in his exalted state, he uttered the Name of God and proclaimed himself Messiah; when in his low mood, he tried to exorcise his demons using practical Kabbalah. Seeking a cure, he met Nathan of Gaza, who persuaded him that Shabbetai Zvi was indeed the Messiah who had arrived to restore Israel. This was the beginning of the Shabbatean messianic movement that long outlived the man himself, who was imprisoned in Constantinople and, when threatened with torture, converted to Islam. He lost the favor of many of his disciples, but others rationalized that his apostasy was a step to his becoming the Messiah.

Shechem: Son of Hamor the Hivite. He raped Dinah, Jacob's daughter (Genesis 34).

Shiphrah: A Hebrew midwife in Egypt, ordered by Pharaoh to kill the Israelite newborn male infants (Exodus 1:15ff.).

Shlumiel: A bungler whose enterprises invariably go awry.

Sideros: A child-killing demon mentioned in the magic bowls dating from the gaonic period, excavated at Nippur.

Simeon bar Yohai (second century): Palestinian sage and teacher. He was a pupil of Rabbi Akiva. He spent many years with his son in a cave evading Roman oppression. His charismatic character and ascetic lifestyle led to many legends about him. He was attributed authorship of the influential kabbalistic Book of Zohar.

Sines, Sisinnios, and Senodoros: The saints whose names protect against the child-stealing demon in Greek versions of the Lilith myth.

Snwy, Snsnwy, Smnglf, or Swny, Sswny, Sngru, and Artiku: The angels whose names protect against the child-stealing demon in Hebrew and Aramaic versions of the Lilith myth.

Solomon (tenth century B.C.E.): King of Israel for almost forty years. Son of David and Bathsheba. The Bible attributes the wealth and peace of his kingdom to his legendary wisdom—he wrote proverbs and songs, solved riddles, spoke the language of flora and fauna, dispensed justice, supervised religious rites, built and dedicated the Temple, and blessed his people. He married many foreign women, a practice that helped him maintain good relationships with his neighbors, but these women sometimes distracted him from his duties. Jewish tradition assumes that his wisdom was divinely inspired, although he also learned magical secrets from Ashmedai, chief of the demons.

Solomon Halevi of Karlin (1738–1792): Hasidic *tzaddik* of Lithuania, who devoted himself so fully and ecstatically to his prayer that his prayers were deemed particularly forceful. He mediated between his followers and God, praying for their needs. He was thought by his followers to be a reincarnation of the first Messiah, but he was killed in the middle of a prayer by a Cossack bullet.

Soranus (of Ephesus) (early second century C.E.): Greek gynecologist, obstetrician, and pediatrician who studied in Alexandria and eventually lived in Rome. His treatises on these and other subjects influenced physicians until the early modern period. His work was translated c. 500 C.E. into Latin, by Muscio, and a Hebrew version (*Sefer ha-toledet*) dates from the fourteenth century. An English translation was made in 1956.

Sore bas Toyvim (latter half of the seventeenth century): If she really existed, she lived in Podolia, Ukraine, and wandered from place to place, writing in her old age a book of *tkhinot* (prayers for women), *Shloyshe she'orim*. The booklet tells of her frivolous youth, for which God punished her with having to wander without a permanent home. She expressed the hope that other women would learn from her experience, acknowledge their errors in time, and have mercy on others. She became a mythical figure in Yiddish literature. However, there is some question as to whether this collection of *tkhinot*, which reveals an extensive knowledge of Hebrew and familiarity with the Zohar, was written by a woman, or by a man, and therefore whether Sore bas Toyvim really existed, or whether she was invented.

Sperling, Avraham Itzhak (1851–1921): Born in Lvov, he spent many years investigating the reasons for Jewish customs and published them in *Ta'amei ha-minhagim ve-makor ha-dinim.*

Tamar: She married Judah's first-born son, Er, but when he died childless, the levirate law required that she marry his brother, Onan. When he, too, died childless and Judah did not give her his third son to marry, she disguised herself as a prostitute and became pregnant from a union with Judah, unknown to him. When she revealed the truth to him, he accepted paternity and declared her righteousness. She gave birth to twins (Genesis 38).

Terah: Father of Abraham (Genesis 11:26).

Verzelya: The child-killing demon in the Ethiopian version of the myth of the demon who attacks women and infants at childbirth.

Vital, Hayyim (1542–1620): A disciple of Isaac Luria in Safed, who wrote down his understanding of Lurianic Kabbalah. He later became rabbi and head of a yeshivah in Jerusalem and lived his last years as rabbi of the Sicilian community in Damascus. He was also a physician and a practical kabbalist, and he wrote down his dreams, his mystical meditations, and stories about his life.

Von Baer, Karl Ernst (1792–1876): Prussian-Estonian embryologist who discovered the mammalian ovum and wrote about this in 1827.

Wijnberg, Rosalie M. (1887–1973): Gynecologist in Amsterdam, who worked in the Portuguese Jewish Hospital and founded the Dutch Association of Women Physicians in 1928. During the Second World War, she was taken to Westerbork Camp and was ordered to sterilize Jewish women who had married non-Jewish men. She bravely refused, and the order was not carried out.

Witcop, Rose (1890–?): Born in Eastern Europe into a religious family, she emigrated as a small child to London's East End. She became an anarchist and campaigned energetically for birth control education.

Yerushalmi, Moses ben Hanokh Altschul (c. 1540–c. 1610): Author of the *Brantspiegel* (first published 1596), a Yiddish ethical tract written for women, which portrayed all the laws and ideals that a virtuous woman should know. Some eighty-eight anecdotes illustrated the lessons given in its seventy-four chapters, covering topics such as the difference between a good and a bad wife, modesty and false pride, how one can talk oneself into Eternal Life, and what a woman should do "when her time comes," which is about the laws of purity and giving birth.

Yishmael: A High Priest mentioned in the Talmud, who had exceptional good looks.

Yohanan: A sage mentioned in the Talmud, who had exceptional good looks.

Zacuto Lusitanus, Abraham (1575–1642): Born in Lisbon to *Marrano* parents, he moved to Amsterdam at the age of fifty and practiced Judaism openly. His *Medici et* *philosophi, praxis historiarum* (Lyon: 1644) was a systematic description of all diseases, including problems in gynecology and obstetrics.

Zahalon, Jacob (1630–1693): Studied medicine in Rome and was Rabbi of Ferrara. He wrote a medical treatise.

Zedekiah: The last king of Judah, a weak ruler, who failed to stave off the Babylonian siege and destruction of Jerusalem. He was taken prisoner, blinded, and sent in chains to Babylonia, where he died.

Zeus: Supreme god of the Greek gods.

Zilpah: Leah's maid, whom Leah offered to Jacob when she found she could no longer bear children. Zilpah bore two of Jacob's sons (Genesis 30:9–13).

Zoroaster: A prophet of ancient Persia, whose sayings are collected in the Avesta. He founded a religion that became the national religion of Persia until the rise of Islam. The Parsees of India adhere to a form of this faith.

SELECTED BIBLIOGRAPHY

CHARMS AND REMEDY BOOKS

Alexander, P.S., "Incantations and Books of Magic," in *The History of the Jewish People in the Age of Jesus Christ, 175 B.C.–A.D. 135*, edited by E. Schürer, translated and edited by G. Vermes, F. Millar, M. Goodman. Revised ed. (Edinburgh: T. & T. Clark, 1986), vol. III, i: 343–379.

Ashkenazi, David Tevle ben Yakov, *Beit David* (Williamsdorf: 1704).

Avida (Zlotnik), Y. "Laḥashim ve-segullot be-aravit ve-yiddish," *Yeda Am* 21–22 (1974):7.

Badehev, Itzhak ben Michael, *Sefer segullah zahav* (Jerusalem: 1894).

Ben-Yaakov, A., *Otzar ha-segullot* (Jerusalem: 1991).

Bernstein, M. "Two Remedy Books in Yiddish from 1474 and 1508," in *Studies in Biblical and Jewish Folklore*, edited by R. Patai, F. L. Lettley, and D. Noy (Bloomington: Indiana University Press, 1960), 289–305.

Betz, H.D., ed., *The Greek Magical Papyri in Translation* (Chicago: University of Chicago Press, 1986).

Binesh, Binyamin, *Sefer amtaḥat Binyamin* (Wilmersdorf: 1716).

Conybeare, F.C., "The Testament of Solomon," *Jewish Quarterly Review* 11 (1899): 1–45.

Davis, E., and D.A. Frenkel, *Ha-kame'a ha-ivri* (Jerusalem: Institute for Jewish Studies, 1995).

Gaster, M., "The Sword of Moses," in *Studies and Texts* (New York: Ktav, 1971), vol. 1.

Ghalioungui, P., *Magic and Medical Science in Ancient Egypt* (London: Hodder and Stoughton, 1963).

Grunwald, M., "Charms and Magic Recipes," *Edot* 1 (1945): 241–248.

Hamoi, A., *Devek me'aḥ* (Izmir: 1870).

Hamoi, A., *Ha'aḥ nafshenu* (Izmir: Reprinted Jerusalem: Bakall, 1981, 1870).

Itzhak ben Eliezer, *Refu'ah ve-ḥayyim me-yerushalayim* (Jerusalem: Bakall, 1974).

Itzhaki, I., *Laḥash ve-kame'a*, (Tel Aviv: Shakked, 1976).

Krispil, N., *Yalkut ha-tzemaḥim*, (Jerusalem: Cana, 1983).

Leibowitz, J.O., and S. Marcus, *Sefer ha-nisyonot: The Book of Medical Experiences attributed to Abraham ibn Ezra*, (Jerusalem: Magnes Press, 1984).

Luntz, Eliahu ben Moshe, *Toldot Adam* (Zolkiew: 1720). *Magic and Superstition in the Jewish Tradition* (Chicago: Spertus College of Judaica, 1975).

Naveh, J., and S. Shaked, *Magic Bowls and Amulets* (Jerusalem: Magnes Press, 1985).

Naveh, J., and S. Shaked, *Magic Spells and Formulae* (Jerusalem: Magnes Press, 1993).

O'Hana, R., *Mareh ha-yeladim* (Jerusalem: 1901). Reprinted by Mea She'arim, Jerusalem, in 1990.

Pallache, H., *Sefer refuah ve-ḥayyim* (Izmir: 1873). *Razi'el ha-malakh* (Israel: Meirav, undated). This is a modern reprinting of *Sefer Razi'el* (Amsterdam: 1701), with additions by the Maggid of Koznitz.

Remedy book, Italy, fifteenth century manuscript, Library of Parma (1706), 1124.

Rozenberg, Y.Y., *Rafael ha-malakh* (Piotrkow: 1911).

Schäfer, P., "Jewish Magic Literature in Late Antiquity and Early Middle Ages," *Journal of Jewish Studies* 41 (1990): 75–91.

Schiffman, L.H., and M.D. Swartz, *Hebrew and Aramaic Incantation Texts from the Cairo Geniza* (Sheffield: Academic Press, 1992), 69ff.

Schrire, T., *Hebrew Amulets* (London: Routledge and Kegan Paul, 1966).

Sefer ha-razim: The Book of Mysteries, translated and edited by M.A. Morgan (Society of Biblical Literature, 1983).

Segullot ve-refu'ot (Yemen: Gross Family Collection, nineteenth century).

Segullot ve-refu'ot, Yiddish (New York: Jesselson Collection, sixteenth or seventeeth century).

Shimmush tehillim (Cracow: 1648).

Simner, Zekhariah ben Yakov, *Sefer zekhirah* (Wilmersdorf: 1729).

Sperling, A.I., *Ta'amei ha-minhagim ve-makor ha-dinim* (Jerusalem: Eshkol, 1961).

Tirshom, Joseph, *Shoshan yesod olam* (c. 1550), Sassoon ms. 290. Prof. M. Benayahu has transcribed the index and a commentary of this manuscript and published these in *Temirin* 1 (1972), 187–269.

Trachtenberg, J., *Jewish Magic and Superstition* (New York: Atheneum, 1982).

Zimmels, H.J., *Magicians, Theologians and Doctors* (London: Edward Goldston & Sons, 1952).

CONTRACEPTION, ABORTION, AND JEWISH MEDICAL ETHICS

Ellinson, G., "Procreation in the Light of Halacha," *Contemporary Thinking in Israel* 3 (1977).

Feldman, D.M., *Marital Relations, Birth Control and Abortion in Jewish Law* (New York: Schocken, 1978).

Jakobovits, I., *Jewish Medical Ethics* (New York: Bloch, 1975).

Rosner, F., and J.D. Bleich, eds., *Jewish Bioethics* (New York: Sanhedrin Press, 1979).

Rosner, F., ed., *Medicine and Jewish Law* (Northvale, NJ: Jason Aronson, 1993), 105–122.

Satlow M.L., *Tasting the Dish: Rabbinic Rhetorics of Sexuality* (Atlanta, GA: Scholars Press, Brown Judaic Studies, 1995).

Steinberg, A., *Jewish Medical Law,* compiled and edited from *Tzitz Eliezer*, translated by D. B. Simons (New York: Bet Shammai, 1989), part IV.

CROSS-CULTURAL STUDIES

Frazer, J.G., *The Golden Bough* (London: Macmillan, 1927). A new abridgment was published in Oxford, by Oxford University Press, in 1994.

Kitzinger, S., *Women as Mothers* (Glasgow: Fontana/Collins, 1981).

Ploss, H.H., and M. and P. Bartels, *Woman*, edited by E.J. Dingwall (London: Heinemann, 1935).

Witkowski, A., *Histoire des accouchements chez tous les peuples* (Paris: 1887).

DIARIES, MEMOIRS, RECORD BOOKS

Abrahams, B.Z., ed., *The Life of Gluckel of Hameln* (London: Horovitz, 1962).

Abrahams, I., ed., *Hebrew Ethical Wills* (Philadelphia: Jewish Publication Society, 1954).

Avron, D., ed., *Pinkas hakasherim shel kehilat Pozna, 1621–1835* (Jerusalem: 1966).

Chagall, B., *First Encounter* (New York: Schocken, 1983).

Cohen, M.R., ed., *The Autobiography of a Seventeenth Century Venetian Rabbi* (Princeton: Princeton University Press, 1988).

Dubnow, Sh., ed., *Pinkas ha-medinah* (Berlin: 1925).

Ger, Abraham, *Sefer brit tamim* (Leeuwarden: 1829), Etz Hayyim Collection 47 D27, Jewish National University Library. This is a mohel's record book.

Goitein, S.D., "Tzeva'ot me-mitzrayim me-tekufat ha-genizah," *S'funot* 8 (1964): 119ff.

Goldman, E., *Living My Life* (New York: Alfred A. Knopf, 1934).

Katzenellenbogen, P., *Yesh manḥilin* (Jerusalem: Makhon Hatam Sofer, 1986).

Katznelson-Shazar, R., ed., *Memoirs of the Pioneer Women of Palestine* (New York: Herzl Press, 1975).

Szwajger, A.B., *I Remember Nothing More* (New York: Pantheon, 1991).

Wetstein, P.H., ed., *Kadmoniyyot me-pinkasa'ot yeshenim* (Cracow: 1892).

Zunser, M.S., *Yesterday: A Memoir of a Russian Jewish Family* (New York: Harper & Row, 1978).

ETHNOGRAPHY

Algeria

Allouch-Benayoun, J., and D. Bensimon, *Les Juifs d'Algerie* (Toulouse: Privat, 1989).

Balkans

Galante, A., *Histoire des Juifs d'Anatolie* (Istanbul: M. Babok, 1937) vol. 1.

Juhasz, E. ed., *Sephardic Jews in the Ottoman Empire* (Jerusalem: The Israel Museum, 1990).

Levy, I.J., *Jewish Rhodes: A Lost Culture* (Berkeley: Judah L. Magnes Museum, 1989).

Molkho, M., "Leida ve-yaldut bein Yehudei Saloniki," *Edot* 2 (1947): 255–269.

Caucasus

"Caucasioni," *The Organ of the Caucasiological Center and the Gapmor Literary Society* 5 (1980).

Chorny, J.J., *Sefer ha-massa'ot be-eretz Kavkaz* (St. Petersburg: 1887), 196, 295–296.

Eastern Europe

Beukers, M., and R. Waale, ed., *Tracing An-sky* (Zwolle: Waanders, 1992).

Sternberg, G., *Stefanesti: Portrait of a Romanian Shtetl* (Oxford: Pergamon Press, 1984).

Zborowski, M., and E. Herzog, *Life Is with People* (New York: Schocken, 1962).

Egypt

Landau, J.M., *Jews in Nineteenth Century Egypt* (New York: New York University Press, 1969).

Ethiopia

Leslau, W., *Falasha Anthology* (New Haven: Yale University Press, 1951).

France

Raphael, F., and R. Weyl, *Les Juifs en Alsace* (Toulouse: Collection Franco-Judaica, 1977).

Georgia

Dayar-Ilem, I., *Seker anthropologi shel ha-kehillah ha-gruzinit be-Ashkelon*, Hebrew University, Sociology and Anthropology Department, Jerusalem, 1974.

Germany

Pollack, H., *Jewish Folkways in Germanic Lands (1648–1806)* (Cambridge: Massachusetts Institute of Technology Press, 1971).

India

Isaac, I.A., *A Short Account of the Calcutta Jews* (Calcutta: 1917).

Kehimkar, H.S., *The History of the Bnei Israel of India* (Tel Aviv: Dayag, 1937).

Slapak, O., *Yehudei Hodu*, (Jerusalem: The Israel Museum, 1995).

Iraq and Kurdistan

Aslan, M., and R. Nissim, *Yehudei Iraq* (Tel Aviv: Ofer, 1982).

Ben-Amri, S., *Ha-shed Tintal* (Herzliya: published by author, 1987).

Brauer, E., *The Jews of Kurdistan*, edited by R. Patai (Detroit: Wayne State University Press, 1993).

Idah, B., "Mahzor ha-ḥayyim be-kerev yehudei Bavel," *Nahardea* 6 (1988): 24.

Sassoon, S.D., *A History of the Jews of Baghdad* (Letchworth: S.D. Sassoon, 1949), 182–183. New edition, New York: AMS Press, 1982.

Israel

Goshen-Gottstein, E., *Marriage and First Pregnancy* (London: Tavistock, 1966).

Yehosha, Y., *Yaldut be-yerushalayim ha-yeshanah* (Jerusalem: R. Mass, 1966).

Yehosha, Y., *Yerushalayim t'mol shilshom* (Jerusalem: R. Mass, 1977) vol. I: 139–142.

Libya

Hacohen, M., *Hagid Mordechai: korot Luv ve-yehudei'ah* (Jerusalem: Ben Zvi Institute, 1979).

Slouschz, N., *Travels in Africa* (Philadelphia: Jewish Publication Society, 1927).

Zouarch, P., ed., *Yahadut luv* (Tel Aviv: Va'ad hakehillot luv be-Israel, 1982).

Morocco

Ben-Ami, I., *Ha'aratzat ha-kadoshim* (Jerusalem: Magnes Press, 1984).

Ben Simhon, R., *Yahadut Marocco* (Lod: Orot Yahadut ha-magreb, 1994).

Goulven, J., *Mellahs de Rabati-Salé* (Paris: 1927), 16–17.

Malka, E., *Essai d'ethnographie traditionelle des Mellah* (Rabat: 1946).

Mathieu, J., "Notes sur l'enfance juive du Mellah de Casablanca," *Bulletin de l'Institut d'Hygiene du Maroc* 7 (1947): 15–49.

Ovadia, D., *Kehillot zafro* (Jerusalem: Mahon le-heker toldot kehillot yehudei Marocco, 1975), vol. III.

Toledano, E., *Brit milah ve-minhagei'ah* (Kiryat Yam: published by author, 1977).

Zafrani, H., *Mille ans de vie juive au Maroc* (Paris: Maisonneuve & Larose: 1983).

Persia

Mizrahi, H., *Yehudei Paras* (Tel Aviv: Dvir, 1959).

Sephardic Communities

Dobrinsky, H., *A Treasury of Sephardic Laws and Customs* (New York: Yeshiva University Press, 1986), 3–30.

Grunwald, M., "Tales, Songs, and Folkways of Sephardic Jews," *Folklore Research Center Studies* 6 (1982): 205, 225–227.

Tunisia

Hadad, B., *Sefer Djerba yehudit* (Jerusalem: Beir ha-otzer ha-ivri, 1979).

Yemen

Brauer, E., *Ethnologie der jemenitischen Juden* (Heidelberg: 1934).

Kappah, Y., *Halikhot Teiman* (Jerusalem: Ben Zvi Institute, 1963).

Nahum, Y.L., *Metz'fonot yehudei Teiman* (Tel Aviv: published by author, 1961).

Zadok, M., *Yehudei Teiman: toldoteihem ve-orḥot ḥayyeihem* (Tel Aviv: Am Oved, 1967).

Zadok, H., *Be-ohalei Teiman* (Tel Aviv: David Ben Nun, 1981).

FOLKLORE

Ausubel, N., ed., *A Treasury of Jewish Folklore* (New York: Crown, 1948).

Ginzburg, L., *The Legends of the Jews* (Philadelphia: Jewish Publication Society, 1913).

Lauterbach, J.Z., "The Naming of Children in Jewish Folklore, Ritual and Practice," in *Studies in Jewish Law, Custom and Folklore* (New York: Ktav, 1970), 30–75.

Patai, R., *On Jewish Folklore* (Detroit: Wayne State University Press, 1983).

Rappoport, A.S., *The Folklore of the Jews* (London: Soncino Press, 1937).

Schauss, H., *The Lifetime of a Jew* (New York: Union of America Hebrew Congregations, 1950).

Shtal, A., *Mishpaḥah ve-giddul yeladim be-yahadut ha-mizraḥ* (Jerusalem: Academon, 1993).

Wassertil, A., ed., *Yalkut minhagim* (Jerusalem: Misrad ha-hinukh ve-ha-tarbut, 1977).

Zlotnik, Y. (Elzet J.L.), "Miminhagei Israel," *Reshumot* 1 (1918): 362–367.

FOLKTALES

Alexander, T., and D. Noy, *Otzaro shel abba* (Jerusalem: Center for Research of Sephardic and Oriental Culture, 1989).

Avitsuk, J., ed., *Ha-ilan she-safag dima'ot (The Tree That Absorbed Tears)* (Haifa: Israel Folklore Archives, 1965).

Baharav, Z., *Shishim Sippurei Am* (Haifa: Israel Folklore Archives, 1964). Reprinted in Israel by Ya'ad in 1977.

Band, A.J., *Nahman of Bratslav: The Tales* (New York: The Paulist Press, 1978), 109–111.

Bar-Hayyim, Z.A., *Sippurim nifla'im* (Jerusalem: Ravid ha-zahav, 1964). Original edition a hundred years earlier.

Bar–Itzhak, H., and A. Shenhar, *Jewish Moroccan Folk Narratives from Israel* (Detroit: Wayne State University Press, 1993).

Ben–Yehezkel, M., ed., *Sefer ha-ma'asiyot*, 4th ed. (Tel Aviv: Dvir, 1977), vol. 4.

Bialik, H.N. and Y.N. Ravnitzky, eds., *The Book of Legends: Sefer ha-aggadah* (New York: Schocken, 1992).

Bin–Gorion, E., *Me-makor Israel* (Bloomington: Indiana University Press, 1976).

Buber, M., *Tales of the Hasidim, Later Masters* (New York: Schocken, 1948).

Buber, M., *Legends of the Baal Shem Tov* (New York: Schocken, 1969).

Buber, M., *Tales of the Hasidim: Early Masters* (New York: Schocken, 1972).

Fus, D., *Sheva havilot zahav* (Haifa: Israel Folklore Archives, 1969).

Kaidanover, Z.H., *Kav ha-yashar* (Frankfurt: 1706).

Levin, M., *Hasidic Stories* (Tel Aviv: Greenfield Press, 1975).

Noy, D., ed., *Folktales of Israel* (Chicago: University of Chicago Press, 1963).

Patai, R., *Gates to the Old City* (New York: Avon, 1980).

Sabar, Y., *The Folk Literature of the Kurdistani Jews* (New Haven: Yale University Press, 1982).

Sadeh, P., *Jewish Folktales* (Garden City, NY: Doubleday, 1989).

Schwartz, H., *Miriam's Tambourine* (Oxford: Oxford University Press, 1988).

Schwartz, H., *Gabriel's Palace: Jewish Mystical Tales* (Oxford: Oxford University Press, 1993).

Schwarzbaum, H., *The Mishle Shualim (Fox Fables) of Rabbi Berekhiah Hanakdan* (Kiron: Institute for Jewish and Arabic Folklore, 1979).

Shenhar, A., and H. Bar–Itzhak, *Sippurei am me-beit she'an* (Haifa: Haifa University, 1981).

Yasif, E., *Sippurei Ben Sira be-yamei ha-beinayim* (Jerusalem: Magnes Press, 1984).

Yona, Y.A., ed., *Judeo-Spanish Ballad Chapbooks of Y.A. Yona* (Berkeley: University of California Press, 1971)

INFERTILITY

Gold, M., *And Hannah Wept* (Philadelphia: Jewish Publication Society, 1988).

Grazi, R.V., *Be Fruitful and Multiply* (Jerusalem: Feldheim, 1994).

HISTORICAL SOURCES

Abrahams, I., *Jewish Life in the Middle Ages* (New York: Atheneum, 1969).

Alsberg, P.A., "Registration of Births, Deaths and Marriages in European Jewish Communities, in Palestine and in Israel," *Archivum* 9 (1959): 101–119.

Basnage, J., *République des Hébreux* (Amsterdam: 1713), vol. II: 340.

Bedarride, I., *Les Juifs en France, en Italie et en Espagne* (Paris: 1861).

Beinart, H., *The Jewish Life of the Conversos* (Jerusalem: Magnes Press, 1981).

Bloom, H.I., *The Economic Activities of the Jews of Amsterdam in the Seventeenth and Eighteenth centuries* (Port Washington, NY: Kennikot Press, 1937), reprinted in 1967.

Bodenschatz, J., *Kirchliche Verfassung der Heutige Juden* (Leipzig: 1748–1749).

Buxtorf, J., *Synagoga Judaica* (Basel: 1603), chap. 2.

Calimani, R., *The Ghetto of Venice* (New York: M. Evans and Co., 1987).

Finkelstein, L., *Jewish Self-government in the Middle Ages* (Philadelphia: Jewish Publication Society, 1924), 245, 351.

Friedman, M.A., *Ribui nashim be-Israel* (Jerusalem: Bialik Institute, 1986).

Goitein, S.D., *A Mediterranean Society* (Berkeley: University of California, 1978), vols. I to III.

Grunwald, M., *Hamburgs Deutsche Juden* (Hamburg: 1904).

Horowitz, E., "The Eve of Circumcision: A Chapter in the History of Jewish Night Life," *Journal of Social History* 23 (1989), reprinted in Ruderman, D.B., ed., *Essential Papers on Jewish Culture in Renaissance and Baroque Italy* (New York: New York University Press, 1992), 554–588.

Hsia, R. Po-Chia, *The Myth of Ritual Murder: Jews and Magic in Reformation Germany* (New Haven: Yale University Press, 1988).

Ilan, T., *Jewish Women in Greco-Roman Palestine* (Tubingen: J.C.B. Mohr [Paul Siebeck], 1995).

Kirchner, J.C., *Jüdische Ceremoniel* (Nürnberg: 1726).

Lowenstein, S.M., "Voluntary and Involuntary Limitation of Fertility in Nineteenth Century Bavarian Jewry," in *Modern Jewish Fertility*, edited by P. Ritterband and P. Hyman (Leiden: E.J. Brill, 1981).

Marcus, J.R., *Communal Sick-Care in the German Ghetto* (Cincinnati: Hebrew University College Press, 1947).

Marcus, J.R., *The Jew in the Medieval World* (New York: Atheneum, 1981).

Melamed, R. L., "Medieval and Early Modern Sephardi Women," in *Jewish Women in Historical Perspective*, edited by J. Baskin (Detroit: Wayne State University Press, 1991).

Pansier, P., *Les Médecins juifs à Avignon aux trièzième, quatorzième et quinzième siècles* (Harlem: Janus, 1910).

Shulvass, M.A., *The Jews in the World of the Renaissance* (Leiden: E.J. Brill, 1973).

Schudt, J., *Jüdische Merkwurdigkeiten* (Leipzig: 1717), vol. II.

Wolf, L., ed., *The Legal Sufferings of the Jews in Russia* (London: T. Fisher Unwin, 1912).

Wurfel, A., ed., *Historische Nachtricht von der Judengemeinde in dem Hofmarkt* (Fürth: 1754).

HISTORY OF MEDICINE

Aristotle, *The Works of Aristotle Translated into English*, edited by J.A. Smith and W.D. Ross: *De generatione animalium*, translated by A. Platt (Oxford: Oxford University Press, 1958) and *The History of Animals*, translated by D.W. Thompson (Oxford: Oxford University Press, 1967).

Asaph Judeaus, *The Book of Medicine*, see Simon, I., *Asaph ha-iehoudi: Médecin et astrologue du Moyen Age* (Paris: Librairie Lipschutz, 1933).

Barkai, R., "A Medieval Treatise on Obstetrics," *Medical History* 33 (1989): 96–119. (A transcript and commentary of Bibliothèque Nationale, Paris, ms. 1120, f.66v–67r.)

Benveniste, Sheshet, *Ha-ma'amar be-toladah* (Oxford University, Bodleian Neub. 2142).

Berlant, M., *Die Glückliche Mutter* (Vilna: 1836).

Blumenfeld-Kozinski, R., *Not of Woman Born* (Ithaca, NY: Cornell University Press, 1990).

Cardoso, Isaac, *Philosophia Libera* (Venice: 1678), book VI.

Castro, Rodrigo de, *Universa muliebrum morborum* (Cologne: 1689).

Cohn, Tobias, *Ma'aseh Tuvya* (Venice: 1708).

Friedenwald, H., *The Jews and Medicine* (Baltimore: Johns Hopkins Press, 1944), vols. I, II.

Isaacs, H., *Medical and Paramedical Manuscripts in the Cambridge Genizah Collection* (Cambridge: Cambridge University Press, 1994).

Katan, H., *Likkutim be-korot ha-nitu'ah be-hityahsut meyuhedet el mekorot ha-yehudiot*, thesis, Hebrew University, Jerusalem, 1982.

Maimonides' Medical Writings: Maimonides' Treatises on Poisons, Hemorrhoids, and Cohabitation, edited and translated by F. Rosner (Haifa: Maimonides Research Institute, 1984), vol. 1.

Maimonides' Medical Writings: Maimonides' Commentary on the Aphorisms of Hippocrates, edited and translated by F. Rosner (Haifa: Maimonides Research Institute, 1987).

Maimonides' Medical Writings: The Medical Aphorisms of Moses Maimonides, edited and translated by F. Rosner (Haifa: Maimonides Research Institute, 1989), vol. 3. Maimonides' sixteenth treatise here is on gynecology and obstetrics, 262–270.

Medical ms. dated 1591, Oxford University, Bodleian Library, ms. 2135.

Meyerhof, M., and D. Joannides, *La Gynecologie et l'obstetrique chez Avicenna (Ibn Sina) et leurs rapports avec celles des Grecs* (Cairo: R. Schindler, 1938).

Preuss, J., *Biblical and Talmudic Medicine*, 2nd ed. (Brooklyn: Hebrew Publication Company, 1983).

Rosner, F., ed., *Sex Ethics in the Writings of Moses Maimonides* (New York: Bloch, 1974).

Rosner, F., *Medicine in the Bible and Talmud* (New York: Ktav, 1977).

Sefer ha-toledet (The Book of Generation), Jews College ms. 253, now British Library, Montefiore ms. 420. This is a medieval Hebrew adaptation of Muscio's (sixth century) Latin text, *Gynecia*, which in turn was a translated version of Soranus's treatise on this topic, written four centuries earlier. Two other manuscripts of *Sefer ha-toledet* are preserved in Rome (Casanatense Library, J.IV.5) and in the Vatican (ms. heb. 366 no. 5). This is transcribed in French in Barkai, R., *Les Infortunes de Dinah: Le livre de la génération* (Paris: Editions du Cerf, 1991).

Shatzmiller, J., *Jews, Medicine and Medieval Society* (Berkeley: University of California Press, 1994).

Soranus, *Gynecology*, translated by O. Temkin (Baltimore: Johns Hopkins University Press, 1956).

Zacutus Lusitanus, Abraham, *Medici et philosophi, praxis historiarum* (Lyon: 1644), book III.

Zahalon, Jacob, *Otzar ha-ḥayyim* (Venice: 1683).

Zikaron ha-ḥolayim, Jews College London, Montefiore ms. 440.

INNOVATIVE APPROACHES TO CHILDBIRTH RITUALS

Adelman, P.V., "The Womb and the Word: A Fertility Ritual for Hannah," in *Four Centuries of Jewish Women's Spirituality*, edited by E.M. Umansky and D. Ashton (Boston: Beacon Press, 1992), 247–257.

Barth, L.M., ed., *Berit Mila in the Reform Context* (New York: Berit Mila Board of Reform Judaism, 1990).

Cohen, A., *Zeved ha-bat* (Jerusalem: Caneh, 1990).

Diamant, A., *The Jewish Baby Book* (New York: Summit Books, 1988).

Feld, M., "Healing after a Miscarriage," in *Four Centuries of Jewish Women's Spirituality*, edited by E.M. Umansky and D. Ashton (Boston: Beacon Press, 1992), 221–222.

Frymer-Kensky, T., "A Ritual for Affirming and Accepting Pregnancy," in *Daughters of the King*, edited by Grossman S. and R. Haut (Philadelphia: Jewish Publication Society, 1992), 290ff.

Leifer, D.I., "Birth Rituals and Jewish Daughters," *Sh'ma*, April 2 (1976). Also in Koltun, E., ed., *The Jewish Woman: New Perspectives* (New York: Schocken, 1976).

Reifman, T. F., ed., *Blessing the Birth of a Daughter: Jewish Naming Ceremonies for Girls* (Englewood, NJ: Ezrat Nashim, 1978).

Schneider, S.W., *Jewish and Female* (New York: Touchstone [Simon and Schuster], 1985).

Strassfeld, S. and M. Strassfeld, eds., *The Second Jewish Catalogue* (Philadelphia: Jewish Publication Society, 1976).

Zonderman, S., "Spiritual Preparation for Parenthood" *Response*, Spring (1985).

JEWISH MYTHOLOGY

Dan, J., "Samael, Lilith, and the Concept of Evil in Early Kabbalah," *Association for Jewish Studies Review* 5 (1980): 19–25.

Graves, R., and R. Patai, *Hebrew Myths* (New York: Doubleday, 1964).

Koltuv, B. B., *The Book of Lilith* (York Beach: Nicolas Hays, 1986)

Patai, R., *The Hebrew Goddess*, 3rd ed. (Detroit: Wayne State University Press, 1990).

JEWISH POETRY COLLECTIONS

Carmi, T., ed. and trans., *The Penguin Book of Hebrew Verse* (Harmondsworth: Penguin, 1981).

Howe, I., and E. Greenberg, eds., *A Treasury of Yiddish Poetry* (New York: Holt, Rinehart, and Winston, 1966).

Schwartz, H., and A. Rudolf, eds., *Voices Within the Ark* (New York: Avon, 1980).

LULLABIES AND WELCOMING SONGS

Attias, M., *Romancot ve-shirei am be-yahadut Sepharad* (Jerusalem: Ben Zvi Institute, 1961).

Avishur, Y., ed., *Women's Folk Songs in Judaeo-Arabic from Jews in Iraq* (Tel Aviv: Iraqi Jews Traditional Culture Center Publication, 1987).

Lasseri, Y., *Ha-shirah ha-yehudit-amamit be-marocco* (Tel Aviv: Ha-Kibbutz ha-me'uḥad, 1986), 25–28.

Maoz, B., "Shirei ha-eres shel yehudei ha-sephardim me-turkiya ve-me-artzot ha-balkan," *Meḥkarei Yerushalayim be-folklor yehudi* 5–6 (1984): 57–70.

Mlotek, E.G., and J. Mlotek, comp., *Pearls of Yiddish Song*, (New York: Education Department of Workman's Circle, 1988).

Ratzhabi, Y., "Shirat ha-ishah ha-yehudit be-teiman," *Yeda Am* 5 (1957): 87–88.

Rubin, R., ed., *A Treasury of Jewish Folksongs* (New York: Schocken, 1964).

Weich-Shahak, S., "Shirim sephardi'im yehudi'im le-brit milah," *Dohan* 12 (1989): 165ff.

PRAYERS

Woman's prayer book manuscript, Mannheim, 1733, Collection of Mr. Itzhak Einhorn.

Woman's prayer book manuscript, Italy, eighteenth century, Collection of Mr. Itzhak Einhorn.

Aaron Berekhiah ben Moses of Modena, *Tefillah derekh si'ah ha-sadeh*, Oxford, Bodleian Library, 8°732.

Aaron Berekhiah ben Moses of Modena, *Ma'avar Yabok* (Vienna: 1857). The first edition was published in Venice in 1626.

Ascher, B.H. *The Book of Life* (London: 1847). This is a shortened, English version of Jacob ben Solomon's *Ma'aneh lashon*.

Azulai, Y.D., *Sefer avodat ha-kodesh* (Pressburg: 1818).

Cardin, N.B. *Out of the Depths I Call to You: A Book of Prayers for the Married Jewish Woman* (Northvale, NJ: Jason Aronson, 1992).

Epstein, Yehiel Michl, *Seder tefillah derekh yesharah*, (Frankfurt an der Oder: 1703).

Epstein, Yehiel Michl, *Kitzur shnei luhot ha-brit* (Jerusalem: Y.L. Garner, 1984). This is an edition of *Shnei luhot ha-brit* by Isaiah ben Avraham Horowitz (1565–1630), first published in Amsterdam, 1649. Epstein's edition was first published in Fürth, 1683.

Frankfort, Simeon ben Israel Judah, *Sefer ha-hayyim* (Amsterdam: 1703).

Hacohen, Eliyahu ben Shlomo Avraham, *Shevet mussar* (Jerusalem: Y. Rubenstein, 1963), part 2, chap. 24. First published in Constantinople in 1712.

Hannover, Nathan Nata, *Sha'arei Tziyyon* (Amsterdam: 1662), *Sha'ar* 5, *tikkun*.

Hurwitz, S., ed., *Mahzor Vitry* (Nürnberg: J. Bulka, 1923).

Jacob ben Isaac Ashkenazi of Yanov, *Tze'enah u-re'enah*, (Amsterdam: 1702/3). Reprinted in Jerusalem by Makhon Hama'or in 1975.

Klirs, T.G., comp., *The Merit of Our Mothers: A Bilingual Anthology of Jewish Women's Prayers* (Cincinnati: Hebrew Union College Press, 1993).

Kol t'khinah (The Voice of Supplication) (Trieste: 1824).

Moellin, Jacob ben Moses, *Sefer Maharil* (Sabionetta: 1556).

Neuda, F., *Stunden der Andacht* (Prague: 1857).

Papo, Eliezer ben Yitzhak, *Sefer beit tefillah* (Bilograd: 1860).

Rosenthal, Dovid Simcha, *A Joyful Mother of Children* (Jerusalem: Feldheim, 1982).

Solomon, Jacob ben Abraham, *Ma'aneh lashon* (Prague: 1615). This has been republished (Tel Aviv: Sinai, 1965).

Weissler, C., "The traditional piety of Ashkenazic women," in *Jewish Spirituality from the Sixteenth Century to the Present*, edited by A. Green (New York: Crossroad, 1987),

245–275. Quoting from *Seder tkhines u-vakoshes* (Fürth: 1762) and *Shloyshe She'orim*, prayers attributed to Sore bas Toyvim, eighteenth century. Also *Neues tkhinos u-vakoshes* (Hamburg: 1729).

Weissler, C., "Mitzvot Built into the Body," in *Jews and their Bodies*, edited by H.E. Schwartz (New York: State University of New York, 1992).

Yerushalmi, Moses ben Hanokh, *Brantspiegel* (Basel: 1602), chap. 35.

Zelig, Shmuel ben Yehoshua, *Sha'arei dim'a* (Jerusalem: 1884).

RABBINIC SOURCES

The Mishnah, translated by H. Danby (Oxford: Oxford University Press, 1949).

The Babylonian Talmud, translated and edited by I. Epstein (London: Soncino Press, 1935–1938), 35 vols. Hebrew editions of the Talmud carry Rashi and Tosafot commentaries.

The Talmud of the Land of Israel (The Jerusalem Talmud), translated by J. Neusner (Chicago: University of Chicago Press, 1982–1986), 33 vols.

The Midrash Rabbah, translated and edited by H. Freedman and M. Simon (London: Soncino Press, 1951), vols. 1–10.

Abraham ben David of Posquières (Ravad), *Ba'alei ha-nefesh* (Brooklyn: 1980), *Sha'ar kedushah*.

Aldabi, Meir, *Sh'vilei emunah* (Warsaw: 1887), part 5.

Anav, Zedakiah ben Abraham ha-rofeh, *Shibolei ha-leket*, edited by S. Mirsky (Jerusalem: Sura, 1966).

Bahya ben Asher, *Bi'ur al ha-Torah*, edited by H. D. Shawal (Jerusalem: Mossad ha-rav Kook, 1967).

Braude, W.G., ed., *Pesikta Rabbati* (New Haven: Yale University Press, 1968).

Buber, S., ed., *Pesikta* (Lyck: 1868).

Caro, J., *Shulḥan arukh*, edited by Z.H. Preisler and S. Havlin (Jerusalem: Ketuvim, 1993). For English translation of abridgment, see Ganzfried, S., *Code of Jewish Law: Kitzur Shulḥan arukh*, translated by H.E. Goldin (New York: Hebrew Publishing Co., 1961).

Chumash with Targum Onkelos, Haphtaroth and Rashi's Commentary, translated by A.M. Silbermann and M. Rosenbaum (Jerusalem: Silbermann, 1984).

Cohen, S.J., ed. and trans., *The Holy Letter: A Study in Medieval Jewish Sexual Morality, Ascribed to Nahmanides* (New York: Ktav, 1976).

Duran, Simon ben Tzemaḥ, *Magen avot* (Livorno, 1785).

Eleazar of Worms, *Sefer ha-roke'ah* (Jerusalem: 1967).

The Fathers According to Rabbi Nathan, translated by A.J. Saldarini (Leiden: E.J. Brill, 1975).

Jacob ben Asher (Tur), *Arba'ah ha-turim* (Vilna: 1900).

Jellinek, A., ed., *Beit ha-midrash* (Jerusalem: Bamberger and Wahrmann, 1938).

Judah ben Samuel of Regensburg (Judah the Pious), *Sefer Hasidim* [Bologna 1538 version], edited and translated by R. Margoliyot (Jerusalem: Mossad harav Kook, 1957). Another version [Cod. de Rossi 1133] of *Sefer Hasidim* was edited by Judah Hacohen Wistinetzki, second edition, and published in Frankfurt in 1924.

Kehati, P., ed., *Pirkei avot* (New York: World Zionist Organization, 1984).

Lampronti, I., ed., *Paḥad Itzhak* (Livorno: 1834). Reprinted in 1962–1966.

Levine, M. Hershel, ed. and trans., *Falaquera's "Book of the Seeker"* (New York: Yeshiva University Press, 1976).

Levy, R., and F. Cantera, eds., *Abraham Ibn Ezra, The Beginning of Wisdom* (Baltimore: Johns Hopkins Press, 1939).

Maimonides, M., *Code of Maimonides: Mishneh Torah* (New Haven: Yale University Press, 1965).

Maimonides, M., *Guide for the Perplexed*, translated by M. Friedlander, second edition (New York: Dover, 1956).

Margalioth, M., ed., *Midrash ha-gadol* (Jerusalem: Rav Kook Institute, 1956).

Midrash tanḥuma, translated by J.T. Townsend (Hoboken, NJ: Ktav, 1989). The Hebrew original was first published in Constantinople in 1522.

Moellin, Jacob ben Moses, *Sefer Maharil* (Sabionetta: 1556).

Neusner, J., ed. and trans., *The Tosefta* (Hoboken, NJ: Ktav, 1981), 6 vols.

Paquda, Bahya ben Joseph ibn, *The Book of Direction to the Duties of the Heart*, edited and translated by M. Mansoor (London: Routledge and Kegan Paul, 1973).

Pirkei de Rabbi Eliezer, edited and translated by G. Friedlander (New York: Hermon Press, 1981).

Portaleone, Abraham, *Shiltei ha-gibborim* (Mantua: 1612).

Sa'adia Gaon, *The Book of Beliefs and Opinions* (New Haven: Yale University Press, 1948).

Siddur Rav Sa'adia Gaon, edited by I. Davidson, S. Assaf, and B.I. Joel. (Jerusalem: Mekitzei Nirdamim, 1941).

Theodor, J., and C. Albeck, eds., *Genesis Rabbah* (Jerusalem: 1964).

Yalkut Shimoni (Jerusalem: 1960), vols. I and II.

SECONDARY SOURCES

Cohen, J., *"Be Fertile and Increase, Fill the Earth and Master It": The Ancient and Medieval Career of a Biblical Text* (Ithaca, NY: Cornell University Press, 1989).

Trier, S.A., ed., *Rabbinische Gutachten über die Beschneidung* (Frankfurt: 1844).

Ulmer, R., *The Evil Eye in the Bible and Rabbinic Literature* (Hoboken, NJ: Ktav, 1994).

Weisberg, J.D., *Sefer otzar ha-brit* (Jerusalem: Makhon Torat ha-brit, 1986), vol. 1.

ZOHAR AND KABBALAH

Bacharach, Naphtali ben Jacob Elhanan, *Emek ha-melekh* (Amsterdam: 1648).

Kaplan, A., *Meditation and the Bible* (York Beach, ME: Samuel Weiser, 1992).

Lachower, F., and I. Tishby, eds., *The Wisdom of the Zohar* (Oxford: Littman Library, Oxford University Press, 1989).

Scholem, G., *Kabbalah* (New York: Meridian, 1978).

Weiss, J., *Studies in Eastern European Jewish Mysticism* (Oxford: Oxford University Press, 1985).

The Zohar (London: Soncino Press, 1931), vols. I–V.

Index of Biblical and Talmudic References

Index of Personalities

General Index

Page numbers in **boldface** indicate photograph or illustration.

abortion, 44, 45–51, 100
  abortifacients, 46, 48–50,
    232nn. 57, 58
  and adultery, 39, 46–47
  and diagnosis of handicap,
    50, 232n. 69
  and the Holocaust, 50–51,
    232n. 67
  for mother's health, 231n.
    41
  and rape, 47–48
  to save mother's life, 46,
    131–132
abstinence, **38,** 39–41
Aden, 71, 188, 194
  See also Moslem lands
adoption, 27–28
adultery, 60, 61, 81, 226n. 45
  and abortion, 39, 46–47
  accusations of, 64,
    178–179
Afghanistan, 153, 186, 190
  See also Moslem lands
afterbirth, 159–160
Algeria, 17, 49, 66, 71
  See also Moslem lands;
    North Africa
Alpha Beta of Ben Sira, The,
  146, 149, 155
Alsace, 35, 153, 154, 189–190
  See also Europe; France
Amtahat Binyamin, 154
amulets, 11, 47, **142, 157**
  to ease delivery, 123–124
  for fertility, 30–31, 35,
    228–229n. 94
  for contraception, 44–45
  to protect pregnancy, **84,**
    89, 90–92
  See also under Lilith; demons

Angel of Death, 129, 185,
  199–200
angel script, 30, 45, 91
angels, 20, 24, 80
  and birth, 116, 118, 123
  and conception, 28, 56, 61,
    72–73
  to guard pregnancy, 90, 91
  See also Lilith, angels protect
    against
anti-Semitism, 39, 104–106,
  108, 177, 244n. 23
Arabic, 80, 146, 190
Aramaic, 22, 49, 63, 123, 145,
  207
Argentina, 206
artificial insemination, 35, 62
Ashkenazi Jews, 16, 83
  and abortion, 48
  and birth, 115, 121–122
  and celebration of birth,
    166, 171, 204–205
  and circumcision, 178,
    181, 183
  and death in childbirth,
    130, 137, 193
  and genealogy, 266n. 9
  and infertility, 10, 31
  and midwives, 101, 109
  and naming, 189–190, 200
  and nursing, 160, 161
  and pregnancy, 70, 88, 91
  and redemption of the
    first-born, 188
  remedy books, 122
  tales of, 63–64, 75, 107
Asian Jews, 163, 167, 182, 200
  and circumcision, 170, 182
  See also Bukhara; India;
    Iraq; Kurdistan; Persia;
    Turkistan
assimilation, 215, 219
Assyria, 42, 123, 154
astrology, 66, 70, 82, 86,

201–202, 266n. 11
atonement, 24, 120, 125
  See also repentance
Austria, 10, 66, 108, 117, 185
  See also Europe
Avignon, Synod of, 105, 164

Babylonia, 56, 80, 133, 137,
  159, 177
  amulets in, 228–229n. 94
  astrology in, 266n. 11
  demons in, 29, 63, 144,
    145, 151, 153
Balkans, 6, 169, 189, 202
  See also Bulgaria; Greece;
    Rhodes; Rumania;
    Turkey
barrenness. See infertility
Beginning of Wisdom, The, 202
Bessarabia, 208
  See also Eastern Europe;
    Moldavia
Bible, 3, 124
  birth records in a, 203
  book, 93, 189–190, 192
  and infertility. (See under
    infertility)
  and circumcision, 175,
    176, 182, 184, 185
  and death in childbirth,
    135, 137
  and magic, 44, 90–91
  and midwives, 102
  and miscarriage, 85, 86, 87
  and postnatal rituals, 175
  and preference for sons, 7
  and wet nurses, 163
  See also under tales; Index
    of Biblical and Talmudic
    References
bigamy, 5, 15, 18
birth, **97, 112, 158**
  caesarean, 130, 132–135,
    186, 251n. 7

327